Synthetic peptides as antigens

The Ciba Foundation is an international scientific and educational charity. It was established in 1947 by the Swiss chemical and pharmaceutical company of CIBA Limited—now CIBA-GEIGY Limited. The Foundation operates independently in London under English trust law.

The Ciba Foundation exists to promote international cooperation in biological, medical and chemical research. It organizes about eight international multidisciplinary symposia each year on topics that seem ready for discussion by a small group of research workers. The papers and discussions are published in the Ciba Foundation symposium series. The Foundation also holds many shorter meetings (not published), organized by the Foundation itself or by outside scientific organizations. The staff always welcome suggestions for future meetings.

The Foundation's house at 41 Portland Place, London, W1N 4BN, provides facilities for meetings of all kinds. Its Media Resource Service supplies information to journalists on all scientific and technological topics. The library, open seven days a week to any graduate in science or medicine, also provides information on scientific meetings throughout the world and answers general enquiries on biomedical and chemical subjects. Scientists from any part of the world may stay in the house during working visits to London.

Synthetic peptides as antigens

Ciba Foundation Symposium 119

1986

JOHN WILEY & SONS
Chichester · New York · Brisbane · Toronto · Singapore

ISBN 0 471 99838 9

Suggested series entry for library catalogues:
Ciba Foundation symposia

Ciba Foundation Symposium 119
x + 307 pages. 64 figures, 36 tables

British Library Cataloguing in Publication Data
Synthetic peptides as antigens.—(Ciba Foundation
  symposium; 119)
  1. Peptides   2. Peptide synthesis   3. Antigens
  I. Series
  616.07'92   QD431

Printed in Great Britain at The Bath Press, Avon

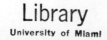

Contents

Symposium on Synthetic Peptides as Antigens, held at the Ciba Foundation,
London, 4–6 June 1985
The subject of this symposium was proposed by P. Dukor and D. G. Braun

Editors: Ruth Porter (Organizer) and Julie Whelan

v

G. L. Ada   Chairman's summing-up   294

Contributors

G. L. Ada (*Chairman*) Department of Microbiology, The John Curtin School of Medical Research, Australian National University, PO Box 334, Canberra City, ACT 2601, Australia

D. Altschuh Institut de Biologie Moléculaire et Cellulaire, CNRS, 15 rue René Descartes, 67084 Strasbourg, France

R. F. Anders Walter and Eliza Hall Institute of Medical Research, Immunoparasitology Unit, Post Office, Royal Melbourne Hospital, Victoria 3050, Australia

S. S. Alkan Pharmaceuticals Division, Department of Research, CIBA-GEIGY Limited, CH-4002 Basle, Switzerland

F. Brown Wellcome Biotechnology Ltd, Langley Court, Beckenham, Kent BR3 3BS, UK

G. Corradin Department of Biochemistry, University of Lausanne, CH-1066 Epalinges, Switzerland

M. J. Crumpton Imperial Cancer Research Fund, PO Box 123, Lincoln's Inn Fields, London WC2A 3PX, UK

A. B Edmundson Department of Biology, 201 Biology Building, University of Utah, Salt Lake City, Utah 84112, USA

G. I. Evan Ludwig Institute for Cancer Research, MRC Centre, Hills Road, Cambridge CB2 2QH, UK

H. M. Geysen Department of Molecular Immunology, Commonwealth Serum Laboratories, 45 Poplar Road, Parkville, Victoria 3052, Australia

S. K. Gupta (*Ciba Foundation Bursar*) National Institute of Immunology, PO Box 4922, New Delhi 110029, India

Ch. Heusser Immunology, Pharmaceuticals Research Department, CIBA-GEIGY Limited, CH-4002 Basle, Switzerland

J. H. Humphrey Department of Medicine, Royal Postgraduate Medical School, Ducane Road, London W12 OHS, UK

A. Klug MRC Laboratory of Molecular Biology, MRC Centre, Hills Road, Cambridge CB2 2QH, UK

P. J. Lachmann Mechanisms in Tumour Immunity Unit, MRC Centre, Hills Road, Cambridge CB2 2QH, UK

E. S. Lennox Celltech Limited, 244–250 Bath Road, Slough SL1 4DY, Bucks, UK

R. A. Lerner Department of Molecular Biology, Research Institute of Scripps Clinic, 10666 North Torrey Pines Road, La Jolla, California 92037, USA

Y. Liu (*Ciba Foundation Bursar*) Institute of Basic Medical Sciences, Chinese Academy of Medical Sciences, 5 Dong Dan San Tiao, Beijing, China

I. McConnell Department of Veterinary Pathology, Royal (Dick) School of Veterinary Studies, Summerhall, Edinburgh EH9 1QH, UK

R. S. Nussenzweig Department of Medical and Molecular Parasitology, New York University Medical Center, 550 First Avenue, New York 10016, USA

V. Nussenzweig Department of Pathology, New York University Medical Center, 550 First Avenue, New York 10016, USA

J. B. Rothbard* Department of Medical Microbiology, Sherman Fairchild Science Building, Stanford University School of Medicine, Stanford, California 94305, USA

M. Sela The Weizmann Institute of Science, Rehovot 76100, Israel

J. J. Skehel National Institute for Medical Research, The Ridgeway, Mill Hill, London NW7 1AA, UK

D. R. Stanworth Rheumatology and Allergy Research Unit, Department of Immunology, The Medical School, University of Birmingham, Vincent Drive, Birmingham B15 2TJ, IL

---

* *Present address:* Imperial Cancer Research Fund, PO Box 123, Lincoln's Inn Fields, London WC2A 3PA, UK.

V. C. Stevens   Department of Obstetrics & Gynecology, Ohio State University, 567 Means Hall, 1654 Upham Drive, Columbus, Ohio 43210-1228, USA

R. J. P. Williams   Inorganic Chemistry Laboratory, University of Oxford, South Parks Road, Oxford OX1 3QR, UK

Introduction

G. L. ADA

Department of Microbiology, The John Curtin School of Medical Research, Australian National University, PO Box 334, Canberra City, ACT 2601, Australia

1986 Synthetic peptides as antigens. Wiley, Chichester (Ciba Foundation Symposium 119) p 1-5

The purpose of this meeting is to discuss peptides, and especially their antigenic properties. The study of the properties of peptides has become a major scientific activity with an increasing emphasis on their potential use as the basis of vaccines against a variety of diseases, but also as a tool for basic research. It must be a great source of satisfaction to Michael Sela, who is with us at this symposium, to see the development of this approach to the study of the immune system which he pioneered a quarter of a century ago.

During this meeting, one question in the back of my mind will be: what is the potential of peptide-based preparations to form the basis of new vaccines? In the first part of the introduction, let me make a few points about vaccines. Vaccines are perhaps the most cost-effective means of combating infectious diseases. There are some fifty different vaccines at present in use, mainly in Western countries, against both human and veterinary diseases. Vaccines against viral diseases have frequently been particularly successful; of these, those composed of live attenuated virus have, in many cases, remarkable records. The most notable example is the eradication of smallpox by vaccination. There are vaccines against five common childhood diseases, so that with one main exception, pertussis, these diseases are largely under control in developed countries. Not so in other countries. Less than 20% of the world's children were vaccinated in 1983, despite the general availability of the vaccines at moderate cost.

There are in addition many diseases against which either no vaccine is available or current vaccines are unsatisfactory. Table 1 lists some of these diseases. Three programmes of the World Health Organization support research on some of them. This table should not be regarded as all-inclusive.

I think it is also appropriate at this meeting to allude to the major differences in the standards of living of people in developed, developing and least-developed countries. Thus, between the developed and least-developed countries, maternal mortality rates differ by about 100-fold, infant mortality rates by

1

TABLE 1 Major diseases (or disease agents) of global public health importance for which vaccines are unavailable or current vaccines are inadequate

A. *WHO Tropical Diseases Programme*
   Malaria, leishmaniasis, trypanosomiasis
   Schistosomiasis, filariasis
   Leprosy (First-generation vaccine under test)

B. *Report of Sub-committee of Global Advisory Committee of Medical Research*

Cytomegalovirus	[a]Respiratory syncytial virus	Gonorrhoea
Herpes simplex	Rabies	[a]*Meningococcus*
[a]Dengue	Rotavirus	Pertussis
[a]Hepatitis A	Chlamydia	[a]*Pneumococcus*
Hepatitis B	*Escherichia coli* enteritis	[a]*Streptococcus*
Influenza	Typhoid, paratyphoid	[a]Tuberculosis

[a] Research on these organisms is now sponsored by the WHO Vaccine Development Programme.

about eight-fold and the health budget per person per year by over 100-fold, the figure for least-developed countries being less than two dollars. I mention this information to give the group, as medically oriented scientists, an indication of the goals we should have in our sights—even though the realization of those goals may be distant.

It is convenient to list the newer approaches to the development of vaccines under four headings (Table 2), but these should not be regarded as mutually

TABLE 2 New approaches to the development of vaccines

1. Construction of recombinant infectious vectors
      Viruses: vaccinia, herpes, adenovirus
      Bacteria: *Salmonella* Ty21a
2. Synthesis of protective antigens in prokaryotes or lower eukaryotes
3. Anti-idiotypes
4. Synthesis of oligopeptides

exclusive. The construction of recombinant, infectious vectors shows great potential and has, in animal models, already shown remarkable promise against some infections, such as rabies. The other three approaches are closely related, being the synthesis of antigens (e.g. proteins/glycoproteins), either as such or as fusion products by bacteria or lower eukaryotes; the production of anti-idiotypes; and the synthesis of oligopeptides which, up to a certain size, most likely involves chemical or enzymic synthesis. The main thrust of this symposium is the peptides and their relationship to the protein of which they represent a part. The peptides that we shall be mainly interested in are epitopes, which, in a simplified way, can also be regarded as anti-idiotypes.

Peptide-based vaccines potentially offer a number of advantages. (1) The first is that they should be safe to use and cause the smallest number of side-reactions. Because of this, it is thought that such preparations should gain wide public as well as official acceptance. (2) The second advantage is the possibility that the best vaccines might contain only those sequences of a protein which would stimulate the most desirable responses. (3) These vaccines should be stable, obviating the need for cold-chains.

Do they have any disadvantages? If we exclude aspects such as cost, the possible need to provide a carrier protein, adjuvants and delivery systems—all of which may be solvable in time, and possibly quite soon—a potential disadvantage is the risk of significant Ir (immune response) gene effects—that is, variation in the immune response of individuals in an outbred population. These may not be of great significance in the immune response to a hormone or a toxin, but with the more complicated infectious agents, evidence is only now being obtained which suggests that this may be of some consequence.

The programme of the symposium has evolved as a result of inputs from a number of people to Ruth Porter, but especially from Mike Crumpton. I would like to thank all for their contributions. The symposium falls fairly comfortably into four segments. The first segments is on the immune response, and John Humphrey, with Peter Lachmann, will deal with the regulation of the immune response. They have a formidable task. Without wishing to pre-empt in any way what they might say, I would like to make three comments. (1) We think of vaccines mainly in terms of infectious disease, but we should bear in mind that infectious diseases can vary tremendously. On the one hand, with an acute infection like influenza, the infectious process can occur and the host recover within a week or so. In such a situation, it has not been very difficult to ascertain the role of different components of the immune response in the prevention of virus infection or recovery from infection. This can be contrasted with chronic diseases such as malaria or schistosomiasis; in the former the parasite exists in different forms in the bloodstream only transiently and there can be recurrent infections, whereas with the latter, after penetration of the skin by cercaria and their maturation, the adult worms may exist *in copulo* in the bloodstream for more than twenty years, apparently impervious to the host's immune system. (2) In most cases, infection can only be prevented by specific antibody and most vaccines are made with the aim of inducing antibody formation, or at least priming for this. In some cases, there is something to be said for a vaccine which substantially limits infection rather than prevents it; for this, generation of a cell-mediated immune response to aid recovery may be desirable. (3) With few exceptions, generation of an appropriate antibody response will involve activation of T as well as B cells. In recent years it has become apparent that these two classes of lymphocytes may preferentially recognize different amino acid sequences in a protein molecule; furthermore, there is evidence, though more limited as yet, that different sequences may activate T helper or T suppressor cells.

In the second section of the meeting we shall be hearing about relationships of epitopes (antigenic determinants) to the parent protein molecules and to the combining sites of immunoglobulins. I anticipate being entranced by some superb examples of computer graphics, but, speaking as a biologist, I would like to know: (1) Are we closer to being able to predict those segments of a protein which, when isolated or synthesized and used as an antigen, will result in the formation of antibody which reacts well with the protein itself? (2) Will we be able to predict whether a given peptide will preferentially react with T or B lymphocytes? If we can formulate some general rules about protein structure and immune reactivity in terms of the constituent peptides by the end of the meeting, this Ciba Foundation Symposium will have been a signal success for that reason alone.

In the third section we shall hear about five examples of work directed to demonstrating the synthesis of peptides and their ability, when presented in an appropriate manner, to generate a protective immune response against an infectious organism or an iso-immunogen. First, I personally am excited by the achievement of Mario Geysen and his colleagues in synthesizing an anti-idiotype or mimotope using as template a monoclonal antibody recognizing a discontinuous epitope. The potential of this approach seems to be quite significant. Two papers are concerned with malaria. Called by some the King of Diseases, it represents, as indicated previously, a substantial challenge. About one-third of the world's population is exposed to the malaria parasite and the development of an effective, safe and cheap vaccine would represent an achievement not far short of smallpox eradication. The two contributions come from laboratories very heavily engaged in this work. Michael Sela will then tell us about the extensive contributions of the Weizmann Institute in the area of synthetic peptides against bacterial toxins. Finally, in this section, we have an unusual presentation—a vaccine against an iso-immunogen, the human chorionic gonadotropic hormone (hCG). I proposed this topic for the meeting for two main reasons. One is that if our attempts to protect people in the third world against major infectious diseases are successful, it will be all the more important to regulate human fertility, and vaccination is potentially one effective way to achieve this. The second reason is that the results that Vernon Stevens will discuss represent about ten years of hard work devoted to one end—to producing a first-generation vaccine. The fact that Phase I trials have now been approved in two developed countries is an indication of the status of the work.

The final section contains three contributions in which peptides are used as haptens to produce antibodies which are then used as probes. There is also the possibility that they may be used as modulators of immune function, as Denis Stanworth will impress upon us.

There have been a number of recent meeting devoted to discussions of peptides. This Ciba Foundation Symposium offers an especially rich feast in an area which has the potential of being of great benefit to mankind.

Regulation of *in vivo* immune responses: few principles and much ignorance

J. H. HUMPHREY

Department of Medicine, Royal Postgraduate Medical School, Hammersmith Hospital, London W12 0HS, UK

Abstract. An attempt is made, based largely on reports of experiments carried out *in vitro*, to piece together the sequence of events between the interaction of antigens with B or T lymphocytes and the immune responses which result. These include stimulation of B lymphocytes to secrete antibody or to become B memory cells, and stimulation of T helper cells and cytotoxic/suppressor T cells to multiply and become functional effector cells. Thymus-independent (T1) stimulation is described of a subpopulation of B cells by poorly degradable immunogens with multiple epitopes, and the generation of B memory cells, as well as stimulation of B cells requiring cooperation with T cells. Stimulation of T helper (T_H) cells by antigens involves first activation by interleukin 1 (IL-1) and then presentation of the antigen at the surface of antigen-presenting cells (usually macrophages, dendritic cells or B cells) in association with class II major histocompatibility complex molecules (MHC II); for extrinsic (foreign) proteins this requires initial capture of the protein, followed by denaturation and/or degradation so as to associate the molecule or fragments with MHC II. Some peptides can become suitably associated without further degradation, whereas T1 antigens may be unable to become associated effectively. T cells so stimulated express receptors for interleukin 2 (IL-2), and secrete various molecules, including factors which stimulate B cells to divide and/or secrete Ig, interferon-γ and IL-2. In turn, IL-2 causes proliferation of T_H and cytotoxic/suppressor T cells. Interferon-γ stimulates the expression of MHC II by macrophages and some epithelial cells and increases the activity of NK (natural killer) cells.

This simplified account embraces many of the experimental observations, but there are sufficient exceptions to make clear that much remains to be discovered even in respect of the interactions of antigen-presenting cells, T cells and B cells *in vitro*. Application of such general principles to predict the outcome of immunization *in vivo* would need also to take into account the microenvironments in lymphoid tissues where antigens are retained, and the flow of lymphocytes through them; how long the antigens persist; and how the immune response is modified by responses already elicited, including the idiotype network. Because such information is not usually available, enlightened guesswork may still be the best guide to practice.

1986 Synthetic peptides as antigens. Wiley, Chichester (Ciba Foundation Symposium 119) p 6-24

Since this symposium has a clearly defined purpose, to consider synthetic peptides as antigens, my contribution will relate to mammals with fully developed immunological systems and I do not propose to discuss birds or immature animals. When I accepted the suggested title I did so under the impression that a number of principles governing the regulation of immune responses were reasonably well established. They had largely been derived from experiments using selected populations of mouse or human cells *in vitro*. Until recently these populations were heterogeneous, but with improved technology allowing much smaller numbers to be examined in limiting dilution experiments, and with the development of T cell and B cell lines and hybridomas, of macrophage cell lines and of means to identify the factors which they secrete, valid general principles have become not easier, but more difficult to discern! However, the only way to provide a useful contribution as a basis for discussion seems to me to be to state some principles briefly and dogmatically, based largely on my reading of the literature.

B cells

Although the response of B cells to antigens is mainly regulated by interaction with T cells, at least some B lymphocyte populations are able to interact directly with antigens, without T cell cooperation. Since this simplifies the problem, I shall discuss B cells first.

Development of B cells

B lymphocytes arise from stem cells in the bone marrow which have the immunoglobulin (Ig) genes in a germline arrangement and express neither intracellular nor surface Ig. The genes for the heavy (H) chain of Ig are rearranged and expressed and cytoplasmic μ chains are produced. This is followed by rearrangement of the light (L) chain genes and both cytoplasmic and membrane IgM are formed. The variety of Ig variable (V) region expression by this early immature or virgin B cell population is enormous, and includes receptors (i.e., surface Ig molecules) which can potentially combine with almost any molecular shape above a certain size (about five amino acids), including self determinants. At this stage, cross-linking of the surface Ig receptors (by antigen or by antibody against surface Ig, including antibody against the idiotype, at very low concentrations) results in the B cells failing to re-express these surface receptors and the effective elimination of these cells (reviewed by Nossal 1983). More mature B cells can also be eliminated by similar cross-linking of their receptors but only at much higher concentrations of the antigens or antibodies responsible. The net result is a population of unstimulated B lymphocytes of which individual cells bear any one of an almost unlimited range of Ig receptors, including a number which can recognize self determinants. Unless stimulated by antigens (or *in vitro* and perhaps *in vivo* by non-specific B cell mitogens), B cells die quite soon. Where and how is still a mystery, but constant renewal of B cells occurs throughout adult life (according to Osmond et al 1981, some 10^8 new B cells are produced in a mouse each day).

If stimulated, the B cells expand clonally to become antibody-secretory cells and/or to become B memory (B_M) cells. During clonal expansion, somatic mutation in the V region genes allows an even wider range of antibody combining sites to be present in the B cell population. Those B cells whose receptors have the highest affinity for epitopes (antigenic determinants) on the stimulating antigen are likely to multiply preferentially (Tonegawa 1983). The class or subclass of Ig secreted was until recently considered to be ordained by an orderly switch from IgD to IgG3, IgG1, IgG2b, IgG2a, IgE and IgA, according to the constant (C) region gene sequence in the genome, but in practice it varies with the nature of the antigen, the subpopulation of B cells involved, and the local environment (e.g. T cells in the gut mucosa can switch B cells preferentially to IgA secretion: Kawanishi & Strober 1983).

B_M cells are small resting lymphocytes with an increased density of surface Ig, which do not secrete Ig unless restimulated by antigen with T cell cooperation. As a population they are long-lived *in vivo*, though whether this is true longevity of individual cells, or the result of constant stimulation to multiply by residual antigen (e.g. in germinal centres—see below) or by anti-idiotypic Ig (which has a combining site closely resembling the epitope of the original antigen) has not been resolved.

Control of B cell proliferation and Ig secretion

Thymus-independent (T1) antigens. There is considerable evidence that a subpopulation of virgin B cells can be stimulated to secrete IgM, IgA and some subclasses of IgG without cooperation with T cells, by some antigens operationally termed thymus-independent or T1 (summarized in Gray et al 1985). These are commonly poorly degradable polysaccharides or polypeptides with repeated epitopes—e.g. bacterial capsular antigens—or, for experimental purposes, haptenated polysaccharides such as Ficoll. Some, notably bacterial lipopolysaccharides, have an inbuilt capacity for stimulating macrophages. They all elicit very rapid antibody responses in athymic (*nu/nu*) as well as normal mice and rats, but only those with macrophage-stimulating activity elicit responses in CBA/N mice, which fail to develop a B cell subpopulation (which normally appears some weeks after birth). Those that elicit responses in CBA/N mice are termed T1-1, and those which do not are T1-2 (Scher 1982).

T1 immunogens all persist in macrophages for long periods of time and are continuously released in small amounts into the circulation. They evoke long-lasting antibody responses, but B_M cells are not normally detectable (this is partly a question of how they are looked for; see below). *In vitro*, resting single B cells generally (though not always—Pike & Nossal 1984) require B cell stimulatory factors, produced by T cells, before antigen stimulation causes their growth and differentiation to Ig secretion. Whether similar factors are produced by macrophages in the case of T1 antigens, or whether direct stimulation by antigen can take place, is not clear.

The difference between T1-1 and T1-2 antigens is probably that both can stimulate a particular subset of B cells in the marginal zone of the spleen white pulp, which is discussed later; but T1-1 antigens, by virtue of their stimulation of macrophages, can stimulate other B cells as well. Persistence of the antibody response is likely to be due to persistence of the antigenic stimulus.

Some other polymeric antigens which are regarded as typically thymus-dependent, such as sheep erythrocytes, have also been found to evoke IgM antibody responses in thymus-deprived or *nu/nu* mice, albeit much smaller and more transient than in euthymic animals (e.g. Kindred 1971, Wortis 1971). Although it has been argued by Coutinho & Möller (1975) that all T1 responses can be accounted for by polyclonal activation of B cells which have concentrated the antigen at their surface, for example, bacterial lipopolysaccharides, this is controversial (Klaus & Humphrey 1975). I suspect that many polymeric antigens with repeated epitopes, whether operationally thymus-independent or not, can stimulate a transient T1 response *in vivo*, though not necessarily *in vitro*. But since most antigens are rapidly degraded and do not continue to circulate, this response is too small and short-lived to be regarded as significant.

A point of some interest is that if T cell 'help' is provided by an artifice such as the injection of allogeneic T cells sufficient to induce a mild graft-versus-host reaction, a typical thymus-dependent antibody response to the T1 antigen is superadded (Klaus & McMichael 1974). The fact that T1 antigens do not elicit T cell help is probably due to their inability to become associated with class II MHC (major histocompatibility complex) antigens and thus to be recognizable by specific T cells (see later).

Thymus-dependent antigens. The majority of B cells, and all B_M cells, have been found to require cooperation with T cells before they can differentiate

towards antibody secretion. The 'help' needed is provided by B cell stimulatory
and differentiation factors, secreted by activated T cells, without which the
interaction of the epitope on the antigen with the Ig receptor on the B cell
surface is ineffective (Howard & Paul 1983). Although growth and differentiation factors are clearly distinguishable, their number, nature and mode of
action have not yet been fully elucidated (Kishimoto 1985). Since the antigen
moiety recognized by the T cell is associated with class II MHC antigens
(see below) and is quite distinct from the epitope (determinant) recognized
by the B cell Ig receptor, it has long been a puzzle to know how specific
cooperation between T and B cells could occur. The probable answer, suggested initially by Benacerraf (1978) and by Unanue (1981), and substantiated
by experiments by Lanzavecchia (1985), is that B cells capture and bind the
whole antigen molecules by means of their Ig receptors specific for a particular
epitope on the antigen, and then 'process' the antigen in much the same
way as do macrophages (outlined below) so as to associate it with their own
surface MHC II molecules in a form which can be recognized by the receptors
on T cells, which were stimulated in the first instance by antigen presented
directly by macrophages. The T cells are now restimulated by the processed
antigen and secrete B cell stimulatory factors, which in turn cause the local
B cells to secrete their anti-epitope antibody. If indifferent (i.e. non-specific)
B cells are also present nearby, they too may be stimulated to secrete their
Ig product. This would account for the non-specific Ig production which *in
vivo* usually accompanies specific antibody stimulation (e.g. Humphrey 1963).
The scheme is illustrated by Fig. 1 (redrawn from Howard 1985).

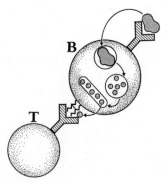

FIG. 1. Model of cooperation between T and B lymphocytes. In this model the T cell has
only one receptor, which recognizes a complex of processed antigen and MHC II moleule on
the B cell surface. Antigen processing is initiated by attachment of native antigen to the Ig
receptor. (Redrawn by permission from Howard 1985 *Nature* vol 314, p 494–495. © 1985 Macmil-
lan Journals Limited.)

B memory cells

In a primary response *in vitro*, B_M cells have never to my knowledge been detected. This may be because they have not been looked for, but it may be because *in vivo*, at least, there is a special mechanism for eliciting them. This involves the stimulation of virgin B cells by antigen complexed with antibody resulting from an early, probably thymus-independent response, which has activated the complement component C3 and become attached to receptors for C3 on follicular dendritic cells in germinal centres of the spleen and other lymphoid tissues (Klaus et al 1980). Such complexes can remain in the germinal centres for many months (Mandel et al 1980). In this microenvironment, which contains few T cells, those virgin B cells (which also bear C3 receptors) whose Ig receptors can recognize the antigen are stimulated to divide and become resting B memory cells with an increased density of surface Ig. However, unless they are restimulated by antigen with T cell cooperation, they do not become Ig-secreting cells. B_M cells can be detected long after the initial stimulation, and are usually regarded as long-lived cells. Although functionally this is so, it is difficult to be sure that their apparent longevity is not due to continual generation of new B_M cells by the antigen retained on follicular dendritic cells in the germinal centres. This may not be the only way in which B_M cells are produced, but it is certainly the most efficient. Once B_M cells with high affinity receptors have been generated it is possible that more may be produced as a result of subsequent stimulation by T-dependent antigen, without germinal centres being involved, but I am not aware that this has been formally tested.

T cells

The precursors of T lymphocytes arise in the bone marrow but undergo subsequent differentiation in the thymus. The T cell receptors for antigen have recently been characterized and the genes coding for them identified. These receptors (Ti) are heterodimers, made up of two glycopeptide chains (α and β) cross-linked by disulphide bonds. They are controlled by multiple genes for V, D, J and C regions, which are joined together in a similar manner to the immunoglobulin genes, and are capable of exhibiting a comparably enormous number of antigenic specificities (see Robertson 1984a,b). More recently, a third gene product (γ), similar to the α and β chains, has been described (Kranz et al 1985). Its function is uncertain, but it may be involved in recognizing class I MHC molecules (see below). Ti heterodimers differ from immunoglobulin molecules by being functionally associated with a further molecule, defined on human T cells by the monoclonal antibody OKT3

(Meuer et al 1984) and usually referred to as T3. This molecule appears to be involved in triggering the T cells to divide. A mouse analogue of the T3 molecule has now been described (Allison & Lanier 1985), so this feature is likely to be general. Also part of the T cell recognition complex are two other components, involved in the recognition of antigens in association with MHC determinants, namely T4 and T8, in T cells recognizing MHC II and MHC I respectively (see below).

Rearrangement of Ti genes from their germline configuration to that characteristic of mature T cells has not been detected in T cell precursors, but occurs within the thymus, so the receptor (Ti) is presumably expressed during differentiation and division there (Snodgrass et al 1985). In the thymus, some 90% of the multiplying T cells die. This is reasonably supposed to be due to elimination of T cells that possess receptors for the 'self' antigens (i.e., molecules which compose the various cells in the thymus or are present in the tissue fluids there). The T cells that emerge from the thymus form a population capable of recognizing an enormous repertoire of antigens, including of course any self antigens not already encountered in the thymus.

A remarkable feature of T cell receptors is that they recognize antigens only when associated with MHC molecules, and that T cells differentiate within the thymus into two distinct lineages: T helper (T_H) cells which recognize antigens associated with class II MHC molecules, and cytotoxic/suppressor (T_C) cells which recognize antigens associated with class I MHC molecules. Each lineage is characterized by well-defined cell surface molecules (T4 and T8, above) recognized by monoclonal antibodies—in humans, T_H by OKT4 and T_C by OKT8. The involvement of these molecules in the recognition of MHC II or MHC I has been put into a neat hypothesis by Reinherz et al (1983), illustrated in Fig. 2. Although the hypothesis is not accepted by everyone, it is at present the simplest.

Proliferation of T cells

Stimulation of T_H and T_C cells occurs somewhat differently. Resting T_H cells with suitable receptors need first to be activated by interleukin 1 (IL-1), produced by macrophages or dendritic cells (see below). They are then stimulated by antigen associated with MHC II molecules on antigen-presenting cells. The antigens may be already present as part of the cell surface, but extrinsic antigens must be taken up and 'processed' in such a way as to become associated with MHC II. The activated T_H cells rapidly develop receptors for interleukin 2 (IL-2) and the capacity to secrete IL-2. This causes non-specific proliferation of the T cells (Smith et al 1980). They secrete B cell differentiation factors and other lymphokines. These include interferon-γ, which in turn has

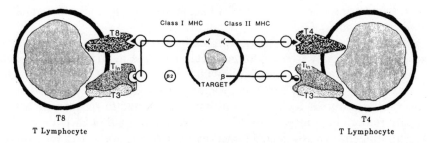

FIG. 2. A model of the human T cell receptor. The specific receptors which enable the T cells to recognize different antigens are shown as Ti_n. These are tightly linked with an invariant molecule T3 involved in the activation of the T cells. T_H cells which recognize antigens in association with MHC II, and T_C cells which recognize antigens in association with MHC I, have additional molecules as part of their receptors, namely T4 and T8 respectively. The target is represented as having on the left-hand side an antigen ⊖ associated with the MHC I α-chain plus β_2-microglobulin and, on the right-hand side, antigen associated with the β- (polymorphic) and the α-chains of MHC II. (Figure taken from Reinherz et al 1983, with permission of E. L. Reinherz and of *Immunology Today*.)

several important effects beside inhibiting the synthesis and assembly of viruses—namely, the stimulation of natural killer (NK) cells and the stimulation of MHC II expression and the down-regulation of MHC I expression by other cell types (Trinchieri & Perussia 1985). In the absence of continuing antigenic (or mitogenic) stimulation, the expanded T_H clones revert to resting T_H cells, and remain in this state for many months or years, available for restimulation.

Cytotoxic T cells appear to have receptors drawn from the same genetic repertoire as helper cells (Rupp et al 1985) but (in mice at least) are stimulated preferentially by antigen associated with the mysterious I-J rather than I-A components of MHC II (Dorf & Benacerraf 1985); and their receptors recognize antigens associated with MHC class I rather than class II molecules. From experiments with model systems *in vitro* most T_C cells appear to require IL-2 released by T_H cells as well as antigen presented in the context of MHC I in order to proliferate—that is to say, they require T_H help. Activated T_C cells can kill target cells expressing the antigen which they recognize, and release interferon-γ (Morris et al 1982) and a lymphocytotoxin (which can act as a non-specific inhibitor of ongoing responses) (Ruddle 1985). T_C have been regarded as the main agents responsible for killing virus-infected cells on which early viral antigens are expressed but, at least for some viruses, NK cells are reckoned to be equally if not more important (Biron & Welsh 1982). Since NK cells are activated by interferon-γ, the link with T cell activation remains nevertheless.

As with T_H cells, *in vitro* experiments and the sequelae of immunization *in vivo* indicate that once the antigenic stimulus has been removed, T_C cells revert to a resting state and persist for long periods as memory cells available for restimulation.

Unfortunately, the generalization presented above has proved to have many exceptions, especially when cultured T cell lines and hybridomas have been examined. For example, some T cells with the T_C phenotype have been found to secrete IL-2 (Moretta 1985) and some with the T_H phenotype have been shown to be cytotoxic for cells, even though restricted to recognizing MHC II. Cultured cell lines may be abnormal. Nevertheless, although T_C cells cyto-toxic for influenza virus-infected targets express T8 and are restricted to MHC I, in measles infection T_C have been found to express T4 and be restricted to MHC II.

Antigen presentation to helper T cells

Although of great importance to the symposium, and sure to be discussed by later contributors, the recent studies of how antigens are presented to T cells cannot be considered in any detail in this overall review. The subject is well reviewed by Unanue (1984). A brief summary goes as follows.

Antigens are presented by cells on which they are or can become associated with the appropriate class II MHC molecules. There is an additional require-ment for resting T cells that they be first activated by IL-1. In normal circum-stances the antigen-presenting cells are macrophages expressing MHC II, or dendritic (interdigitating, Langerhans) cells which constitutively express large amounts of MHC II molecules and can also secrete IL-1 (Sauder et al 1984), or B cells. Most studies have been done with macrophages and B cells and cell lines derived from them.

If the antigen is not already on the cell surface, it must be taken up by the presenting cell and then altered in some way so as to become associated with the MHC II molecule on the cell membrane. This alteration is commonly termed 'processing', and involves the unfolding and/or partial digestion of the antigen—at least in the case of globular proteins and glycoproteins. Whether carbohydrate antigens of the T1 kind discussed earlier are able to be 'processed' has not been tested, but it is a fair guess that they cannot be and that this is why T cells do not recognize them. The 'processed' antigens seem to associate with MHC II molecules at the surface of the presenting cell in some preferred stable configuration which is recognized by the T cell receptor (Ti). How this occurs is not known. Several workers have attempted to isolate or even detect the postulated complexes, but the only claim to have succeeded of which I am aware is by Babbitt et al (1985). They have shown that a selected peptide from hen egg-white lysozyme (HEL 46–61), which is immunogenic in mice expressing the HLA molecule I-A^K but not in those expressing I-A^D, associates selectively during equilibrium dialysis *in vitro* with purified solubilized preparations of I-A^K but not I-A^D isolated from a hybridoma cell line bearing I-A$^{D/K}$.

Comparable studies of 'processing' by B cells lead to similar conclusions, with the difference that B cells do not normally provide the IL-1 required to activate resting T cells and that they capture antigen via their Ig receptors, as already mentioned.

The presentation of antigens to cytotoxic T cells has not been examined by similar methods. However, since T$_C$ cells normally recognize antigens already expressed in the membrane of the presenting cells, 'processing' is presumably not required—even though there may be preferred ways in which MHC I and different antigenic determinants are recognized together.

Features neglected in this outline of the immune response

The preceding broad outline of the features involved in the stimulation of B and T cells summarizes what may occur in principle, even if the principles are rather shaky. It omits many factors which will decide what actually happens in practice, especially when extrinsic antigens are to be administered *in vivo*. Some of these additional considerations are listed below.

1. The route of administration and distribution of the antigen will affect which antigen-presenting cells take it up and what sorts of T or B cells encounter it, and its structure will determine for how long it persists.

2. The microenvironments in which lymphocytes encounter the antigen will affect which kinds are stimulated. Since subsets of B and T lymphocytes circulate through preferred microenvironments, 'homing' of lymphocytes will be important. Some of these factors were discussed in an earlier symposium (Ciba Foundation 1981).

3. Once an early thymus-independent antibody response has occurred (which can be within 1–2 days), any free antigen is likely to be complexed with antibody. This will accelerate its uptake by granulocytes and macrophages, including the majority which do not express MHC II, and the complexes may activate complement. Activation of complement causes the release of vasoactive materials as well as activating granulocytes and macrophages to release prostaglandins and leukotrienes, which affect the flow and distribution of lymphocytes.

4. The idiotype network operates in all immune responses to a greater or lesser extent, and anti-idiotype and anti-anti-idiotype (etc.) antibodies and specific T cells will undoubtedly act to regulate the later stages of an immune response—either negatively or positively (e.g. Geha 1983, 1984).

5. T$_H$ and T$_C$ cells have receptors for a variety of peptide and other

hormones, β-adrenergic agents, acetylcholine and histamine, the effects of which upon their function are largely unknown (Besedovsky et al 1983), but may be involved in the fine regulation of their behaviour.

Despite their relevance to the interpretation of immunological principles when put into practice, studies of the fate and distribution of antigens *in vivo* are nowadays out of fashion. The older literature has been summarized (Humphrey 1982). Other than pointing out these areas of ignorance and the complications they may introduce, I shall not enlarge upon them, but will mention instead some factors which could help us to devise effective peptide immunogens.

What sorts of immune response are wanted?

I assume that for prevention of the attachment of virus or bacteria or even protozoal parasites to their host cells, antibody that would block the sites on the microbes involved in attachment would be valuable. I also suppose that antibody may under some circumstances be involved in eliminating infected cells, either by complement-mediated lysis or by opsonization for killing by K (killer) cells. An adequate specific antibody level and a supply of B memory cells are therefore needed.

I also assume that both T_H and T_C cells are required to help B memory cells, to produce interferon-γ (and activate NK cells), and to kill cells expressing early viral or other microbial antigens. So a supply of T memory cells ready to be activated is also needed.

From the principles of the regulation of immune responses outlined here, it is apparent that antigens must be presented in such a way that they are effectively taken up by macrophages (i.e. not lost by excretion, nor rapidly removed by irrelevant cells such as granulocytes or hepatocytes) and can also be processed so as to be recognized by T cells. They must presumably also be stable to enzymes which would destroy the immunogenic configuration. This seems inevitably to involve attachment of the antigen to a carrier molecule. The obvious choice of carrier would be one that is already known to be an effective and not too toxic immunogen, such as tetanus or diphtheria toxoids, which have 'adjuvanticity'—namely, a separate and distinct affinity for other cell surface components such as gangliosides—or keyhole limpet haemocyanin (KLH) in humans, though other carrier molecules have been used. Whether it will ever be possible to predetermine the mode of attachment of a peptide antigen, or to design the peptide so as to facilitate its association with MHC II, I do not know.

It seems likely that the choice of carrier could determine by what cells the antigen is presented, although little is known about this. For example, if a carrier were selectively taken up by dermal Langerhans cells and transported by them to the T cell areas of the draining lymph nodes, it might preferentially stimulate T cell-dependent responses rather than antibody responses. Although considerations of this kind may explain why dermal infections (e.g. with vaccinia virus) or intradermally injected antigens are more effective than antigens delivered by other routes at stimulating T cells, little or nothing is known about the detailed intracellular fate of the antigens (see e.g. Humphrey 1982).

Various means have been devised for targeting antigens towards macrophages and inducing macrophage-activating properties by associating the antigens with adjuvants, or by incorporating them into liposomes or causing them to form micelles. For example, conjugation with long-chain fatty acids (Hopp 1984) or with muramyl dipeptide (Arnon et al 1983) or non-covalent association with glycoside micelles (Morein et al 1984) cause larger and more prolonged antibody responses in experimental animals than result from injecting similar amounts of the immunogen alone. However, since no information is available about where and for how long such immunogens survive, no amount of general principles is likely to explain why or how the effects are obtained. Enlightened guesswork seems still to be the best guide to practice.

REFERENCES

Allison JP, Lanier LL 1985 Identification of antigen receptor-associated structures on murine T cells. Nature (Lond) 314:107-109

Arnon R, Shapira M, Jacob CO 1983 Synthetic vaccines. J Immunol Methods 61:261-273

Babbitt BP, Allen PM, Matsueda G, Haber E, Unanue ER 1985 Binding of immunogenic peptides to Ia histocompatibility molecules. Nature (Lond) 317:359–361

Benacerraf B 1978 A hypothesis to relate the specificity of T lymphocytes and the activity of I region-specific Ir genes in macrophages and B lymphocytes. J Immunol 120:1809-1812

Besedovsky HO, del Rey AE, Sorkin E 1983 What do the immune system and the brain know about each other? Immunol Today 4:342-346

Biron CA, Welsh RM 1982 Activation and role of natural killer cells in virus infections. Med Microbiol Immunol 170:155-172

Ciba Foundation 1981 Microenvironments in haemopoietic and lymphoid differentiation. Pitman, London (Ciba Found Symp 84)

Coutinho A, Möller G 1975 Thymus-independent B-cell induction and paralysis. Adv Immunol 21:114-191

Dorf ME, Benacerraf B 1985 I–J as a restriction element in the suppressor T-cell system. Immunol Rev 81:7-19

Geha RS 1983 Presence of circulating anti-idiotype-bearing cells after booster immunization with tetanus toxoid (TT) and inhibition of anti-TT antibody synthesis by auto-anti-idiotypic antibody. J Immunol 130:1634-1639

Geha RS 1984 Idiotypic determinants on human T cells and modulation of human T cell responses by anti-idiotypic antibodies. J Immunol 133:1846-1851

Gray D, Chassoux D, MacLennan ICM, Bazin H 1985 Selective depression of thymus-independent anti-DNP antibody responses induced by adult but not neonatal splenectomy. Clin Exp
Immunol 60:78-86

Hopp TP 1984 Immunogenicity of a synthetic HBsAg peptide: enhancement by conjugation
to a fatty acid carrier. Mol Immunol 21:13-16

Howard JC 1985 Immunological help at last. Nature (Lond) 314:494-495

Howard M, Paul WE 1983 Regulation of B-cell growth and differentiation factors. Annu Rev
Immunol 1:307-331

Humphrey JH 1963 The nonspecific globulin response to Freund's adjuvant. Coll Int Cent Natl
Rech Sci 116:401-407

Humphrey JH 1982 The fate of antigens. In: Lachmann PJ, Peters DK (eds) Clinical aspects
of immunology, 4th edn. Blackwell Scientific Publications, Oxford, p161-186

Kawanishi H, Strober W 1983 Regulatory T-cell in murine Peyer's patches directing Ig-A specific
isotype switching. Ann NY Acad Sci 409:243-257

Kindred B 1971 Immunological unresponsiveness of genetically thymus-less (nude) mice. Eur
J Immunol 1:59-61

Kishimoto T 1985 Factors affecting B cell growth and differentiation. Annu Rev Immunol 3:133-
158

Klaus GGB, Humphrey JH 1975 Concepts of B lymphocyte activation. Transplant Rev 23:105-118

Klaus GGB, McMichael AJ 1974 The immunological properties of haptens coupled to thymus-
independent carrier molecules. II. The influence of the graft-versus-host reaction on primary
antibody responses to hapten-coupled polysaccharides and proteins. Eur J Immunol 4:505-511

Klaus GGB, Humphrey JH, Kunkl A, Dongworth DW 1980 The follicular dendritic cell: its
role in antigen presentation in the generation of immunological memory. Immunol Rev 53:3-28

Kranz DM, Saito H, Heller M, Takagaki Y, Haas W, Eisen H, Tonegawa S 1985 Limited diversity
of the rearranged T-cell gene. Nature (Lond) 313:752-755

Lanzavecchia A 1985 Antigen-specific interaction between T and B cells. Nature (Lond) 314:537-
539

Mandel T E, Phipps RP, Abbot A, Tew JG 1980 The follicular dendritic cell: long term antigen
retention during immunity. Immunol Rev 53:29-59

Meuer SC, Acuto O, Hercend T, Schlossman SF, Reinherz EL 1984 The human T-cell receptor.
Annu Rev Immunol 2:23-50

Morein B, Sundquist B, Hoglund S, Dalsgaard K, Osterhaus A 1984 Iscom, a novel structure
for antigenic presentation of membrane proteins from enveloped viruses. Nature (Lond)
308:457-460

Moretta A 1985 Frequency and surface phenotype of human T lymphocytes producing interleukin
2. Analysis by limiting dilution and cloning. Eur J Immunol 15:148-155

Morris AG, Lin Y–L, Askonas BA 1982 Immune interferon release when a cloned cytotoxic
T-cell line meets its correct influenza-infected target cell. Nature (Lond) 295:150-152

Nossal GJV 1983 Cellular mechanisms of immunological tolerance. Annu Rev Immunol 1:33-62

Osmond DG, Fahlman MTE, Fulop GM, Rahal DM 1981 Regulation and localization of lymphocyte production in the bone marrow. In: Microenvironments in haemopoietic and lymphoid
differentiation. Pitman, London (Ciba Found Symp 84) p68-82

Pike BL, Nossal GJV 1984 A reappraisal of 'T-independent' antigens. 1. Effect of lymphokines
on the response of single adult hapten-specific B lymphocytes. J Immunol 132:1687-1695

Reinherz EL, Meuer SC, Schlossman SF 1983 The delineation of antigen receptors on human
T lymphocytes. Immunol Today 4:5-8

Robertson M 1984a Receptor gene rearrangement and ontogeny of T lymphocytes. Nature (Lond)
311:305

Robertson M 1984b T-cell antigen receptor: the capture of the snark. Nature (Lond) 312:16-17

Ruddle N 1985 Lymphotoxin redux. Immunol Today 6:156-159

Rupp F, Acha-Orbea H, Hengartner H, Zinkernagel R, Joho R 1985 Identical V_β T-cell receptor genes used in alloreactive cytotoxic and antigen plus I–A specific helper T cells. Nature (Lond) 315:425-427

Sauder DN, Dinarello CA, Morhenn VB 1984 Langerhans cell production of interleukin-1. J Invest Dermatol 82:605-607

Scher I 1982 The CBA/N mouse strain: an experimental model illustrating the influence of the X-chromosome on immunity. Adv Immunol 33:1-64

Smith KA, Lachman LB, Oppenheim JT, Favata MF 1980 The functional relationship of the interleukins. J Exp Med 151:1551-1556

Snodgrass HR, Kisielow P, Kiefer M, Steinmetz M., Von Boehmer H 1985 Ontogeny of the T-cell antigen receptor within the thymus. Nature (Lond) 313:592-595

Tonegawa S 1983 Somatic generation of antibody diversity. Nature (Lond) 304:575-581

Trinchieri G, Perussia B 1985 Immune interferon: a pleiotropic lymphokine with multiple effects. Immunol Today 6:131-135

Unanue ER 1981 The regulatory role of macrophages in antigenic stimulation. Part II. Symbiotic relationship between lymphocytes and macrophages. Adv Immunol 31:1-136

Unanue ER 1984 Antigen-presenting function of the macrophage. Annu Rev Immunol 2:395-428

Wortis HH 1971 Immunological responses of 'nude' mice. Clin Exp Immunol 8:305-317

DISCUSSION

Lachmann: You discussed a new model of T–B cell cooperation (see Lanzavecchia 1985), and I wonder what you think about the physiological importance of antigen presentation to T cells by antigen-reactive B cells. The basis of this model is the finding that EBV-transformed antigen-specific B cell lines are much better presenters of antigen than are B cell lines of irrelevant specificity. I might add that EBV-transformed B cell lines of irrelevant specificity are, in turn, much better antigen presenters to T cells than are resting B cells (Vyakarnam & Lachmann 1984). Is it possible that one of the reasons why an antigen-reactive B cell presents antigen so well is that the antigen activates it to secrete growth and differentiation factors? I would like to see controls of antigen presentation using non-antigen-reactive B cells that have been activated in some other way. I also can't quite see how, *in vivo*, the antigen-reactive B cell and the antigen-reactive T cell will come together as a frequent enough event to start an immune response.

Humphrey: Either the cells have to meet, as you say, or factors have to be released which act at a distance or stick to other cells, so that B cells, when they pass by, later on, will encounter those factors. Antigen-specific soluble helper factors released by T cells have been described. I suppose that a T cell which recognized PPD (purified protein derivative of tuberculin) could produce a factor which could help a B cell that had bound haptenated PPD via the hapten.

As you have pointed out, B cells appear not to have receptors for PPD, but they could bind it indirectly.

Klug: In this new model of T and B cell interaction, when the antigen is processed by the B cell the pieces of protein presented to the T cell presumably need not be the same as the part of the protein initially presented to the B cell Ig receptor. In other words, this model allows two antigenic determinants to be recognized, so that there is the possibility that the B cell is recognizing one determinant and the T cell is reacting to another. Isn't that the strength of the new model?

Humphrey: That is correct. There would presumably be a number of different fragments of the antigen expressed on the B cell and it would depend on some T cell recognizing one of the fragments if T–B cell cooperation is to take place. I imagine that a determinant on the antigen adopts some preferred configuration in association with the MHC II (Ia) determinant, and that it is the combination which is recognized by the T cell. There is little direct evidence of how this happens.

Liu: What is thought to be the nature of the association between Ia antigen and the antigenic determinant? Is it antigen-specific, or is it just a physical connection?

Humphrey: This is the question. Bob Schwartz (1985) has produced compelling but indirect evidence from the study of presentation to mouse T cells of various cytochromes, which differ little from one another, that mice of different strains recognize different cytochromes according to whether or not they express particular genes for their MHC II chains. His findings are consistent with the idea that meaningful presentation of these antigens to T cells depends upon association with MHC II, and that different sites on the cytochromes associate differently. I mentioned in my paper that Unanue and his colleagues have some evidence for specific associations *in vitro* (Babbitt et al 1985).

Sela: On the question of whether T and B cells have to recognize the same antigenic determinant, I would like to remind you that the early work of Benacerraf and his colleagues (Levine et al 1963) in the guinea-pig showed that whatever the epitope that was attached to the carrier, so long as the carrier was polylysine, certain strains would not respond. This has nothing to do with antigenic specificity. The capacity to respond was strictly dependent on the nature of the carrier. This was done before the B and T cells were known, but you could now say that some epitope on the carrier would be recognized by the T cell and have to interact with the B cell. In our own work with mice, we knew that any hapten attached to branched polyalanine would not produce an antibody response in SJL mice, whether we used DNP, penicillin or the 'loop' of lysozyme. On the other hand, SWR mice would not respond to any hapten attached to branched polyproline (Mozes & Sela 1974). In view of these results, when we consider what might be important for a synthetic vaccine in the future, the nature of the polymeric carrier may be crucial; and this may depend on MHC.

Humphrey: This is the whole point of the new model. The 'carrier' is what is responded to by the T cell. The question was how the B cell captures the carrier. This model is a mechanism by which the hapten-specific cell doesn't have to capture the carrier, except via the hapten (see Lanzavecchia 1985).

Lachmann: There are excellent carriers that B cells don't seem to recognize, however—of which PPD may be a good example.

Anders: Lanzavecchia gave no evidence of the fine specificity of the collaborating T and B cells; there was no proof that they were seeing the same epitope.

Humphrey: That is true. This work was done with B cell clones specific for tetanus toxoid (TT) which stimulated two TT-specific T cell clones, but whether the latter each recognized the same epitopes is not evident.

Corradin: This is the best model available to explain T–B cell collaboration (antibody production), in conjunction with the notion that the T cell recognizes denatured antigens and the B cell recognizes native antigens. How can the two cells recognize each other, if the B cell cannot process antigens? The fact that the antigen is recognized by Ig and then processed tells you that the epitopes recognized by T and B cells can be different.

Ada: Is the role of the antibody to protect the particular epitope, while it is in the B cell?

Corradin: I would say that its role is to capture the antigen and then to process it and present it on the surface such that it can interact with any antigen-specific T cell.

Lerner: We may be about to beg the important chemical question here. Regardless of what happens in antigen processing, the clonality of the situation is determined before processing, by the original antigenic hit. We can't escape the essential protein-chemical questions just by assuming that the antigen is broken down.

V. Nussenzweig: This is an important issue in relation to all synthetic vaccines. A vaccine will be more effective if the native antigen can boost the immune response. Suppose the vaccine consists of a peptide coupled to, say, diphtheria toxoid or tetanus toxoid, which is used as the carrier. According to this model, a boost will occur only if the synthetic epitope is processed, expressed again on the cell surface, and the T cell recognizes it. The processing of the diphtheria or tetanus toxoid is irrelevant to the encounter with the native antigen.

Humphrey: The studies of the detailed presentation of antigens or fragments to T cells, of which I am aware, used T cell clones selected for their ability to be stimulated by antigens taken up by antigen-presenting cells *in vitro*. Thus, the clones selected would most probably have been those which recognize degraded antigen. There must be occasions where degradation of an antigen is not required. It is not uncommon to raise antibodies which are specific for the tertiary configuration of a protein antigen. For example, some monoclonal antibodies against human Ig react only with Ig in its native (folded) configuration (Nik Jaafar et al 1983). Unless the antigens were thymus-independent, the response must have required T cell help, and the Ig must presumably have been associated with MHC II in native form.

Another example, perhaps even more striking, was the demonstration 20 years ago that rabbits immunized with soluble antigen–antibody complexes (of the same allotype) could make antibodies which were reactive with the complexes but not against the antigen or antibody alone (Henney et al 1965).

Lennox: An area of ignorance which you touched on is the question of how one directs type-specific immune responses; that is, directing the desired IgG class. In vaccine production, that is of prime importance.

Humphrey: The surprising observation is that in the presence of gut-associated T cells, IgM-expressing B cells promptly switch to IgA production, which implies that gene expression can be affected by external influences (Kawanishi & Strober 1983). Sometimes selective stimulation of a particular Ig class can be due to preferential help from T cells. We know that helper or suppressor T cells can recognize B cells by virtue of their idiotype. I suppose that T cells may specifically help or suppress B cells which express not only idiotypes but allotypes and even class-specific markers on their immunoglobulin. There is evidence that helper cells and suppressor cells may regulate IgE production, for example. But a distinct variable may be the subpopulation of B cells that respond. In humans, and mice and rats, there is a B cell subpopulation in the marginal zone in the white pulp of the spleen which express IgM but not IgD. It has been studied extensively in rats by Ian MacLennan and his colleagues in Birmingham. These B cells secrete IgG2c and IgM predominantly. If B cells expressing IgD are eliminated by administering anti-IgD from birth onwards, the response to various immunogens of those cells which do not express IgD is unimpaired, but the antibodies elicited are IgG2c, IgM and IgA, rather than the more usual IgG2a and IgG1 (Gray et al 1982, Bazin et al 1985). The biological relevance of this subpopulation of B cells is evident from the effect of splenectomy, which removes most of them. After splenectomy, humans give a greatly diminished antibody response to a model T1-2 immunogen, namely DNP-Ficoll (Amlot & Hayes 1985). Experiments in mice and rats have led to similar conclusions (Amlot et al 1985).

Ada: You discussed the generation of memory cells. We want a vaccine to generate long-lived memory cells. Is it persistence of antigen that determines the longevity? We know that antigens don't always persist. Vaccinia virus does not persist for long, but you can get long-lived memory to vaccinia virus.

Humphrey: It has never been formally shown that persistence of B cells does not depend upon continuous antigenic stimulation. The best evidence was from an Australian study in which rhesus-negative women had had rhesus-positive babies and had then had hysterectomies. Their IgM disappeared rapidly but the IgG level remained detectable for years, in the absence of stimulation by rhesus antigen. What keeps the B cells producing this IgG is, of course, akin to the question of why there are such things as normal levels of immunoglobulin, or of B cells or T cells. I suspect that it is the result of continuous generation of non-specific stimulatory factors by macrophages and by T cells in local environments, and that there is a basal level of, say, interferon and probably also of interleukin 2 production. Since IL-2 is rapidly picked up by its receptors, you wouldn't be able to detect it.

Alkan: How do we know that B cell memory exists?

Humphrey: It exists functionally. You can take a population of B cells after priming with antigens bearing some particular epitope, supply T cell help specific for a different carrier moiety, transfer the two cell populations to an irradiated mouse and then stimulate with the original epitope attached to the second carrier. If unprimed B cells are used there is no or a negligible antibody response, but when primed B cells—i.e., B memory cells—are supplied, there is a rapid IgG antibody response specific for the original epitope (e.g. Klaus & Humphrey 1977). This type of experiment was devised by N.A. Mitchison. What it shows is that the B cell population of a primed animal contains an increased number of cells able to respond to the particular epitope (with suitable T cell help) and they remain increased for a long time after the original priming.

REFERENCES

Amlot PL, Hayes AE 1985 Impaired human antibody response to the thymus-independent antigen, DNP-Ficoll, after splenectomy. Lancet 1:1008-1011

Amlot DL, Grennan D, Humphrey JH 1985 Splenic dependence of the antibody response to thymus-independent (T1-2) antigens. Eur J Immunol 15:508-512

Babbit BP, Allen PM, Matsueda G, Haber E, Unanue ER 1985 Binding of immunogenic peptides to Ia histocompatibility molecules. Nature (Lond) 317:359-361

Bazin H, Platteau B, MacLennan ICM, Johnson GD 1985 B-cell production and differentiation in adult rats. Immunology 54:79-88

Gray D, MacLennan ICM, Bazin H, Khan M 1982 Migrant $\mu^+\delta^+$ and static $\mu^+\delta^-$ lymphocyte subsets. Eur J Immunol 12:564-569

Henney CS, Stanworth DR, Gell PGH 1965 Demonstration of the exposure of new antigenic determinants following antigen–antibody combination. Nature (Lond) 205:1079-1981

Kawanishi H, Strober W 1983 Regulatory T-cell in murine Peyer's patches directing Ig-A specific isotype switching. Ann NY Acad Sci 409:243-257

Klaus GGB, Humphrey JH 1977 Generation of memory cells. I. The role of C3 in the generation of B memory cells. Immunology 33:31-40

Lanzavecchia A 1985 Antigen-specific interaction between T and B cells. Nature (Lond) 314:537-539

Levine BB, Ojeda A, Benacerraf B 1963 Studies on artificial antigens. III. The genetic control of the immune response to hapten–poly-L-lysine conjugates in guinea pigs. J Exp Med 188:953-957

Mozes E, Sela M 1974 The role of the thymus in a genetically controlled defect of the immune response at the carrier level. Proc Natl Acad Sci USA 71:1574-1577

Nik Jaafar MI, Lowe JA, Ling NR, Jefferis R 1983 Immunogenic and antigenic epitopes of immunoglobulins. V. Reactivity of a panel of monoclonal antibodies with subfragments of human Fcγ and abnormal paraproteins having deletions. Mol. Immunol 20:679-686

Schwartz RH 1985 T-lymphocyte recognition of antigen in association with gene products of the major histocompatibility complex. Annu Rev Immunol 3:237-61

Vyakarnam A, Lachmann PJ 1984 Migration inhibition factor secreting human T-cell lines reactive to PPD: a study of their antigen specificity, MHC restriction and the use of Epstein-Barr virus-transformed B-cell lines as requirement for antigen-presenting cells. Immunology 53:601-610

Raising antibodies by coupling peptides to PPD and immunizing BCG-sensitized animals

P. J. LACHMANN*, L. STRANGEWAYS*, A. VYAKARNAM* and G. EVAN†

*Mechanisms in Tumour Immunity Unit and †Ludwig Institute for Cancer Research, MRC Centre, Hills Road, Cambridge CB2 2QH, UK

Abstract. The use of PPD (purified protein derivative of tuberculin) as a carrier has several significant advantages. It provides very powerful T cell help and it gives rise to virtually no antibody response against itself. This is particularly useful if it is intended to go on to make monoclonal antibodies, where the presence of a large amount of anti-carrier antibody is a nuisance! Furthermore, unlike most comparably powerful adjuvant systems, it can be used in man.

PPD coupling has been used to raise antibodies to haptens and to raise T cell responses to tumour cells. It is here reported that small peptides coupled to PPD will give rise to good titres of anti-peptide antibody. For peptides that contain no cysteine, coupling has been achieved by attaching succinimidyl 4-(N-maleimidomethyl) cyclohexane-1-carboxylate (SMCC) to the α-amino group of the peptide and N-succinimidyl 3-(2-pyridyl-dithio) propionate (SPDP) to the PPD and allowing an uncleavable bond to form between them.

Data on immunization with the leucotactic nonapeptide of the α chain of the complement component C3 and with some oncogene-related peptides have been obtained.

1986 Synthetic peptides as antigens. Wiley, Chichester (Ciba Foundation Symposium 119) p 25-57

It is now some twenty years since the hapten carrier effect on antibody formation and the linked recognition by T cells and B cells of antigens was first described (Mitchison 1971). At the core of this phenomenon lay the observation that a whole group of smaller antigenic determinants to which good antibodies can be formed are not on their own immunogenic. These are the haptens of classical immunology. It therefore became clear that the capacity to react with an immunoglobulin receptor on a B cell was not in itself an efficient stimulus for the induction of antibody formation. It was further recognized that if these haptens were coupled to an immunogenic molecule that could be recognized by T cells (the carrier) an anti-hapten response could be obtained, and that this required a T cell response solely to the carrier. Since with very few exceptions, such as the phenyl arsonate (ARS) hapten, it was shown that the commonly used small molecular weight chemical haptens could not act as carriers, it was recognized that the immune system was asymmetrical and that there were groups of compounds that were well recognized by B cells which could not be recognized by or stimulate a response in T cells (at least of the helper subtype). It has less commonly been appreciated that this asymmetry occurs also in the other direction and that there are molecules that can be recognized by helper T cells and act as carriers which do not give rise to antibodies, at least under normal conditions of immunization. The most striking example of what may thus be described as a T cell hapten is the protein component (purified protein derivative or PPD) of tuberculin.

PPD elicits delayed-type hypersensitivity (DTH) reactions in animals and humans who have previously encountered the tubercle bacillus, either as a result of infection or as a result of immunization with Bacillus Calmette-Guérin (BCG). Skin reactivity to PPD is widely used in this way as a diagnostic *in vivo* test to detect previous exposure to tubercle bacilli. Even the repeated intradermal injection of tuberculin in a Mantoux test does not itself give rise to tuberculin sensitivity, so the test can be used on multiple occasions. It is this property of eliciting T cell immunity without the capacity to induce it that justifies the name 'T cell hapten' for tuberculin.

In the mouse, but not in man, PPD is a polyclonal B cell mitogen (Sultzer & Nilsson 1972), though the effect even in mice is not powerful enough for us to demonstrate it after *in vivo* injection of tuberculin. Nor is antibody formation to PPD itself seen after PPD injection even into BCG-immunized animals.

Purified protein derivative of tuberculin (PPD)

PPD is prepared from the culture supernatants of *Mycobacterium tuberculosis* by ultrafiltration, heating to 100 °C and precipitation of protein with trichloroacetic acid (Seibert 1940).

The PPD used in these studies was generously donated by the Central Veterinary Laboratory in Weybridge and the batch used for the majority of the work, including all the most recent work, is Batch 298. This material is water-soluble and dark-brown in colour. It is not readily soluble in salt solutions above 0.5 M. The stock solutions are made up at 20 mg/ml in water and are then centrifuged in a Beckman J-21 centrifuge at 15 000 r.p.m. for 20 minutes. The pelleted material is rejected. The supernatant, on the basis of its Biuret reaction, has a protein concentration of 16 mg/ml. It gives a characteristic optical density spectrum with peaks at around 230 and at 260 nm. The extinction at 260 nm is around 2.6 for a solution of 1 mg/ml. Although this preparation is clearly not a single substance, its protein content—the material that is iodinated by the iodogen method—is predominantly a component of $M_r 10\,000$. It is very difficult to remove the contaminating coloured material. Passage over a Sepharose–Con A column removes some material but few iodine counts and little biological activity. Treatment with ribonuclease similarly has no effect.

An alternative source of PPD is the Statens Seruminstitut in Copenhagen. Their material is supplied as a solution of 1 mg PPD/ml phosphate-buffered saline and is colourless. Its properties are generally similar to those of the Weybridge PPD. Autoradiographs of the polyacrylamide gel electrophoresis patterns of radioiodinated samples of both PPDs are shown in Fig. 1.

Although PPD itself is not so far fully characterized, a closely related product obtained from tubercle bacilli rather than from their culture medium has been crystallized and sequenced by Kuwabara (1975). This peptide has

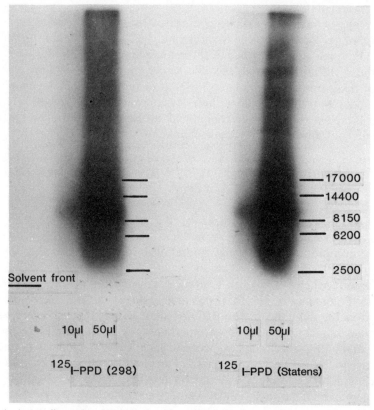

FIG. 1. Autoradiographs of polyacrylamide gels (15%) after electrophoresis of radioiodinated samples of two PPD preparations.

an M_r of 9700 and contains four lysines, two tyrosines and one intra-chain disulphide bond: the sequence gives no obvious clue to its peculiar immunological properties.

Coupling PPD to other materials

PPD behaves as a conventional protein in its chemical reactions using common coupling procedures reacting with lysine or tyrosine residues, such as 4-hydroxy-3-iodo-5-nitrophenylacetic acid (NIP)–azide coupling (Brownstone *et al* 1966), binding to diazotized polyaminostyrene (PAS), and iodination using the iodogen procedure.

For uncharacterized coupling to other proteins, glutaraldehyde has been used. For this purpose the glutaraldehyde is re-distilled to ensure freedom from polymers, as described by Gillett & Gull (1972) and is used at a final concentration of 0.06%.

For more defined and soluble conjugates the most successful technique has been to thiolate PPD using *N*-succinimidyl 3-(2-pyridyldithio) propionate (SPDP, Pharmacia) as described by the manufacturers. By offering five groups per mole of PPD it has been possible to get coupling of between two and three of the groups. The thiolated PPD, after reduction, can be coupled to succinimidyl 4-(*N*-maleimidomethyl) cyclohexane-1-carboxylate (SMCC, Pierce) attached to the other component to be conjugated. The reactions are carried out substantially as recommended by the manufacturers.

Evidence that the protein component of PPD is the material giving DTH in vivo

[125]I-labelled PPD was insolubilized by diazotization to polyaminostyrene (Amos & Lachmann 1970). This insolubilized and radioactive PPD was highly effective in inhibiting macrophage migration in the peritoneal exudate cells of BCG-sensitized guinea-pigs and in eliciting DTH *in vivo* in such animals. Furthermore, when ^{125}I-labelled PAS-PPD was injected subcutaneously into either a BCG-positive or BCG-negative guinea-pig, the radiolabel was retained at the skin site of the BCG-positive animal much longer than in the normal animal (Table 1). These experiments demonstrate that the protein portion of the PPD which can be diazotized and iodinated is indeed the antigen giving rise to DTH *in vitro* and *in vivo*. Furthermore, they demonstrate that the technique of coupling a material (in this case PAS) to tuberculin, and giving it to a BCG-positive animal, causes this material to be localized and retained at the site of injection. This is one property which is important in enhancing antigenicity (see Humphrey, this symposium).

TABLE 1 Retention of ^{125}I-labelled PAS-PPD in the skin of BCG-positive and BCG-negative guinea-pigs

| | Radioactivity recovered (c.p.m.) | |
Time after injection	BCG-positive guinea-pigs	BCG-negative guinea-pigs
One day	48 243 (80.4%)	21 278 (35.5%)
Two days	25 691 (42.8%)	854 (1.4%)

[125]I-labelled PAS-PPD (approx. 60 000 c.p.m.) was injected subcutaneously into each site of BCG-positive or BCG-negative guinea-pigs.

In conjunction with Dr T. D. Kellaway, we raised antisera by injecting PPD in complete Freund's adjuvant into BCG-positive rabbits that reacted by immunoprecipitation with high concentrations of PPD. Such antisera however failed to precipitate ^{125}I-PPD in a Farr assay, showing that they reacted not with the protein (which was responsible for DTH) but with non-iodinatable impurities in the PPD preparation.

Previous experience with immunization using PPD as a carrier

Anti-NIP immunization

In our initial experiments we studied antibody formation to the synthetic hapten, NIP. It was shown (Lachmann & Amos 1970) that NIP-PPD gave rise to antibodies only in guinea-pigs that had been previously rendered tuberculin-sensitive by immunization with BCG or by giving complete Freund's adjuvant, and that the prior injection of PPD into a normal animal in fact reduced even the low background response. The effect showed carrier specificity and the amount of anti-NIP antibody obtained was substantial (Table 2).

TABLE 2 The use of PPD as a carrier in the production of anti-NIP antibody in guinea-pigs primed with hapten (0.5 mg NIP-chicken globulin) four weeks before challenge

| Challenge antigen (300 μg) | Units of antibody[a] | | |
	No carrier priming	Primed with PPD (20 μg)	Primed with BCG
NIP-PPD	8.2	3.4	>70
NIP-bovine serum albumin	—	7.9	1.4

[a]Ten units of antibody give 30% binding of 10^{-8} M NIP-CAP (N-(4-hydroxy-5-iodo-3-nitro-phena-cetyl)aminocaproic acid).
(From Lachmann & Amos 1970.)

The PPD carrier system was also extensively explored by immunizing individual lymph nodes *in vivo* in sheep bearing efferent lymphatic cannulae (Hopkins et al 1981). These experiments were aimed at demonstrating that the repeated stimulation of a single node which was cannulated so that all cells passing through it were lost to the animal would lead to the abrogation of systemic cellular immunity to the carrier. In the present context, the results demonstrated high levels of antibody formation in both lymph and serum. The experiment illustrated in Fig. 2 compares anti-NIP immunization into

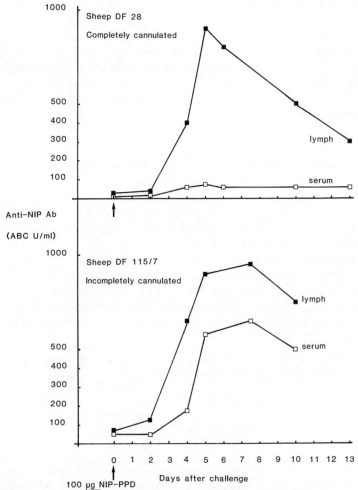

FIG. 2. Effect of immunization with NIP-PPD (100 μg) into a sheep lymph node, either completely or incompletely cannulated. (From Hopkins et al 1981, with permission of the authors.)

a completely cannulated node—where no antigen reaches the rest of the animal and where all the lymphocytes draining the stimulated node are removed—with immunization into a node where only one of two efferents had been cannulated. In the former case antibody was formed only in the lymph and was relatively short-lived; in the latter case antibody was found both in lymph and in plasma and the response lasted longer. The longer response can plausibly be attributed to the effect of the recirculating, PPD-reactive T cells.

The use of Con A-PPD to raise antibodies to cell surface antigens

We next explored whether coupling PPD to cell surfaces could allow antibody formation and cellular immunity to be induced to weak surface antigens, in particular to the tumour-specific transplantation antigens of methylcholan-threne-induced sarcomas in mice (Lachmann & Sikora 1978, Lachmann et al 1981, Vyakarnam et al 1981). It was found that coupling PPD chemically to cell surfaces reduced the immunogenicity of the cells in normal (BCG-negative) animals, presumably because of chemical damage to the tumour antigens. To overcome this problem PPD was coupled to concanavalin A (Con A) and the conjugate fractionated by G75-Sephadex affinity chromatography, which binds only the Con A that still has intact carbohydrate-binding sites. Only a small percentage of Con A-PPD was recovered, but the material could be bound to cells and turned out to be a powerful adjuvant. We were able to demonstrate both a high titre of antibody formation to the syngeneic cells and greatly enhanced tumour rejection. The latter could be shown using a Winn assay to be due not to antibody but to a T cell-mediated reaction. There is thus every reason to believe that immunization using a PPD carrier not only induced antibodies to the groups coupled to it but could also greatly enhance the T cell reactivity to the bound antigen. This ability to generate T cell reactivity is another condition to which importance is attached in vaccines (see Humphrey, this symposium).

We then asked whether, as had been supposed, the effect of BCG immunization was to induce helper T cells reactive to PPD or whether there were other, as yet not understood, mechanisms. For this purpose a series of anti-PPD T cell lines were grown and subsequently cloned (Sia et al 1984). All turned out to be of the helper phenotype (OKT4-positive); no suppressor/cytotoxic T cells (OKT8-positive) were encountered.

All T cell lines were assayed for their capacity to provide help *in vivo* to enable normal mice to make anti-NIP antibody in response to the injection of NIP-PPD. For this purpose the mice were previously given NIP-primed B cells. Whereas the T cells varied in the extent to which they were capable of giving this help, the 'best' clone of T cells (11C6) was highly effective

TABLE 3 Anti-NIP antibody responses of C57BL/10 mice given different numbers of PPD-reactive T cells (clone 11C6) and then injected with NIP-PPD

T cells transferred	NIP-binding capacity of serum (units/ml)[a]
—	12
2×10^5	375
2×10^6	496
10^7	1004

[a]Means of assays on three mice. Ten units of antibody give 30% binding of 10^{-8} M NIP-CAP. (Data from Sia et al 1984.)

in giving rise to anti-NIP antibody formation (Table 3). This T cell clone was also able to induce, in a naive mouse immunized with PPD-coupled tumour cells, the same capacity to reject tumours as is seen in a BCG-positive animal (Table 4). These experiments therefore demonstrate not only that it is solely the generation of helper T cells reactive to PPD which is required as the consequence of previous immunization with BCG, but also that the same helper T cells, which can help a B cell make anti-NIP antibody, can also help other T cells to generate an anti-tumour response.

A limited clinical trial of this method has been carried out, immunizing patients who have had squamous carcinomas of the lung resected with their own tumour cells coupled with Con A-PPD (Lachmann et al 1985). In this study no antibodies have so far been detected; indeed, the immunogenicity of these cells is not well established. The clinical results of the trial were statistically insignificant, though suggesting some improvement in survival. The trial demonstrated, however, that repeated injection of PPD-coupled cells to a BCG-positive person is free from any harmful side-effects, over a period of up to five years.

TABLE 4 The rejection of MC6A tumours in C57BL/10 mice immunized with tumour cells coupled to PPD through Con A and given PPD-reactive T cells (clone 11C6)

T cells transferred	Antigenic ratio at Day 9 after tumour challenge[a]
—	1.06
—(BCG-positive mice)	3.02
10^5	1.24
10^6	4.16
10^7	3.50

[a]The antigenic ratio is the mean diameter of tumours in unimmunized mice divided by the mean diameter of tumours in immunized mice.

Raising antibodies to Trypanosoma brucei

In conjunction with Dr Richard Le Page and Miss Karen Clegg, we have examined whether Con A-PPD enhances the immunogenicity of the surface antigens of *T. brucei*. Good enhancement of the response to this already quite highly antigenic organism was found in BCG-positive mice (Fig. 3). In these experiments the adjuvanticity of Con A-PPD was compared with the effect of *Bordetella pertussis*—itself a good adjuvant in mice. The results show one unexpected, and so far not further explored, observation, namely that *B. pertussis* is an effective adjuvant—for this antigen, at least—only in BCG-sensitized mice. The reason for this is not clear and it is not known whether *B. pertussis* and *M. tuberculosis* cross-react as T cell antigens.

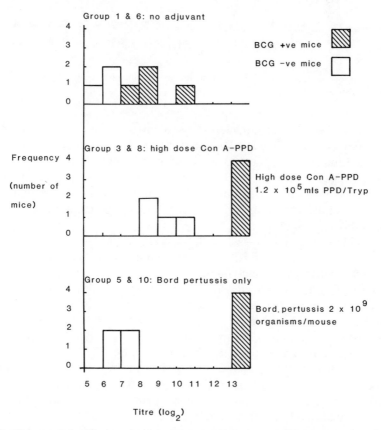

FIG. 3. Histograms showing immune lytic titres of sera from mice immunized intraperitoneally with 5×10^6 *Trypanosoma brucei* organisms at weekly intervals for four weeks. (Unpublished results, K. Clegg, R. Le Page & P.J. Lachmann 1981.)

Immunization with PPD conjugates of peptides

The putative leucotactic nonapeptide of the C3 α chain

Analysis of the proteolytic fragmentation of the complement component C3 in different laboratories has shown that two closely related fragments of the α chain differ in the ability to induce leucocytosis in rabbits. Thus the C3d-k fragment (Meuth et al 1983) is active whereas the physiological C3d,g fragment (Davis et al 1984) is not. Sequence studies showed that these fragments differ in that C3d-k has an extra nine amino acids. Fig. 4 shows the amino acid

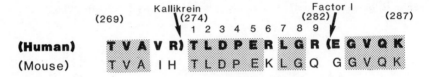

FIG. 4. Amino acid sequences of the putative leucotactic nonapeptide from the α chain of C3 of man and mouse.

sequence of the relevant nonapeptide and surrounding regions in man and mouse (Fey et al 1984, de Bruijn & Fey 1985). The differences between the mouse and human nonapeptides are clearly very small. The human peptide was synthesized for Dr A. E. Davis in Boston and we have attempted to raise antibodies to it in rats. It seems unlikely that the rat and mouse sequences will be much different, so the difference 'across' which immunization is being attempted is very small.

The human nonapeptide—which has no side-chains that can be used for coupling—was coupled to SMCC through the α-amino group of the N-terminal amino acid and this was then coupled to SPDP-derivatized PPD. A number of AO × LOU rats immunized with the PPD–nonapeptide conjugate all made good titres of antibody (Table 5, upper). Antibodies to this peptide were assayed by the Farr test. For this purpose the nonapeptide was radiolabelled, again through its α-amino group, using the Bolton & Hunter reagent. The Farr test has advantages over the frequently used ELISA (enzyme-linked immunosorbent assay) technique, in that it measures the reaction with the peptide in solution rather than with the potentially aggregated material on a microtitre plate, and is capable of giving quantitative estimates of the concentration of antibody and of its affinity.

The antibodies to the nonapeptide can be used to probe α-chain fragments of C3 on Western blots (Fig. 5); they also agglutinate erythrocytes coated with C3bi (EAC3bi; Table 5, lower). The antibody therefore has the appro-

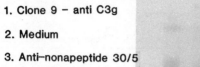

Reduced 5–12% PEG 4000 cut of NHS run on a 10% SDS–polyacrylamide gel, blotted and probed with:

1. Clone 9 – anti C3g

2. Medium

3. Anti–nonapeptide 30/5

4. Anti–nonapeptide 4/3

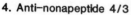

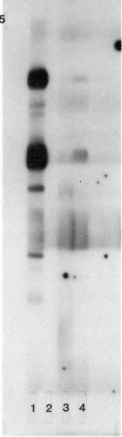

FIG. 5. Western blot of α chain fragments of C3 probed with rat anti-human nonapeptide antibody.

priate anti-C3 activity. Attempts to make monoclonal antibodies to the human nonapeptide are still in progress.

Oncogene peptides (see also Evan et al, this symposium)

Two synthetic peptides from the c-*myc* oncoprotein sequence were obtained from Cambridge Research Biochemicals Ltd. Mice were immunized either

TABLE 5 Results of immunizing BCG-positive AO × LOU rats with the putative human leucotactic nonapeptide coupled to PPD:30 μg of conjugate intravenously at two-weekly intervals, five times (1985 experiments) and 50 μg of conjugate in complete Freund's adjuvant followed by 50 μg intravenously at 10-day intervals, twice (1984 experiments)

Antibodies assayed by Farr test				
Animals	% specific binding (using 1.5×10^{-8} M ^{125}I-nonapeptide)			
	1/10	1/100	1/1000	1/10 000
Rat no. 2 (30/5/84)	52%	16.4%	5.7%	3%
Rat 0R (29/4/85)	34.6%	6.8%	6.4%	1.7%
Rat 1R (29/4/85)	36.4%	5.9%	3.1%	0.8%
Rat 2R (29/4/85)	45.5%	13.4%	3.3%	2%
Normal rat serum	0%			

Antibodies assayed by agglutination of EAC3bi	
Animal	Titre of agglutination
Rat 1 (14/5/84)	1/729
Rat 2 (14/5/84)	1/243
Rat 3 (14/5/84)	1/243

TABLE 6 Results of immunizing BCG-positive and BCG-negative BALB/c and B10 mice with two synthetic peptides from the c-myc sequence, conjugated with PPD or KLH, assayed by the ELISA technique

Conjugate	Mice	Half-maximal titres[a]	OD_{max} (1/200–1/400)
Peptide 1			
Peptide–KLH	BCG-negative	0, 0, 0, 0, 0, 0	0
	BCG-positive	0, 0, 0, 0, 0, 0	0
Peptide–PPD	BCG-negative	0, 0, 0	0
	BCG-positive	3200,>12 800, 0, 0, 3000, 0	$\begin{cases} 5000 \text{ (responder mice)} \\ 38 \text{ (all mice)} \end{cases}$
Peptide 2			
Peptide–KLH	BCG-negative	0, 0, 0	<0.2 (all mice)
	BCG-positive	0, 0, 0, 0, 0, 0	<0.2 (all mice)
Peptide–PPD	BCG-negative	0, 0, 0, 0, 0	0.3 (all mice)
	BCG-positive	0, 0, 0, 0, 0, 0	0.4–0.8 (BALB/c)
			0.5–0.9 (B10)

[a]0 = <1/100.

with PPD–peptide conjugates prepared by the SMCC/SPDP technique or with KLH (keyhole limpet haemocyanin)–peptide conjugates prepared with glutaraldehyde. Table 6 shown the antibody responses obtained, measured by the ELISA technique. These peptides are not highly antigenic. None of the animals responded to either KLH-coupled peptide. To one of the PPD-coupled peptides (peptide 1:Lys-His-Lys-Leu-Glu-Glu-Leu-Arg-Asn-Ser-Lys-Ala; the C-terminal peptide), three out of six of the BCG-primed mice gave high titres and three did not respond. To the other peptide (peptide 2: Ala-Glu-Glu-Glu-Lys-Leu-Ile-Ser-Glu-Glu-Asp-Cys), no animal has so far responded to a significant titre; though here too, although the responses are weak, those to the PPD conjugate in the BCG-positive mice are significant, whereas in the BCG-negative animals and in those given the KLH conjugate the responses are totally negative.

Antibody formation to PPD and to KLH was tested on Ouchterlony plates in the mice given the various conjugates. There was a strong line against KLH in the appropriate sera but none against PPD.

A similar comparison has been made with a peptide derived from the erb-B oncogene (Met-Lys-Cys-Ala-His-Phe-Ile-Asp-Gly-Pro-His-Cys) (also supplied by Cambridge Research Biochemicals Ltd). Here again (Table 7), a much higher titre was obtained by immunizing BCG-positive mice with the PPD conjugate than by immunizing even with substantially larger doses of a KLH conjugate.

Ubiquitin

Finally, good results were obtained, in conjunction with Dr H. J. Thogersen, by immunizing BCG-primed rabbits with a conjugate of PPD with the polypeptide ubiquitin, which is associated with intracellular protein degradation. (Table 8). This is of interest, since it had proved impossible to make antibodies to this peptide in four BCG-primed rabbits using a KLH conjugate and immunizing in complete Freund's adjuvant.

TABLE 7 Results of immunizing BCG-positive and BCG-negative BALB/c mice with erb-B peptide 0078 conjugated with PPD or KLH, assayed by the ELISA technique

Conjugate	Mice	Half-maximal titres[a]	Geometric mean titre
Peptide-KLH	BCG-negative	500, 400, 0, 0, 100, 700	$\begin{cases} 344 \text{ (responders)} \\ 49 \text{ (all)} \end{cases}$
Peptide-PPD	BCG-negative	200, 150, 300	208
	BCG-positive	4000, 7000, 800	2819

The peptide–KLH conjugate was injected intraperitoneally (20 μg peptide) first in complete Freund's adjuvant, then after 3–4 weeks in incomplete Freund's adjuvant and after two weeks in incomplete Freund's adjuvant. The peptide–PPD conjugate (approx. 4 μg peptide) was injected in incomplete Freund's adjuvant, the injections spaced as for the KLH conjugate.
[a]0 = <1/100.

TABLE 8 Results of immunizing four BCG-primed NZW rabbits with four intramuscular injections of 40 μg ubiquitin–PPD conjugate (1:1 by weight, coupled with glutaraldehyde), assayed by the ELISA technique

Rabbit	Half-maximal titre
1	2500
2	4600
3	4800
4	5200

No detectable anti-ubiquitin antibody was made by four BCG-primed NZW rabbits immunized with ubiquitin–KLH (500 μg) injected once in complete Freund's adjuvant followed by five injections in incomplete Freund's adjuvant.

Ubiquitin was prepared by the method of Ciechanover et al (1982).

Discussion and conclusions

The use of PPD as a carrier in tuberculin-sensitive animals has been shown to provide a peculiarly powerful mechanism for immunizing against a variety of antigens. These include small chemical haptens; cell surface antigens on tumour cells and on trypanosomes; proteins; and small synthetic peptides. For the tumour antigens it has been possible to show that not only antibody formation but also T cell immunity to the coupled antigen is generated at an enhanced level. The technique has been shown to be effective in rabbits, guinea-pigs, sheep, rats and mice. It has been used in man to immunize against tumours and has been shown to be without harmful effects, although the immune response elicited could not be evaluated. Experiments on immunizing human beings with PPD-protein conjugates are now planned; the first antigen to be used will be the high molecular weight fraction of bee venom.

For the oncogene peptide-PPD conjugates the response was compared to that given to conventional KLH–peptide conjugates and found to be substantially higher. In some instances where the KLH conjugate failed altogether, the PPD conjugate nevertheless produced good antisera.

Why this particular carrier system should be so highly effective is not known. Certainly it is advantageous to inject antigens into the sites of DTH reactions, and to use a carrier to which the animal shows a strong pre-existing T cell sensitivity may have an advantage in this regard. Among other effects the DTH reaction causes retention of antigen at the site of injection with a much slower rate of release than would otherwise occur. However, the major part of the adjuvant effect requires associative recognition and is not seen when PPD is simply mixed with the antigen (Lachmann & Sikora 1978). It does therefore seem that the 'help' provided by a carrier molecule that elicits a really powerful T cell response may be of particular importance in boosting the B cell response to a physically linked and associatively recognized antigen. The amount of anti-NIP formed in response to NIP–PPD in animals injected with cloned helper T cells was increased sharply by increasing the number of helper T cells given, over a wide range. This demonstrated that the amount of T cell help remains the limiting factor in the response even when large numbers of cloned T helper cells are present. A further reason why antibody responses to conjugates having PPD as a carrier may be particularly good is that PPD itself is a very ineffective B cell antigen. This may prevent various forms of antigenic competition that might inhibit the immune response to the coupled antigen.

It may also be significant that PPD given to BCG-positive animals seems not to give rise readily to suppressor cells. Neither in man nor in mouse have we been able to find a suppressor T cell among any of the lines and clones grown. Whether this is a property peculiar to PPD or a result of the method of sensitization with living organisms, or both, is undetermined.

Whatever the mechanism, the combination of the powerful adjuvant effect with the absence of a requirement to use precipitates or oily emulsions which may give rise to permanent granulomas makes the use of PPD an attractive technique with which to approach the development of human vaccines based on synthetic peptides. In the UK and in much of Europe the population is offered BCG vaccination and is therefore largely PPD-sensitive, and the injection of PPD into humans is a routine procedure. It is therefore also a method that will be relatively simple to introduce.

Acknowledgements

The authors would like to thank the Cancer Research Campaign for supporting some of the work described. They are also most grateful to Mr R. G. Oldroyd and Miss R. Glover for technical assistance, and to Mrs Margaret Cumpsty and Dr Sarah Coppendale for help with the manuscript.

REFERENCES

Amos HE, Lachmann PJ 1970 The immunological specificity of a macrophage inhibition factor. Immunology 18:269

Brownstone A, Mitchison NA, Pitt-Rivers R 1966 Chemical and serological studies with an iodine-containing synthetic immunological determinant 4-hydroxy-3-iodo-5-nitrophenylacetic acid (NIP) and related compounds. Immunology 10:465-479

Ciechanover A, Elias S, Heller H, Hershko A 1982 'Covalent affinity' purification of ubiquitin-activating enzyme. J Biol Chem 257:2537-2542

Davis AE III, Harrison RA, Lachmann PJ 1984 Physiologic inactivation of fluid phase C3b: isolation and structural analysis of C3c, C3d,g (α2D) and C3g. J Immunol 132:1960-1966

de Bruijn MHL, Fey GH 1985 Human complement component C3: cDNA coding sequence and derived primary structure. Proc Natl Acad Sci USA 82:708-712

Evan GI, Hancock DC, Littlewood T, Pauza CD 1986 Characterization of the human c-*myc* protein using antibodies prepared against synthetic peptides. This volume, p 245-259

Fey G, Domdey K, Wiebauer K, Whitehead AS, Odink K 1984 Structure and expression of the C3 gene. In: Müller-Eberhard HJ, Miescher PA (eds) Complement. Springer-Verlag, Berlin, p 9

Gillett R, Gull K 1972 Glutaraldehyde—its purity and stability. Histochimie 30:162-167

Hopkins J, McConnell I, Lachmann PJ 1981 Specific selection of antigen reactive lymphocytes into antigenically stimulated lymph nodes in sheep. J Exp Med 153:706-719

Humphrey JH 1986 Regulation of *in vivo* immune responses: few principles and much ignorance. This volume, p 6-19

Kuwabara S 1975 Amino acid sequence of tuberculin-active protein from *Mycobacterium tuberculosis*. J Biol Chem 250:2563-2568

Lachmann PJ, Amos HE 1970 Soluble factors in the mediation of the co-operative effect. In: Miescher PA (ed) Immunopathology, vol VI. Schwabe, Basel, p 65

Lachmann PJ, Sikora K 1978 Coupling PPD to tumour cells enhances their antigenicity in BCG-primed mice. Nature (Lond) 271:463-464

Lachmann PJ, Grant RM, Freedman, LS, Sikora K, Bleehen NM 1985 A preliminary trial of a novel form of active immunotherapy in squamous cell carcinoma of the lung. Br J Cancer 51:415-417

Lachmann PJ, Vyakarnam A, Sikora K 1981 The heterogenization of tumour cells with tuberculin. I. The coupling of tuberculin to cell surfaces using Con-A as ligand. Immunology 42:329-336

Meuth JL, Morgan EL, DiScipio RG, Hugli TE 1983 Suppression of T lymphocyte function by human C3 fragments. I. Inhibition of human T cell proliferative responses by a kallikrein cleavage fragment of human iC3b. J Immunol 130:2605

Mitchison NA 1971 The carrier effect in the secondary response to hapten–protein conjugates. II. Cellular cooperation. Eur J Immunol 1:18

Seibert F B, DuFour EH 1940 Purified protein derivative. Am Rev Tuberc Pulm Dis 41:59

Sia DY, Lachmann PJ, Leung KN 1984 Studies in the enhancement of tumour immunity by coupling strong antigens to tumour cells ('heterogenization of tumours'). Helper T cell clones against PPD help other T cells mount anti-tumour responses to PPD-coupled tumour cells. Immunology 51:755-763

Sultzer BM, Nilsson BS 1972 PPD tuberculin—a B cell mitogen. Nature New Biol 240:198

Vyakarnam A, Lachmann PJ, Sikora K 1981 The heterogenization of tumour cells with tuberculin. II. Studies of the antigenicity of tuberculin-heterogenized murine tumour cells in syngeneic BCG positive and BCG negative mice. Immunology 42:337-348

DISCUSSION

Crumpton: When you raise antibodies against tumour cells using the con-canavalin A (Con A)-binding fraction conjugated to PPD, do you know the nature of the antigen(s) mediating humoral and cellular immunity? One would like to know whether it is carbohydrate or protein.

Lachmann: We were using the MC6A tumour of Sikora et al (1977), and the specific transplantation antigen is thought to be a recombinant retroviral glycoprotein, gp70 (Lennox et al 1981).

Lennox: The appearance of the MC6A-specific transplantation antigen is *associated* with gp70, but the direct experiment of isolating a 6A-specific gp70, immunizing with it and showing that it is a protective immunogen, has not been done. We did immunize with other independent tumours which contain this antigen and got protection against 6A. If other tumours are selected by a positive cross-reaction with a monoclonal antibody that sees the gp70 of 6A, we can show cross-protection against 6A challenge. By that argument, the tumour-specific antigen might be the gp70.

Humphrey: When you transferred anti-PPD T cell clones, was this to normal or irradiated mice? In other words, were the B cells unstimulated?

Lachmann: We can use the recipient animal's unstimulated B cells but then two or more injections of NIP-PPD are required to obtain anti-NIP antibody. The experiments shown in Table 3 were done by transferring NIP-reactive B cells into the test mice from other mice previously immunized with NIP-chicken globulin.

Anders: How effective might PPD be if used as a carrier to immunize populations such as some in Papua New Guinea, in which tuberculosis and leprosy are endemic? There is a lot of tuberculosis in individuals immunized with BCG and, in some areas, Mantoux reconversion rates are high.

Lachmann: Most people exposed to tuberculosis have positive Mantoux reactions, whether they are protected or not. The normal, exposed population contains a small percentage with tuberculin 'anergy', as defined by a negative Mantoux test. A proportion of these have overwhelming or miliary tuberculosis (negative anergy), a proportion have sarcoidosis (positive anergy), and others have no clear cause for their anergy. Unless specific tests for T helper activity to PPD have been done, anergy due to failure of effector mechanisms (where a positive test can be obtained by injecting corticosteroids into the skin with the PPD) must also be distinguished from failure to generate the T helper cells. I imagine that most of a population that is much exposed to mycobacteria would have particularly high tuberculin sensitivity, rather than the reverse.

Gupta: We also found that if we immunize mice with the β subunit of human chorionic gonadotropin (hCG) or luteinizing hormone-releasing hormone (LHRH) linked to tetanus toxoid as carrier, BCG potentiates the antibody response.

We are trying to make monoclonal antibodies against $H_{37}Rv$ by immunizing with a mycobacterial sonicate or with different preparations of PPD obtained from the mycobacteria. In general, we obtained a very poor antibody response against $H_{37}Rv$. How can one stimulate an immune response against PPD or related antigens, in order to make monoclonal antibodies reactive against $H_{37}Rv$?

Lachmann: The heated, denatured material is not, in our hands, appreciably antigenic for B cells. Others are now immunizing with more native mycobacterial products to obtain antibodies cross-reacting with PPD. I have tested one candidate monoclonal (kindly supplied by Dr J. Ivanyi, MRC Tuberculosis & Related Infections Unit) and am not so far convinced that it reacts with PPD since, when used on an affinity column, it does not remove PPD activity.

Giving antigens together with BCG is different from the procedure I have described to you. If antigen is injected into any delayed-type hypersensitivity reaction, there is an adjuvant effect (Dienes & Schoenheit 1929). The effect of giving PPD conjugates requires associative recognition; it doesn't work if PPD is simply mixed with the antigen. The hapten must be linked to the carrier, therefore.

Gupta: Monoclonal antibodies have been raised using antigen 5 isolated from *Mycobacterium tuberculosis* (Daniel et al 1984).

Lachmann: The newer PPDs, made from unheated material and not denatured, are probably different, and strain-specific antibodies have been described (Editorial 1984). We don't mind if the material we use as a carrier is not strain-specific, and the heated PPD is a good carrier. If the aim is to develop better diagnostic tests for tuberculosis, the more characterized tuberculoproteins might give rise to more suitable, strain-specific antibodies.

Klug: Why is PPD so special? If you had started with another protein, boiled it and so on, and stimulated cells with the parent protein, would you not have got the same result as with this non-homogeneous mixture of peptides?

Lachmann: Gell & Benacerraf (1959) have shown that heat-denatured proteins are better at eliciting DTH than at raising antibodies. This may be a general feature of denatured proteins and have to do with the fact that T cells preferentially recognize extended amino acid sequences of processed antigens. But PPD is an unusually powerful T cell antigen; and it doesn't immunize against itself. You have to give the whole organism to get PPD sensitivity.

Klug: Have you purified your PPD preparation to see if the M_r 10 000 protein is the effective one?

Lachmann: Purification is not easy, but if we couple PPD to polyaminostyrene, this picks up a small percentage of protein which is diazotizable and works well as a carrier.

Williams: PPD contains two tyrosines. Have you attempted to find out whether you have labelled both, or one, and could you separate the three differently modified proteins possibly present? If we want to discover why PPD works, it would be nice to know whether either one of the two tyrosines was sufficient (i.e. both residues are equivalent), whether they are inequivalent, or whether both are necessary. The separation might be easy to do on a column.

You said that you often combine PPD through the N-terminus of the peptide. Some of the peptides that you conjugated with PPD contain cysteines, so you could have used those groups for combination. If you were to couple through cysteine, and so alter the availability of groups in the protein, so as to reveal different sites, would it make any difference to antigenicity? Often the N-terminus is an interesting antigenic site in itself.

Lachmann: We haven't done much along this line. We assume that our PPD has the same composition as Kuwabara's protein, but we don't know. The iodination is of one residue per molecule, probably randomly. When we diazotize we offer thousands of diazonium groups to one PPD molecule, so if it is sterically possible, links would form to both tyrosines. Coupling has been done both ways round. The C3 peptide has no cysteine and no other suitable coupling group apart from its amino group. We were interested in showing that coupling SMCC to the N-terminal α-amino group can be made to work. It would be equally interesting to couple with the two reactive groups the other way round. Where the peptide has a cysteine residue, it is easy to put SMCC onto the PPD and to couple that to the cysteine. We coupled Fab fragments to carriers, using the SH group from the reduced intra-chain disulphide.

Lerner: Mike Oldstone has made a detailed study of coupling peptides in different orientations (i.e. N→C versus C→N). The orientation makes a great deal of difference to the success of some immunizations.

Sela: In our work (Schechter et al 1970, 1971, Schechter 1972) we discussed peptides bound either via the amino terminus or via the carboxy terminus to the protein carrier. The portion sticking out is always immunodominant. The two epitopes are almost non-cross-reactive. When one looks to see how big an epitope is, one might conclude that it is a tetrapeptide or a pentapeptide, but this is generally wrong, because the last amino acid on either side is important—not because of its chemical nature but because it blocks the positive or negative charge. For a tetra-alanine hapten attached through its carboxyl group, trialanine amide binds as well as tetra-alanine, whereas when the attachment is through the amino group, acetyl-trialanine binds as strongly as tetra-alanine.

Geysen: The direction of coupling probably makes no difference to antibody induction, providing the charges on both ends are blocked at any one time. With the amide or the acetylated version, the direction of coupling does not affect the antibody response to the peptide. In most cases, of course, the peptide one is working with is taken from the centre of a protein, so normally no charge is seen at either end.

Rothbard: As the complete sequence of the tuberculin-active protein is known (Kuwabara 1975) and Savrda has determined that a hexadecapeptide within this protein can elicit the delayed-type allergic reaction in guinea-pigs (Savrda 1983), I wonder whether one could substitute this or other peptides for PPD in Dr Lachmann's system.

Lerner: An interesting point is that you can make antibody to 'self' pieces of protein, such as the C3 fragment. Likewise, M.S. Brown and J.L. Goldstein (personal communication)) made an antibody in rabbits to human low density lipoprotein (LDL), even though human and rabbit LDL turned out to have the same sequence in this region of the protein. There are many examples of this now. It seems that one may be tolerant to the folded state of one's own proteins but not to pieces of the proteins. So long as a particular piece is not exposed to the external environment, so that antibody would be adsorbed, it seems to be quite easy to make antibodies to proteins which ordinarily would be considered 'self'.

McConnell: You have said that you never get antibodies to PPD and that it fails to prime on its own. Doesn't that prove the new model for T cell priming (Lanzavecchia 1985)? There are no B cells with antibody receptors to first capture and concentrate antigen for presentation to T cells and therefore PPD does not prime.

Lachmann: Presentation of PPD probably has little to do with B cells. We have cloned PPD-reactive T cells in mice using only adherent antigen-presenting cells.

McConnell: How does T–B cell interaction work in the hapten–carrier system, then?

Lachmann: Some of the older models must also be right! The APC must be able to process the antigen; perhaps the EBV-transformed B cell secretes the right lymphokine factors constitutively. There is no necessity for an antigen-reactive B cell to be present in order to clone T cells, although the T cell must be stimulated by antigen associated with class II MHC molecules.

Humphrey: The problem is how the B cell, which has receptors recognizing the peptides in some configuration, comes to be in the neighbourhood of the T cell which is now switched on by PPD (plus MHC II) and producing differentia-tion factors. Would you expect a large non-specific Ig response as well as the specific response, because of the general activation of PPD-responsive T cells?

Lachmann: If PPD is given alone without a hapten on it, there may well be some production of Ig. As to what happens, I imagine it is a little like an affinity column. The APC have PPD bound on them; the T cell reacts with the PPD/class II MHC sites and is stimulated to secrete lymphokines, and the coupled peptide is available on the APC surface. When a peptide-reactive B cell comes close by, it finds itself in a medium full of lymphokines and is 'helped' to differentiate. Furthermore (and this has been studied by Ian McConnell and his colleagues), lymphocyte traffic is much altered. When PPD is injected into the drainage area of a cannulated lymph node in a BCG-positive animal, lymphocyte traffic through that node increases up to fivefold, and the node may enlarge to the size of a golfball in a sheep; so that the chance of the right T lymphocyte passing through is great. If PPD is injected five times over three weeks, enough of the animal's PPD-reactive T cells have passed through that reactive lymph node and been drained by the cannula that the animal no longer gives a positive test to PPD (Hopkins et al 1981).

Humphrey: I am still puzzled by the problem of bringing B cells with Ig receptors specific for the peptide into contact or close association with T cells which are stimulated to respond to PPD, unless one allows that the B cells have captured PPD via the peptide in the conjugate.

McConnell: It has been shown that there is a cap of lymphocytes with the T helper phenotype around the germinal centre in the node. Presumably, this is where the T–B cell interactions take place and where B cells may present antigen. In a hapten–carrier system using NIP-PPD, perhaps anti-NIP-reactive cells capture the NIP-PPD via anti-NIP receptors and are then stimulated by PPD-reactive T cells.

Lachmann: An explanation involving processing via the hapten will not serve for the cloned helper T cells that react only with the carrier and have never seen the hapten, and are capable of producing an even better anti-hapten antibody response *in vivo* than does preimmunization with hapten–carrier. There must be non-specific processes involved.

Ada: Does the increased traffic of lymphocytes cause tissue destruction in the lymph nodes, with the extra production of lymphokines by T cells?

McConnell: You don't see tissue destruction in the nodes, but there is extensive cell proliferation in the T cell-dependent areas.

Corradin: The B cell has to process antigens, for the simple reason that T cells recognize peptides and B cells recognize native structures. We also know that for antibodies to be produced *in vitro*, a thousand times less antigen is needed than for T cell proliferation. The problem is to visualize antigen presentation by macrophages with a thousand times less antigen, without a specific focusing mechanism, as in the case of B cells.

Liu: I would like to speculate as to why PPD should stimulate T cells rather than B cells. Generally speaking, the antigens recognized by T cells are somehow processed, whereas B cells recognize predominantly the native antigens. When you prime an animal with BCG, B cells (which recognize mainly native antigens) and T cells (that recognize mainly denatured antigens) will both be stimulated; when you boost with PPD, which is a denatured protein, the T cell response will predominate. Perhaps it is the immunization procedure you used, rather than the unique chemical properties of PPD, that makes the immune response T cell-dominated.

Lachmann: That may well be so.

McConnell: Another reason why PPD may act as such a good carrier is that perhaps there are no 'suppressor' determinants on PPD which are recognized by T suppressor cells. There is evidence for this for lysozyme. Suppressor cells and antibody recognize determinants in the same region of the molecule. Since

PPD is not recognized by antibody, perhaps there isn't a suppressor determinant on it.

Lachmann: This is what we suggest from our T cell cloning data, but there is a substantial and confusing literature on suppressor T cells generated in response to tubercle bacilli. Whether this response is determinant-specific, or dependent on the conditions of immunization, will not be known until the chemistry of PPD is better understood. Anergy to tuberculosis has been claimed to be due to suppressor cells, so *M. tuberculosis* may be capable of generating suppressor cells that act on PPD sensitivity; but they don't seem to be stimulated by injecting PPD into BCG-stimulated animals in the conditions we are studying.

Alkan: An observation obtained using *M. tuberculosis* (killed bacteria) as carrier gave the converse results to those presented (Alkan et al 1976). When we coupled haptens to mycobacteria and injected them into animals we induced not an antibody response but a T cell response to haptens. We did this with several haptens and in all cases obtained a T cell response to the hapten. The hapten-specific B cell response was always negligible.

Lachmann: That is presumably due to the Wax D of the mycobacterium (which contains the muramyl dipeptide), which acts at a different stage of the immune response. I am interested to learn that you can get T cell reactivity to small haptens. Can you then use the haptens as carriers? If you immunize a poly-L-lysine non-responder guinea-pig with DNP in the way you describe, and then give both NIP and DNP on poly-L-lysine, can you produce antibodies to NIP? Alan Munro and I (unpublished experiments) did this many years ago, sensitizing to DNP by painting the skin with dinitrofluorobenzene, and got no anti-NIP antibody at all.

Alkan: This hasn't been done with DNP. But when we coupled azobenzenearsonate to mycobacteria, it induced in guinea-pigs hapten-specific delayed-type hypersensitivity. Later we showed that those animals were primed for helper T cells. In other words, they gave a secondary antibody response to another hapten, DNP coupled to azobenzenearsonate-L-tyrosine. Also, one could culture lymph node cells of primed animals with hapten–carrier (protein) conjugates and observe hapten-specific proliferation of T cells (Alkan et al 1972). These experiments have since been repeated in mice (unpublished observations).

Altschuh: Dr Lachmann, can you explain why a good immune response can be obtained by injecting free peptides, without any carrier? This has been done with peptides less than 15 residues long (Young et al 1983, Atassi & Webster 1983).

Lachmann: If the peptide is big enough to serve as a carrier, it should be effective at immunizing on its own. If it does not have a carrier determinant, it will act only as a hapten. I agree that 15 residues is impressively small. It used to be said that 3000 molecular weight (or about 25 residues) is about the smallest complete antigen.

Evan: We have managed to get good, high titre responses against a 10-amino acid peptide, unlinked to a carrier. This peptide contains cysteine residues, and we took the precaution of reducing it just before immunizing with it.

Ada: I think Michael Sela produced an antibody to polyproline at one stage.

Sela: The smallest peptides with which we obtained good antibody formation were arsanylated trityrosines (Levin et al 1974). My question here would be: you have a small, well-defined chemical substance that you immunize with. How do you know the extent to which this small molecule binds *in vivo* to a protein? We tried to prove that the arsanylated tyrosine peptides did not bind to a serum protein, and had some evidence for it (Borek et al 1967).

Lachmann: p-Azobenzenearsonate is an exception in that it does act as a carrier. It tells us something about T cell receptors, that this small molecule is almost alone among small chemical haptens in so doing. Immunization with azobenzenearsonate conjugated to poly (γ-D-glutamic acid) gives rise to antibodies to the large poly (γ-D-glutamic acid) moiety (which acts as hapten) while the smalll arsonate moiety acts as carrier (Alkan et al 1971).

Sela: The p-azobenzenearsonate hapten is not unique. Schlossman (1972) and his colleagues, using the dinitrophenyl– oligolysine series, found a sharp cut-off point of size (hepatapeptide) below which the oligomer would not be immunogenic. This must have something to do with peptide structure, so that when one more amino acid is added, the resulting peptide transconforms into a different shape which reacts differently.

Lerner: In a diversity-generating system like the immune system, anything that can happen, will, if the system is pushed hard enough. You need to look at trends. You can raise antibodies to free peptides, but in general this is difficult to do. When antibodies are obtained to free peptides of about 15 amino acids, no doubt a little bit of the immunogen sticks to something so as to mimic a carrier state.

Crumpton: One wants to know what happens to a peptide of this size or smaller when put into an animal and, in particular, its physical state. If it is aggregated and presented as a polymer, then this is an entirely different picture from presentation as free peptide. My prediction is that if you adsorb a 15-amino acid or smaller peptide onto the surface of a glass bead or particle, so that you make it polymeric, then this will be very much better as an immunogen.

Sela: This has been done by adsorption on charcoal.

Crumpton: A crucial requirement is the presence of two determinants which fulfil the carrier and hapten functions and which are spatially disposed in a way permitting T cell–B cell interaction. In a study by Julia Levy of peptides derived from oxidized ferrodoxin, two distinct peptides induced T and B cell immunity when joined by a bridge of more than five but less than 10 glycyl residues (Levy et al 1972, Waterfield et al 1972). In contrast, no immunity was induced when one peptide was attached to itself via a dodecaglycyl bridge. These results indicate a requirement not only for bivalency but also for two different epitopes.

Ada: Was either of the peptides studied by Dr Levy known to react preferentially with T cells, or were they chosen for another reason?

Crumpton: No; the peptides were chosen on the basis that they reacted with antisera against oxidized ferrodoxin. Your question stimulates the further question of whether T and B cells see the same or different structures. In a number of studies, it has been observed that immunologically active peptides, which were identified by reacting with antisera raised against the native protein, also induced cell-mediated reactions in animals primed with the whole protein. These results argue in support of the same epitope being recognized by B and T cells. Superficially, this interpretation is contrary to that derived from Julia Levy's experiment (see above) using two copies of the same peptide attached through a bridge. The requirement for induction of immunity may, however, differ from that for interaction with antigen receptor.

Ada: In relation to possible vaccines, two general questions seem to have emerged so far. One question is whether one should link a T cell peptide with a B cell peptide, and whether this is a practical thing to do. The second concerns the mechanism of presentation of such a complex.

Sela: We did the following experiment with Baruj Benacerraf (Schwartz et al 1976a). A linear polymer of alanine and glutamic acid was used. The immune response to it was under genetic control: some strains of mice were responders and some were non-responders. With a polymer of three amino acids, alanine, glutamic acid and 10% tyrosine, the genetic control was different. One strain (SJL) gave good responses to the antigen containing tyrosine but did not respond to the peptide lacking tyrosine. We knew that the kinetics of the polymerization of the tyrosine monomer was the slowest, in the preparation of the synthetic terpolymer. We, therefore, took the Ala,Glu polymer and attached a pentatyrosine to one end of it. The non-responding strain became able to respond, even though the specificity of the antibody was still Ala,Glu. This relates to the topic we are discussing, because the tyrosine peptide must have been recognized, probably by T cells, whereas antibody production was still to the Ala,Glu peptide, and thus the specificity of the B cell must have been the same. But it seems strange to refer to a pentapeptide as a carrier and a polymer as the epitope!

Lerner: We know that we can take any protein, put it into vaccinia virus as a carrier and make all the antibody we want. Or we can express the protein in a bacterium. The important point is that using synthetic chemistry we can treat vaccines as chemicals. Perhaps it is possible to add a tyrosine residue and improve the antigenicity. This is the important point, that you can do such things to synthetic immunogens, and treat them as chemicals. This makes them very different from ordinary vaccines, which are whole proteins, where it is more difficult to do these chemical manipulations.

Corradin: We need to determine the principles which tell us why a peptide is immunogenic. For example, attachment to the cell membrane is important, because you may need a multivalent interaction with the T cell. Another feature is recognition by the T cell. We could think of the peptide as having two parts: one part has to interact with the macrophage membrane and another part has to interact with the T cell receptor. The peptide has to stay in the macrophage cell membrane for a certain time. Using cytochrome *c* peptides we find that some peptides stick to macrophages better than others. Evidently, certain groups in those peptides interact better with the lipid bilayer. So perhaps we have to make amphipathic peptides, where part of the molecule is hydrophobic and the other part hydrophilic, to activate T cells.

Ada: Can you distinguish between peptides remaining on the membrane, or being taken inside the cell and then re-expressed on the surface?

Corradin: I would say that we don't need peptide internalization for activation of T cells, but the peptide has to interact with the membrane. The question is whether special groups or configurations favour this interaction.

Sela: If you dipalmitylate a small peptide, which provides a 'hook', it becomes a good immunogen by itself (i.e. without a carrier). Probably once you have attached the two palmitic acid residues to the molecule, the resulting conjugate can form a micelle or can hook onto the membrane.

In relation to the macrophage, we had two peptides of identical composition, tyrosyl-tyrosyl-glutamyl-glutamic acid and tyrosyl-glutamyl-tyrosyl-glutamic acid. When they were attached to carriers, Tyr-Glu-Tyr-Glu was thymus-independent, whereas Tyr-Tyr-Glu-Glu was thymus-dependent (Schwartz et al 1976b). They don't cross-react. The thymus-independent peptide sticks to macrophages for longer and penetrates little, whereas the thymus-dependent peptide sticks for a short while, gets inside, and is digested very quickly.

Stanworth: The work of Petrov and his associates (Kabanov et al 1984), who are using artificial polyelectrolytes (e.g. copolymers of acrylic acid and pyrrolidone) as antigen carriers, is interesting in this respect. Conjugation of T cell-dependent antigens to such polymers apparently renders them T cell-independent, and results in enhanced antibody responses, for example to common vaccines like tetanus toxoid.

Evan: What about the idea of either conjugating a synthetic peptide of interest to a lectin, or sticking a palmityl group 'hook' on it, then fixing it on to cells removed from a subject and using that as an immunogen in that subject? Would this have any advantages, in that the peptide would be presented on the cell in the right context?

Sela: This is the question of whether it is worthwhile attaching a hapten to a 'guided missile' that would bring it selectively to the specific immunocyte; this could be an anti-idiotypic antibody, for example.

Crumpton: Dr Corradin and Professor Sela have identified the problem of how peptides can be retained on the surface of macrophages. Professor Sela has given us a clue, in that attachment of a palmityl group may be one way of holding a peptide on the cell surface. There is an acylating enzyme within cells that attached a fatty acid residue to many membrane-associated proteins, including the 'heavy' chain of class I antigens, and the α invariant chains of class II antigens. The significance of acylation with respect to biological function is not clear. Given this situation, it is conceivable that during antigen processing, peptides are acylated, and thereby are retained on the cell surface. We need to study the molecular nature of the epitope on the surface of the antigen-presenting cell in order to answer this question.

Skehel: One property of a peptide required for presentation might be simply that it should stick to cell membranes. However, in the presentation of intracellular proteins this is not sufficient; the molecules have to get through the cell membranes to be expressed. Rather than acylation, the problem of presentation in these cases is how to transfer proteins across membranes.

Ada: We are thinking of peptides here, of course, rather than proteins.

Crumpton: I don't see this as a large problem. If you accept that degradation of the protein antigen takes place in a membrane-bound vesicle, such as a lysosome, then, as judged from our knowledge of the biosynthesis of cell surface proteins, anything which becomes associated with the inner surface of the membrane enclosing the vesicle will end up on the cell surface, if the vesicle fuses with the plasma membrane. Conceivably, peptide acylation takes place within the vesicle mediating degradation such that the peptide becomes attached to the vesicle's inner surface. Fusion of the vesicle with the plasma membrane will result in the peptide being expressed on the outer surface of the cell.

Skehel: There are instances where non-membrane, non-secreted proteins, such as the nucleocapsid protein of influenza virus, are the major determinants recognized by T cells. Such proteins are not normally found in intracellular vesicles, but, for recognition, all or part of them has to be expressed at the cell surface. So, in some way they have to get across the cell membrane.

Humphrey: Part of the answer depends on the significance attached to the binding of peptide fragments to paraformaldehyde-treated presenting macrophages. If paraformaldehyde treatment of these cells prevents acylation, some peptides must be presented to cloned T cell lines simply by soaking the presenting cells in peptide and washing them; so no processing is involved. However, the peptides with which the cloned T cell lines that had been selected react contained a hydrophobic stretch of amino acids (Unanue 1984, p 407), so there may be a hydrophobic interaction (and adding tyrosine might help too). One kind of adjuvant that has been reasonably successful has been fatty acids, attached to two peptides.

Stevens: We have tried adding dipalmitic acid to some reproductive hormone antigen peptides to enhance immunogenicity. Our findings suggest that success may relate to the degree of hydrophilicity or hydrophobicity of the peptide. Very hydrophilic peptides coupled to fatty acids yield immunogens with no enhanced ability to elicit antibody production. They are very soluble even with the fatty acids on them, particularly larger peptides. The chemistry of a particular peptide may be important in determining whether it is made more immunogenic by this type of alteration.

Lachmann: There is a danger of being too mechanistic about antigen presentation. It is necessary but not sufficient that antigens 'integrate' with MHC class II antigens. Antigen presentation *in vivo* can be abrogated by chronic ultraviolet light irradiation of animals (Greene et al 1979, Letvin et al 1980a,b). Exactly what happens to their APC is far from obvious, especially since it is only the skin which is irradiated. The antigen-presenting cell probably has to do something other than just being MHC class II antigen-positive and having antigen stuck to it.

Humphrey: It has to produce interleukin 1, for example!

Ada: May we return briefly to the model of T–B cell cooperation discussed earlier (Lanzavecchia 1985) and ask how important it is in the overall context of antigen presentation.

Alkan: It is a beautiful model. In this model, the determinant recognized by the B cell is indeed different from the determinant that it presents to the T cell. The specific uptake of antigen by the EBV-transformed B cell (via its surface Ig) can be inhibited with free antibody made by the same B cells. Therefore presentation is also prevented. However, if you allow the B cell to take up antigen, and hence to process and present it, you can no longer prevent the interaction of T cells with B cells by means of the free antibody. So I think the epitope that is being recognized by the presenting B cell is different from the one it presents to T cells.

Ada: So you need a bivalent determinant, in other words.

Alkan: Yes.

Corradin: The antigen presented to T cells is a peptide (i.e. a different structure), so it could be the same amino acid sequence with a different tertiary structure from the native molecule. Dr Lanzavecchia has not determined exactly what peptide is being recognized, and he doesn't know what sequence in the native structure of the antigen is recognized by the antibody. You may assume that it is different, but we don't know.

Alkan: I agree with you, and therefore I think I should present another model, in which we know the epitopes recognized by B and T cells very well. Lanzavecchia (1985) does not know the precise epitope recognized by each cell. Some years ago we were working with the simple hapten already mentioned, azobenzenearsonate linked to a single tyrosine (Alkan et al 1971, 1972). It has an M_r of about 500. This small molecule (ABA-T) induces only a T cell response; no B cell responses can be detected. One can take macrophages from normal animals, pulse them with the antigen, and wash thoroughly. T cells can see the antigen presented by these macrophages and will proliferate. One can prevent the interaction of T cells and antigen-pulsed macrophages by anti-Ia antibody. However, one cannot prevent it using a monoclonal anti-ABA antibody (Fong et al 1979).

On this question of whether the antigenic determinants recognized by the T cells and B cells are identical or have to be different, or do they have to be linked, I can only say that when monovalent antigen (ABA-T) is injected into animals there is no antibody response induced because T and B cells cannot collaborate if the epitopes are not linked (Alkan et al 1972) (Fig. 1). However, the T cell response to ABA-T is always present. When two epitopes DNP–ABA-T are linked with a flexible, non-immunogenic bridge (6-aminocaproic acid) one gets a T cell response to ABA-T and a B cell (antibody) response to the DNP hapten.

We also asked the question whether or not two identical haptens would be immunogenic. When ABA-T–ABA-T was linked with a rigid bridge (proline), this symmetrical molecule induced both T and B cell responses *in vivo*. In summary, you can link ABA-T to any hapten you like and as a rule you get T cell responses only to the carrier site (ABA-T) and B cell responses to the other (haptenic) site (DNP, ABA or poly(γ-D-glutamic acid)). Thus, I think the immune response is asymmetric in general; the antigen is taken up by accessory cells and the epitopes after processing are recognized by the T cell. These epitopes are different from those recognized by B cells. Otherwise you would have a problem, namely antibodies (or B cell receptors) competing with T cell receptors. In these conditions, T cells and B cells could not communicate.

Ada: Otherwise you could make antibody to DNP just with B cells.

Alkan: I mean that antibody made by the B cell will block the presentation of that epitope to T cells, so you would have a total block of the immune response to T-dependent antigens.

Corradin: People have said that you cannot block T cell proliferation by antibodies, but you can, if you do the right experiment. We (Corradin & Engers 1984) selected T cell clones which recognize the epitope 23–28 of

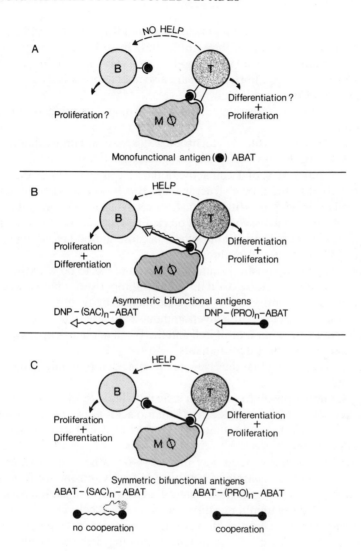

cytochrome *c*, and we made two monoclonal antibodies which recognize more or less the same epitope, with affinities of $\sim10^9M^{-1}$ and $\sim10^7M^{-1}$. When we combine macrophages, antigen plus T cells, and the first of these antibodies, we block T cell proliferation. If we combine the same mixture using the second monoclonal antibody we cannot block proliferation. There is a hundredfold difference in binding constants here. So the reason why many people failed to block T cell proliferation might be twofold. They perhaps didn't check for the specificity of their T cells and monoclonal antibodies; and they did not worry about the affinity constant of their antibodies. If we have macrophages with multivalent binding, we need an antibody with a very high binding constant in order to displace the equilibrium. We are also able to block helper T cells with the same high affinity antibody.

Williams: Are you referring to the cytochrome *c* peptide or the whole cytochrome?

Corradin: This is denatured cytochrome *c*. So we could argue that the T cell recognizes a peptide and the B cell recognizes the native structure to avoid blockage, by antibodies, of T cell activation or T cell help. If the T cell and B cell both recognize the native structure, the B cell product (antibodies) may block T cell proliferation. With two distinct recognition structures, one denatured and the other native, you cannot block T cell activation. Thus, there may be a danger with anti-peptide antibodies, because antibodies of high affinity might actually block T cell proliferation.

Lennox: The point you are raising, Dr Corradin, has to do with the issue of whether the T cell repertoire overlaps the B cell repertoire; that is, whether T cells can respond to antigens that are responded to by B cells. This is distinct from the issue of whether, in a given immune response, when you present a whole protein to an animal, the T cell and the B cell in microscopic interaction see the same or different determinants.

Corradin: I am saying that they can see the same determinants, if the antigen is denatured.

Ada: I was under the impression that in an individual reaction, if you give the immune system a simple peptide, say 15 amino acids long, the B cell sees one part of it and the T cell sees another part; they do not see exactly the same part. Is that still the view?

Lennox: That is the general way it works—or rather, that's what we all believe. You want two separate pieces, one for T cells and one for B cells. So if one is talking about designing a vaccine, that is what one should focus on.

Lachmann: A large number of different clones of B cells can recognize one hapten in an immune response. However the hapten is expressed on the APC, it is able to interact with many different combining sites on B cells.

Williams: When we use the word 'structure' in this discussion, we are using it in two different senses. One 'structure' is the primary sequence and the other is the conformational structure that a molecule may or may not have. When Dr Ada says that a 15-membered peptide appears different when looked at by a T cell or a B cell, do we know for sure that it is different parts of the sequence, rather than different structures of the same sequence?

Ada: I don't think we know that; but they are seeing different things, whether structure or sequence.

Sela: It's worth distinguishing between two separate issues. First, we are not absolutely clear, when we discuss the antibody response to a certain antigen, whether the B cell and the T cell recognize different areas of the molecule which cooperate. The other question is: can the B cell and the T cell independently recognize the same peptide, or the same area? We know that at the antibody level, native lysozyme does not cross-react with denatured lysozyme, and that lysozyme does not cross-react with lactalbumin, even though they are quite similar in their sequence. But at the T cell level, in terms of pure delayed-type hypersensitivity, there is a strong cross-reaction. It is worth remembering that even when we discuss the same sequences, the same part of the molecule, it is possible that the B cell and the T cell see it differently.

Lerner: No cell reads sequence; it all comes down to shapes in the end!

Ada: Let us assume, by and large, that for a given peptide the T and B cell are seeing something a bit different. Then the question arises of whether the Lanzavecchia type of model is an important mechanism of antigen presentation by the B cell, compared with earlier ideas of presentation by macrophages or dendritic cells; or is this an *in vitro* artifact?

Lachmann: The work of Letvin et al (1980a,b) suggests that you can cripple an animal's immune responsiveness by specifically inactivating its antigen-presenting cells with UV light while leaving its T and B cell function largely unaffected; so the B cell presentation model cannot account fully for what seems to occur *in vivo*.

Ada: Is it generally thought, then, that this is an intriguing model but it may not be quantitatively important in the overall response to an antigen?

Crumpton: The model deals with the *in vitro* situation. You can get T cells to present peptides to T cells *in vitro*, but this does not mean that *in vivo* T cells present antigens to other T cells.

REFERENCES

Alkan SS, Nitecki D, Goodman JW 1971 Antigen recognition and the immune response: the capacity of L-tyrosine-azobenzenearsonate to serve as a carrier for a macromolecular hapten. J Immunol 107:353-358

Alkan SS, Williams EB, Nitecki DE, Goodman JW 1972 Antigen recognition and the immune response. Humoral and cellular immune responses to small mono- and bifunctional antigen molecules. J Exp Med 135:1228-1246

Alkan SS, Trefts PE, El-Khateeb M 1976 Induction of T cell response to haptens coupled to mycobacteria. J Immunol Methods 10:197-206

Atassi MZ, Webster RG 1983 Localization, synthesis and activity of an antigenic site on influenza virus hemagglutinin. Proc Natl Acad Sci USA 80:840-844

Borek F, Stupp Y, Sela M 1967 Formation and isolation of rabbit antibodies to a synthetic antigen of low molecular weight. J Immunol 98:739-744

Corradin G, Engers HD 1984 Inhibition of antigen-induced T-cell clone proliferation by antigen-specific antibodies. Nature (Lond) 308:547-548

Daniel TM, Gonchoroff NJ, Katzmann JA, Olds GR 1984 Specificity of *Mycobacterium tuberculosis* Antigen 5 determined with mouse monoclonal antibodies. Infect Immun 45:52-55

Dienes L, Schoenheit EW 1929 The reproduction of tuberculin hypersensitiveness in guinea pigs with various protein substances. Am Rev Tuberc Pulm Dis 20:92-105

Editorial 1984 New tuberculins. Lancet 1:199-200

Fong S, Chen P, Nitecki DE, Goodman JW 1979 Macrophage–T cell interaction mediated by immunogenic and non-immunogenic forms of a monofunctional antigen. Mol Cell Immunol 25:131-142

Gell PGH, Benacerraf B 1959 Studies on hypersensitivity. II. Delayed hypersensitivity to denatured proteins in guinea pigs. Immunology 2:64-70

Greene MI, Sy MS, Kripke M, Benacerraf B 1979 Impairment of antigen- presenting cell function by ultraviolet radiation. Proc Natl Acad Sci USA 76:6591-6595

Hopkins J, McConnell I, Lachmann PJ 1981 Specific selection of antigen-reactive lymphocytes into antigenically stimulated lymph nodes in sheep. J Exp Med 153:706-719

Kabanov VA, Petrov RV, Khattov RM 1984 Soviet Scientific Reviews Section D Physicochemical Biology 5:1-46 (Gordon & Breach, New York)

Kuwabara S 1975 Amino acid sequence of tuberculin-active protein from *Mycobacterium tuberculosis*. J Biol Chem 250:2563-2568

Lanzavecchia A 1985 Antigen-specific interaction between T and B cells. Nature (Lond) 314:537-539

Lennox ES, Lowe AD, Cohn J, Evan GA 1981 Specific antigens on methylcholanthrene-induced tumours of mice. Transplant Proc 13:1759-1761

Letvin NL, Fox IJ, Greene MI, Benacerraf B, Germain RN 1980a Immunologic effects of whole body ultraviolet (UV) irradiation. II. Defect in splenic adherent cell antigen presentation for stimulation of T cell proliferation. J Immunol 125:1402-1404

Letvin NL, Greene MI, Benacerraf B, Germain RN 1980b Immunologic effects of whole-body ultraviolet irradiation: selective defect in splenic adherent cell function *in vitro*. Proc Natl Acad Sci USA 77:2881-2885

Levin H, Becker M, Sela M 1974 Antigenicity of *p*-azobenzenearsonate-containing oligopeptides in rabbits. Eur J Biochem 44:271-278

Levy JG, Hull D, Kelly B et al 1972 The cellular immune response to synthetic peptides containing sequences known to be haptenic in performic acid-oxidized ferredoxin from *Clostridium pasteurianum*. Cell Immunol 5:87-97

Schechter I 1972 Mapping of the combining sites of antibodies specific to polyalanine chains. Ann NY Acad Sci 190:394-419

Schechter B, Schechter I, Sela M 1970 Antibody combining sites to a series of peptide determinants of increasing size and defined structure. J Biol Chem 245:1438-1447

Schechter I, Clerici E, Zazepitzki E 1971 Distinct antigenic specificities of alanine peptide determinants attached to protein carriers via terminal amino or carboxyl groups. Eur J Biochem 18:561-572

Schlossman SF 1972 Antigen recognition: the specificity of T cells involved in the cellular immune response. Transplant Rev 19:97-111

Schwartz M, Waltenbaugh C, Dorf M, Cesla R, Sla M, Benacerraf B 1976a Determinants of antigenic molecules responsible for genetically controlled regulation of immune responses. Proc Natl Acad Sci USA 73:2862-2866

Schwartz M, Hooghe RJ, Mozes E, Sela M 1976b Role of antigenic structure in cell to cell cooperation. Proc Natl Acad Sci USA 73:4184-4186

Savrda J 1983 Synthesis and biological assays of peptides from a tuberculin-active protein. Infect Immun 40:1163-1169

Sikora K, Stern P, Lennox E 1977 Immunoprotection by embryonal carcinoma cells for methylcho-lanthrene-induced murine sarcomas. Nature (Lond) 269:813-815

Unanue EL 1984 Antigen-presenting function of the macrophage. Annu Rev Immunol 2:395-428

Waterfield D, Levy JG, Kilburn DG et al 1972 The effect of haptenic peptides from performic acid oxidized ferredoxin from *Clostridium pasteurianum* and protein carrier–hapten conjugates on the immune response of macrophages and lymphoid cells from animals immunized against oxidized ferredoxin. Cell Immunol 3:253-263

Young CR, Schmitz HE, Atassi MZ 1983 Antibodies with specificities to preselected protein regions evoked by free synthetic peptides representing protein antigenic sites or other surface locations: demonstration with myoglobin. Mol Immunol 20:567-570

Selection by site-directed antibodies of small regions of peptides which are ordered in water

H. JANE DYSON, KEITH J. CROSS, JOHN OSTRESH, RICHARD A. HOUGHTEN, IAN A. WILSON, PETER E. WRIGHT and RICHARD A. LERNER

Department of Molecular Biology, Research Institute of Scripps Clinic, 10666 North Torrey Pines Road, La Jolla, California 92037, USA

Abstract. High resolution nuclear magnetic resonance has been used to study a short peptide which corresponds to the antigenic region of a larger peptide immunogen. This work shows that there is a strong conformational preference for a Type II β-turn in solution. This observation has implications for the nature of the immunogenicity and antigenicity of peptide antigens as well as for the more general question of protein-folding mechanisms.

1986 Synthetic peptides as antigens. Wiley, Chichester (Ciba Foundation Symposium 119) p 58-75

The site-directed nature of anti-peptide antibodies is the essential feature which distinguishes them from all other antibodies (Lerner 1982, 1984). These antibodies have proved useful for finding the protein products of genes, determining the orientation of proteins in membranes, locating sites of virus neutralization, and carrying out structure–function studies on enzymes (Lerner 1982, 1984). But probably the most important feature of such antibodies is the role they are beginning to play in understanding some of the major questions in protein chemistry. As has happened so often in science, a simple experiment has led to a paradox, the resolution of which has ramifications far beyond the original experiment.

The central question, which we term the 'disorder–order' paradox, can be stated as follows: how does an antibody to a short synthetic peptide, always assumed to be in a highly disordered state, react with the more ordered version of the same sequence in the folded protein? This paradox can be resolved if the target site on the protein approaches disorder or, alternatively, if peptide in solution or on a carrier approaches a state of order. There is already considerable evidence to suggest that antigenic sites in proteins may correspond to regions of high atomic mobility (Lerner 1984, Artymiuk et al 1979, Moore

& Williams 1980, Westhof et al 1984, Tainer et al 1984, Williams & Moore 1985, Tainer et al 1985, Hirayama et al 1985) and thus the paradox is relaxed in this direction. Relaxation of the paradox in the other direction requires that, during induction of an immune response, peptides have conformational preferences.

To test the idea that some small peptides are ordered in water, we use anti-peptide monoclonal antibodies reactive with both large peptides and the intact protein to select the favoured recognition units from the larger peptide sequences. The conformations of these units are then studied by high field nuclear magnetic resonance (NMR) spectroscopy. In this paper we present studies of a nonapeptide selected as the immunodominant site of a 36 amino acid-long synthetic immunogen by several monoclonal antibodies which also recognize the native structure from which the immunogen was derived, influenza virus haemagglutinin (Wilson et al 1981, 1984). This nonapeptide (YPYDVPDYA, or peptide I) shows a conformational preference in water solution for a Type II reverse turn (β-turn), an observation unusual in itself, which suggests that in this case the immune system has selected a sequence which is to some extent structured in solution. In addition, if the above finding can be generalized, anti-peptide antibodies might provide reagents of sufficient precision for an immunological approach to the protein-folding problem (Sachs et al 1972a,b, Anfinsen & Scheraga 1975, Wetlaufer 1981, Teale & Benjamin 1976, Celada et al 1978).

Results

Assignment of resonances

The first step of any ^{1}H NMR study in peptide or protein conformation is to assign resonances to specific amino acid protons. In the case of the haemag-glutinin nonapeptide this task was complicated by the presence of several residues of the same type (three Tyr, two Pro, two Asp) and by pronounced cis–trans isomerism about the Tyr-1–Pro-2 peptide bond, which causes dou-bling of most resonances in the spectrum (Fig. 1). Complete spin system assign-ments were achieved by two-dimensional scalar correlated spectroscopy (Aue et al 1976, Bax & Freeman 1981) in both D_2O and H_2O. The phase-sensitive COSY spectrum (Marion & Wüthrich 1983, Rance et al 1983) of the peptide in D_2O is shown in Fig. 2. This spectrum identifies connectivities between all of the non-exchangeable proton resonances. Amide proton resonances were assigned from NH–αCH connectivities in a COSY spectrum measured in water (Fig. 3) using the 'jump-return' method (Guittet et al 1984). These spectra provide complete first-stage resonance assignments—that is, complete spin system assignments. Second-stage assignments to specific amino acids

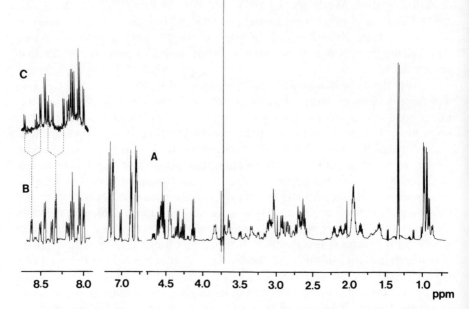

FIG. 1. Resolution-enhanced 500 MHz NMR spectrum of peptide I (YPYDVPDYA) at 278K.
A. Aliphatic and aromatic region. Peptide concentration approximately 10 mM in D_2O adjusted
to pH 4.15 with 0.1 M NaOD and 0.1 M DCl solutions in D_2O.
B. Amide proton region. Peptide concentration approximately 5 mM in 90% H_2O/10% D_2O.
The spectrum was acquired using a 'jump-return' sequence (Plateau & Guéron 1982). Chemical-
shift scale (ppm, parts per million) refers to both B and C.
C. Amide proton region of spectrum of peptide I with Asp-4 > 90% enriched with [15]N. The
spectrum shows splitting of the Asp-4 (*cis*) and Asp-4 (*trans*) NH resonances due to $^1J_{NH}$ coupling.

require information on the spatial and sequential relationship of the residues,
which can be obtained from nuclear Overhauser effect (NOE) experiments,
both one-dimensional and two-dimensional (NOESY) (Jeener et al 1979)
experiments. The evidence which led to the specific assignments is summarized
below:

(i) Tyr-1 is readily assigned, since it has no NH resonance. The amide
protons of N-terminal residues exchange so rapidly with H_2O that a separate
resonance cannot be observed.

(ii) Tyr-8 is assigned by comparison of the COSY spectra of the 9-mer
YPYDVPDYA and a 7-mer which lacks the Ala-9 and Tyr-8 residues.

(iii) Tyr-3 is identified by NOEs to Pro-2 and Asp-4.

(iv) The spin systems of Asp-4 and Asp-7 were unambiguously assigned
by substitution of ^{15}N-labelled Asp at position 4 (Fig. 1C).

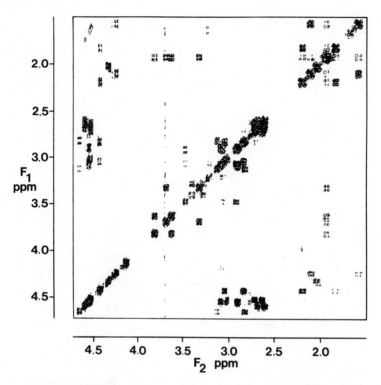

FIG. 2. Portion of the aliphatic region of a phase-sensitive, double quantum filtered COSY spectrum (Rance et al 1983) of peptide I in D_2O solution at 278K.

(v) Pro-2 is assigned from NOEs to the Tyr-1 αCH and Tyr-3 NH resonances.

(vi) Pro-6 is identified by an NOE to the Val-5 αCH resonance.

The specific resonance assignments for the *trans*-Pro-2 peptide are summarized in Table 1. Assignments for the minor *cis*-Pro-2 state are less complete. However, this form of the peptide is of less interest since no conformational preferences are evident for it.

Conformational substates of the nonapeptide in solution

The NMR experiments provide strong evidence that this peptide preferentially adopts a Type II β-turn (reverse turn) in water solution. The temperature dependence of the amide proton resonances (Fig. 4) shows that the Asp-4 NH is protected from solvent, as would be expected in a β-turn involving residues 1–4. Spectra are independent of peptide concentration, indicating

TABLE 1 Assignment of resonances of peptide I[a]

		298K		278K	
		trans	*cis*	*trans*	*cis*
Tyr-1	α	4.44	3.506	4.442	3.493
	β	3.03	3.00	3.061	3.10
	β	2.885	2.92	2.839	2.94
	2,6	7.154	7.016	7.159	7.012
	3,5	6.878	6.875	6.870	6.861
Pro-2	α	4.44		4.441	
	β	2.18		2.20	
	β	1.82		1.84	
	γ	1.93		1.93	
	δ	3.677	3.41	3.72	3.42
	δ	3.256	3.30	3.339	3.24
Tyr-3	α	4.575	4.669	4.534	4.668
	β	3.06	3.154	3.034	3.14
	β	3.03	2.842	3.029	2.83
	2,6	7.111		7.107	7.11
	3,5	6.807		6.797	6.81
	NH	7.788	8.191	7.992	8.365
Asp-4	α	4.624		4.607	
	β	2.63		2.608	
	β	2.71		2.677	
	NH	8.242	8.490	8.320	8.605
Val-5	α	4.365	4.383	4.333	4.361
	β	2.05		2.050	
	γ	0.963	0.963	0.976	0.976
	γ	0.919	0.894	0.935	0.905
	NH	7.937	7.896	8.117	8.188
Pro-6	α	4.284	4.313	4.259	4.291
	β	2.12		2.11	
	β	1.62		1.59	
	γ	1.94		1.93	
	δ	3.809		3.834	
	δ	3.643		3.644	
Asp-7	α	4.57		4.523	
	β	2.63		2.626	
	β	2.71		2.707	
	NH	8.280	8.330	8.449	8.504
Tyr-8	α	4.55		4.560	
	β	3.09		3.100	

TABLE 1 (continued)

		298K		278K	
		trans	*cis*	*trans*	*cis*
Tyr-8 (*contd*)	β	2.920		2.916	
	2,6	7.111		7.115	
	3,5	6.817		6.806	
	NH	7.941	7.972	8.135	8.155
Ala-9	α	4.146		4.127	
	β	1.320		1.323	
	NH	7.898	7.928	8.038	8.052

[a] Spectra obtained for 10 mM solutions of peptide I in D_2O (all resonances except amide resonances) and in H_2O (amide resonances). The pH for each solution (uncorrected meter readings) was 4.10 ± 0.05. Dioxan was used as internal standard.

that intermolecular association is unimportant. Further evidence for the reverse turn is obtained from NOEs between the Tyr-3 NH resonance and the resonances of the Asp-4 NH and Pro-2 αCH protons. The latter NOE to Pro-2 establishes a Type II β-turn (Wüthrich et al 1984). Another possible

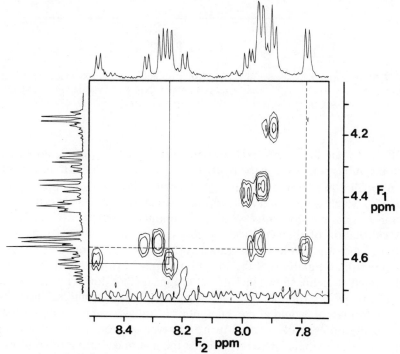

FIG. 3. Portion of COSY spectrum of peptide I in H_2O solution.

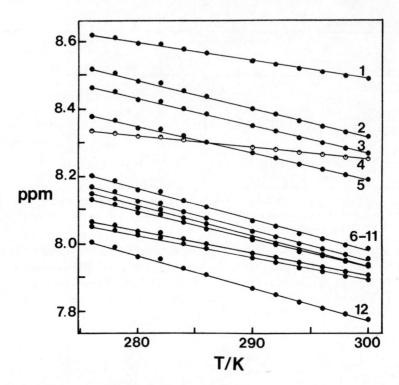

FIG. 4. Temperature dependence of chemical shift of amide proton resonances of peptide I.
1. Asp-4 (*cis*) 2. Asp-7 (*cis*) 3. Asp-7 (*trans*) 4. Asp-4 (*trans*) 5. Tyr-3 (*cis*) 6. Val-5 (*cis*) 7.
Tyr-8 (*cis*) 8. Tyr-8 (*trans*) 9. Val-5 (*trans*) 10. Ala-9 (*cis*) 11. Ala-9 (*trans*) 12. Tyr-3 (*trans*).

NOE, between the Asp-4 NH and the Pro-2 αCH, is often observed in
proteins, but is not visible in the peptide. The percentage NOE to be expected,
given the distance between the two protons in a classical β-turn, is much less
than 1%, which is not observable in these circumstances. The strong conformational preference for a reverse turn is maintained from pH 7 to pH 2.

A calculation of the statistical weights of the three classical rotamers at
each residue was made using values of the $^3J_{C\alpha H\text{-}C\beta H}$ coupling constants
obtained from simulations of the spectra of peptide I (*trans* form). The results
of this calculation are shown in Table 2. It appears that, for Tyr-1, the population of the *gauche* rotamer g^+g^- is insignificant. Model-building shows that
this conformation would force energetically unfavourable steric crowding
between the atoms involved in a β-turn of the type we propose and the aromatic
ring of Tyr-1. We therefore conclude that the β-turn conformation represents
a high proportion of the population of the *trans* form of the peptide.

TABLE 2 Side-chain rotamer statistical weights for peptide I

Residue		$^3J_{obs}$ [a]	Statistical weight of rotamer [b]		
			g⁻t [c]	tg⁺ [c]	g⁺g⁻
Tyr-1	αβ'	7.5	57%	43%	0%
	αβ"	8.8			
Tyr-3	αβ'	6.1	34%	28%	38%
	αβ"	6.6			
Asp-4	αβ'	6.7	42%	35%	23%
	αβ"	7.4			
Asp-7	αβ'	6.9	40%	37%	23%
	αβ"	7.2			
Tyr-8	αβ'	5.8	52%	25%	23%
	αβ"	8.3			
			g⁺	g⁻	t
Val-5	αβ	7.6	56%		44%

[a] $^3J_{obs}$ is the experimentally derived CαH-CβH coupling constant.
[b] Calculated from $^3J_{obs}$ using standard methods (Bystrov 1976).
[c] Note that g⁻t and tg⁺ cannot be distinguished experimentally.

Discussion

Our present NMR studies have established the existence of a stable Type II β-turn (Fig. 5) in a short linear peptide in water; that is, the peptide exists in a partially ordered state. We are unaware of any other well-authenticated examples of highly favoured reverse turns for unprotected linear peptides in aqueous solution.

In the present case, the stable reverse turn is in a peptide which is the site selected by the immune system as the immunodominant region of a larger

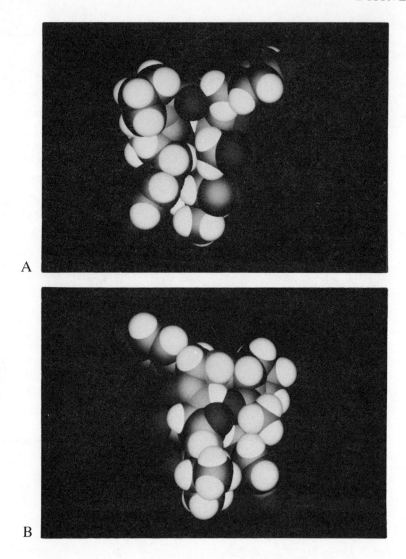

FIG. 5. Computer graphics simulation of portion of peptide I, showing the Type II β-turn structure and the NOEs observed.

A. 'Front' view of first five residues of peptide. Tyr-1 is at lower left, Val-5 at lower right.

B. 'Back' view: Tyr-1 is at lower right, Val-5 at lower left. Note the hydrogen bond visible in the centre of the picture.

C. Same view as B. Backbone representation showing NOEs observed.

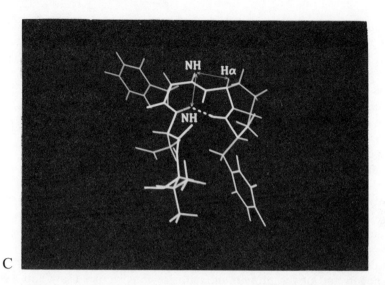

C

peptide antigen. Aside from its application in the study of the immunogenicity and antigenicity of peptides, this observation bears significantly on several fundamental issues, notably the mechanism of protein folding. There have been several previous immunological approaches to the folding problem (Sachs et al 1972a,b, Anfinsen & Scheraga 1975, Wetlaufer 1981, Teale & Benjamin 1976, Celada et at 1978). Stable local structures, which may be different from those in the final folded protein, can be recognized by antibodies, and have been postulated as initiation sites in folding (Sachs et al 1972a,b, Teale & Benjamin 1976, Celada et al 1978). Also, on theoretical grounds, reverse turns have been suggested as intermediates in protein folding (Anfinsen & Scheraga 1975). The experimental observation described herein may thus link the immunological and theoretical approaches to protein folding.

The majority of previous immunological studies of protein folding have utilized anti-protein, rather than anti-peptide, antibodies. Most antibodies prepared against intact proteins bind to determinants formed by residues which are in proximity only in the folded state (Crumpton 1974), making determination of the exact residues to which the antibody binds a formidable biochemical problem. Furthermore, antibodies which bind to the final state may not be the best reagents for studying the process of folding, which is inherently dynamic. Anti-peptide antibodies have several advantages for studying protein folding. Since they are site-directed reagents, they may be used in concert with the newer peptide synthesis methodologies (Houghten 1985) to reduce the problem to a small number of amino acids and determine binding specificity to a high degree of precision. This, in turn, reduces the complexity of subsequent NMR experiments used to investigate conformational preferences in solution. Since small sequences are studied, structures can be detected which might otherwise be masked or altered in large peptides. Finally, as mentioned above, these antibodies may allow the problem to be studied in the correct direction: since during the folding the protein moves from a disordered to a more ordered state, reagents which bind to peptide immunogens may have a better chance of detecting critical folding intermediates.

The main immunological question raised by this work is whether the presence of a stable reverse turn in an immunogen is important for relaxation of the disorder–order paradox. The diversity of the immune system makes generalization from a single observation difficult: until we study more examples, this question must remain open. Interestingly, Schmidt et al (1985) recently pointed out the importance of sequences with high (calculated) probability of forming reverse turns (Kuntz 1972) in the immunogenicity of synthetic peptides corresponding to sequences in the pili of uropathogenic *Escherichia coli*.

Antibody binding may itself influence the conformation of the peptide immunogen and of the protein antigen. Previous studies using anti-protein antibodies have suggested that interaction with the antibody may introduce order into a peptide (Teale & Benjamin 1976, Celada et al 1978, Crumpton & Small 1967, Conway-Jacobs et al 1970, Schechter et al 1971). The conformation of the immunogenic peptide in solution, as demonstrated in the present work, and that of the cognate site in the crystal structure of the protein (Wilson et al 1984) are different, suggesting that one or both conformations must be altered when the peptide or protein is bound to the antibody. To explore this question we are at present engaged in determining the conformation of the synthetic immunogen when bound to a monoclonal anti-peptide antibody, using both NMR and crystallography.

Our current view of ways in which the disorder–order paradox can be resolved is as follows. It seems that there may be a convergence between the postulates that the site in the protein to which antibody binds is mobile and that the immunogenic peptide may be partially ordered. However, the immune system is diverse, and we would not expect the behaviour of all anti-peptide antibodies to be the same. We would expect in some cases a greater requirement for flexibility in the protein target, whereas at other times a greater proportion of ordered structures in the immunogen will be required.

Acknowledgements

We would like to thank Dan Bloch for help with computer graphics simulations, Mark Rance for invaluable help with NMR techniques and Gail Donnan for technical assistance. We acknowledge financial support from NIH Grant No. A119499–01 (R.A.L. and I.A.W.). This is publication number MB-3999 from Scripps Clinic.

REFERENCES

Anfinsen CB, Scheraga HA 1975 Experimental and theoretical aspects of protein folding. Adv Prot Chem 29:205-300

Artymiuk PJ, Blake CCF, Grace DEP, Oatley SJ, Phillips DC, Sternberg MJE 1979 Crystallographic studies of the dynamic properties of lysozyme. Nature (Lond) 280:563-568

Aue PW, Bartholdi W, Ernst RR 1976 Two-dimensional spectroscopy. Application to nuclear magnetic resonance. J Chem Phys 64:2229-2246

Bax A, Freeman R 1981 Investigation of complex networks of spin–spin coupling by 2-dimensional NMR. J Magn Resonance 44:542-561

Bystrov VF 1976 Spin–spin coupling and the conformational states of peptide systems. Prog NMR Spectrosc 10:41-81

Celada F, Fowler AV, Zabin I 1978 Probes of β-galactosidase structure with antibodies. Reaction of anti-peptide antibodies against native enzyme. Biochemistry 17:5156-5160

Conway-Jacobs A, Schechter B, Sela M 1970 Extrinsic Cotton effect and immunological properties of the p-azobenzenearsonate hapten attached to a helical amino acid copolymer. Biochemistry 9:4870-4875

Crumpton MJ 1974 Protein antigens: the molecular bases of antigenicity and immunogenicity. In: Sela M (ed) The antigens. Academic Press, New York, vol 2:1-78

Crumpton MJ, Small PA 1967 Conformation of immunologically active fragments of sperm whale myoglobin in aqueous solution. J Mol Biol 26:143-146

Guittet E, Delsuc MA, Lallemand JY 1984 Real two-dimensional NMR solvent suppression technique. J Am Chem Soc 106:4278-4279

Hirayama A, Takagaki Y, Karush F 1985 Interaction of monoclonal anti-peptide antibodies with lysozyme. J Immunol 134:3241-3247

Houghten RA 1985 A general method for the rapid solid phase synthesis of potentially unlimited numbers of peptides: exact sequence specificity in peptide antigen/antibody interaction. Proc Natl Acad Sci USA, in press

Jeener J, Meier BH, Bachmann P, Ernst RR 1979 Investigation of exchange processes by two-dimensional NMR spectroscopy. J Chem Phys 71:4546-4553

Kuntz ID 1972 Tertiary structure in carboxidase. J Am Chem Soc 94:8568-8572

Lerner RA 1982 Tapping the immunological repertoire to produce antibodies of predetermined specificity. Nature (Lond) 299:592-596

Lerner RA 1984 Antibodies of predetermined specificity in biology and medicine. Adv Immunol 36:1-44

Marion D, Wüthrich K 1983 Application of phase sensitive two-dimensional correlated spectroscopy (COSY) for measurements of ^{1}H–^{1}H spin–spin coupling constants in proteins. Biochem Biophys Res Commun 113:967-974

Moore GR, Williams RJP 1980 Comparison of the structures of various eukaryotic ferricytochromes c and ferrocytochromes and their antigenic differences. Eur J Biochem 103:543-550

Plateau P, Guéron M 1982 Exchangeable proton NMR without base-line distortion, using new strong-pulse sequences. J Am Chem Soc 104:7310-7311

Rance M, Sørensen OW, Bodenhausen G, Wagner G, Ernst RR, Wüthrich K 1983 Improved spectral resolution in COSY ^{1}H NMR spectra of proteins via double quantum filtering. Biochem Biophys Res Commun 117:479-485

Sachs DH, Schechter AN, Eastlake A, Anfinsen CB 1972a Antibodies to a distinct antigenic determinant of staphylococcal nuclease. J Immunol 109:1300-1310

Sachs DH, Schechter AN, Eastlake A, Anfinsen CB 1972b An immunological approach to the conformational equilibria of polypeptides. Proc Natl Acad Sci USA 69:3790-3794

Schechter B, Conway-Jacobs A, Sela M 1971 Conformational changes in a synthetic antigen induced by specific antibodies. Eur J Biochem 20:321-324

Schmidt MA, O'Hanley P, Schoolnik GK 1985 Gal-Gal pyelonephritis *Escherichia coli* pili linear immunogenic and antigenic epitopes. J Exp Med 161:705-717

Tainer JA, Getzoff ED, Alexander H et al 1984 The reactivity of anti-peptide antibodies is a function of the atomic mobility of sites in a protein. Nature (Lond) 312:127-134

Tainer JA, Getzoff ED, Paterson Y, Olson AJ, Lerner RA 1985 The atomic mobility component of protein antigenicity. Annu Rev Immunol 3:501-535

Teale JM, Benjamin DC 1976 Antibody as an immunological probe for studying the refolding of bovine serum albumin. II. Evidence for the independent refolding of the domains of the molecule. J Biol Chem 251:4609-4615

Westhof E, Altschuh D, Moras D et al 1984 Correlation between segmental mobility and the location of antigenic determinants in proteins. Nature (Lond) 311:123-126

Wetlaufer DB 1981 Folding of protein fragments. Adv Prot Chem 34:61-92

Williams RJP, Moore GR 1985 Protein antigenicity, organization and mobility. Trends Biol Sci 10:96-97

Wilson IA, Wiley DC, Skehel JJ 1981 Structure of the haemagglutinin membrane glycoprotein of influenza virus at 3 Å resolution. Nature (Lond) 289:366-373

Wilson IA, Niman HL, Houghten RA, Cherenson AR, Connolly ML, Lerner RA 1984 The structure of an antigenic determinant in a protein. Cell 37:767-778

Wüthrich K, Billeter M, Braun W 1984 Polypeptide secondary structure determination by nuclear magnetic resonance observation of short proton–proton distances. J Mol Biol 180:715-740

DISCUSSION

Geysen: The so-called disorder–order paradox hinges on an assumption that has not been demonstrated, namely that the immune repertoire is very extensive. If in fact it is very limited, the paradox disappears.

Lerner: Absolutely. We, together with Sydney Brenner, have pointed out the potential limitation of the immunological repertoire (see Wilson et al 1985). The idea is as follows. The immune system has evolved its repertoire to 'see' the conformations of sequences that are parts of real proteins. Therefore all the other conformers are irrelevant, because the immune system is biased against them. You may ask about antibody to DNP or phosphocholine; the answer is that these are cross-reactions. If we really knew what the antibody to DNP or phosphocholine was against, we would learn that it was an antibody to some sequence in a protein which is also capable of binding to these relatively hydrophobic organic chemicals.

Geysen: In our recent paper (Geysen et al 1985a) we showed what an anti-peptide response looked like. It was far less than a stochastic response. We argued that the immune repertoire was very limited, to the point where it saw only very few conformations of the particular peptide. We have seen this with every peptide that we have studied in this way.

Lerner: It is hard to understand why a hyperimmune rabbit, say, can't see many different regions of these 20 amino acid-long peptides; but then, how is it that at the level of the intact animal the immune system can discriminate a single amino acid change, even though the sequence on both sides is shared? That is the issue, and again it comes down to shapes.

Ada: To put your view very simply, you think you have two different forms of a peptide both reacting with antibody, and you are asking whether both bind to the same binding site.

Lerner: We have a single antibody and we know two states of the antigen. We know the state in the folded protein, from X-ray crystallography, and we now know the state of a major conformer in solution. We don't know what the conformer is in the binding pocket of the antibody.

Sela: Why should one have to assume that the immune repertoire is unlimited? Why not assume that the peptide which can exist in a million different conformations has just a few which are thermodynamically highly stable, and they appear most of the time, and lead to most of the immune response.

Lerner: You have just solved the folding problem!

Sela: The picture I have always had is that the part of a crystallized protein which is extremely rigid will be difficult to mimic with small peptides (for immunological cross-reactions either way), but those areas that have a high mobility or flexibility will be the areas where the chance of getting antibodies to a protein that will cross-react with the peptide, or vice versa, will be highest. If there were a million different forms in existence, the chances would be smaller, so obviously there is a limited number of preferred conformations.

Lerner: I agree with what you say, but it is not enough to have movement, because if the structure is so different, the entropic cost of the antibody binding will be large. I would like to hear whether the NMR spectroscopists believe that a peptide in water has a few (10–20) conformers.

Crumpton: There is a fallacy in these arguments, and a need for an important qualification. We talk about using peptides for immunization, but we don't use free peptides; we inject peptides attached to carriers, which is entirely different. While I accept that a peptide in aqueous solution has flexibility, it has nothing like the same flexibility when attached to the carrier. In fact it will have preferred conformations which will be determined by the point of attachment, the degree of flexibility of the link, and the interaction of the peptide with the surrounding area of the carrier. Thermodynamics tells us that the peptide will orient itself on the carrier, in order to bury the maximum number of hydrophobic groups. As a result, the number of conformational states that the peptide assumes on the carrier (i.e. presents to the immune system) is very much smaller than you have in a completely flexible situation.

Lerner: But why should *a priori* the adoption of shape by a peptide on a carrier mimic that in the protein?

Crumpton: I agree that this is an important consideration. If we accept that proteins are not rigid molecules but possess segmental mobility, as described by Dr Klug, then surely it is possible to make an antibody against a shape of the peptide that is also expressed among the collection of shapes generated by flexibility of the corresponding portion of the whole protein.

Lerner: You are saying that a peptide in a heterologous protein environment folds in a way that mimics the protein that it was derived from. The extension to that argument is that peptides in general, when given a chance to hydrogen-bond or undergo hydrophobic interactions, with any heterologous protein, tend to fold correctly.

Crumpton: One point of disagreement between us concerns the frequency with which antibodies against synthetic peptides react with a conformational determinant of the whole protein. My impression is that this is a relatively infrequent event. This is based upon my experience with raising antibodies against the constant regions of the T cell antigen receptor (unpublished work), and that of colleagues with antibodies against the EGF receptor (Gullick et al 1985). I would argue that that is to be expected, in view of the problems that arise from using peptides on carriers. How do you see the role of the carrier? Do you see the peptide as being completely flexible?

Lerner: No, I do not.

Ada: I think we accept that the carrier can be important in restricting the amount of conformational change that can occur.

Stanworth: We have experimental evidence (Burt et al 1985) strongly supporting what Mike Crumpton is saying. We put synthetic ε-chain peptides on keyhole limpet haemocyanin (KLH) as carrier and produce anti-peptide antibodies which react with native rat IgE. The same peptides on bovine serum albumin (BSA) as carrier give as good an anti-peptide response, but these anti-peptides do not react with native rat IgE.

Geysen: In our studies, the anti-peptide response is evaluated from the reaction with all the peptides differing from the parent peptide by a single amino acid substitution. In this way the contact residues are determined. Evaluation of the response obtained from a peptide that is (1) indiscriminately coupled to sites on the same protein, resulting in varying local environments for the peptide, (2) absorbed to aluminium hydroxide as the carrier, and (3) coupled in the reverse orientation to that in (1), suggests that in each case the response is very similar and independent of the way in which the peptide was presented. This was interpreted by us to suggest that the immune repertoire is restricted (Geysen et al 1985a).

Lachmann: Antibody formation involves a great deal of selection. When you talk about the repertoire, you are really counting the winners. You cannot tell how many separate antibody clones 'entered the race'; but you do know that by the time those which react best have been selected, only a small number are left. I don't think that tells you anything about the potential repertoire.

Lerner: The difference between anti-peptide antibodies and anti-protein antibodies is that with the latter, the experiments are always circular. Take neutralization as an example. You make a battery of antibodies, say monoclonals, and screen for neutralization; you pick the winners, and you say that monoclonals are wonderful because you have a whole group of those that neutralize virus. We, in contrast, pick a stretch of residues, because it seems interesting, and make polyclonal or monoclonal antibodies to it. Let us say that, at the end, we find that this set of antibodies only react with the proteins in Western blots; so you say that for your purposes these antibodies are not as good as 'ordinary' antibodies. But that is because with anti-protein antibodies you have biased the experiment by throwing everything else away. The difference between a site-specific technology, which ours is, and a highly randomly selective technology, where the assay in the end decides the result, is responsible for the discrepancy between the two kinds of antibodies.

Rothbard: I wonder, Richard, whether your finding that this peptide adopts a reverse turn is fortuitous, or perhaps evidence that turns are logical sites of continuous epitopes. John Nestor first proposed that predicted turns are sensible choices for synthetic peptides which will be used as immunogens (Nestor et al 1985). We used some of his concepts in our choice of peptides in our work on gonococcal pilin (Rothbard et al 1984, 1985). Obviously, if you want to generate anti-peptide sera that cross-react with the intact protein, either the peptide has to resemble the protein, or the protein has to unfold to look like the peptide. I believe that turns have greater likelihood of being present in a linear peptide than either α-helix or a strand of a β-pleated sheet.

I also would like to stress that anti-peptide sera invariably cross-react with the intact protein with lower affinity than anti-protein antibodies. This is consistent with the possibility that there is a loss of binding energy due to the induction of a particular conformation.

Lerner: We don't think there would be enough energy for the antibody to put the extended chain conformation into a Type II reverse turn.

Sela: It is not only very difficult to generalize, but it's dangerous too. In my paper I shall give an example of how, from the same protein, you can make half a dozen synthetic peptides; all of them evoke good antibody responses. Some antibodies don't cross-react with the protein at all; several cross-react one order of magnitude worse; and one cross-reacts as strongly as the original protein. So I wouldn't predict anything *a priori*!

V. Nussenzweig: We shall present data on a peptide which contains many asparagines and prolines, residues which occur frequently in β-turns. This peptide represents the immunodominant epitope of the sporozoite antigen of *Plasmodium falciparum* very well. It is amazing how well the anti-peptide antibodies appear to recognize the native configuration of the protein. But in several instances we have prepared anti-peptide antibodies which failed to react with the native protein.

Corradin: In your paper on flexibility, Dr Lerner, you and your co-workers didn't show inhibition of the antibody reaction with the native protein (Tainer et al 1984). You showed only that there is binding on a plastic plate and precipitation of the iodinated protein. We know that iodination can denature protein. Native, unlabelled protein was not used to inhibit the antigen–antibody interaction.

Lerner: We have now done this, in experiments with Mario Geysen.

Corradin: What is the affinity between the native protein and the peptides? That is the important point.

Geysen: We have examined antisera raised against 12 different native proteins and scanned them against a complete set of hexapeptides from each of the sequences (Geysen et al 1985b). In that way, because we went from anti-whole protein sera, we identified 310 unique regions of those proteins which were immunogenic. When a survey of those hexapeptides was made using structure-prediction algorithms, with all their limitations, we were unable to demonstrate a preference for the immune response against any given structure, α-helix or β-sheet. What did stand out was a bias *against* β-turns. The one secondary structure in a protein that the immune response didn't like to see was the β-turn. These data reflect the anti-protein response, which is closer to the real situation.

Skehel: If you look at the antigenic sites of intact proteins, many antibodies recognize residues in β-turns.

Geysen: We are not saying you can't get any, but if you look at enough immunogenic epitopes, you find that β-turns are represented less than they ought to be on a purely random chance basis.

Lerner: In my view, it is foolish to vote. We shall next be reduced to voting for which are the most immunogenic amino acids. If we get 20 different votes we should quit!

REFERENCES

Burt DS, Hastings GZ, Stanworth DR 1985 Use of synthetic peptides in the production and characterization of antibodies directed against predetermined specificities in rat immunoglobulin E. Mol Immunol, in press

Geysen HM, Barteling SJ, Meloen RH 1985a Small peptides induce antibodies with a sequence and structural requirement for binding antigen comparable to antibodies raised against the native protein. Proc Natl Acad Sci USA 82:178-182

Geysen HM, Mason TJ, Rodda SJ, Meloen RH, Barteling SJ 1985b Amino acid composition of antigenic determinants: implications for antigen processing by the immune system of animals. In: Lerner RA et al (eds) Vaccines 85. Cold Spring Harbor Laboratory, Cold Spring Harbor, NY, p 133-137

Gullick WJ, Downward J, Parker PJ, Whittle N, Kris R, Schlessinger J, Ullrich A, Waterfield MD 1985 Proc R Soc Lond B Biol Sci, in press

Nestor JJ, Moffatt JG, Chan HW 1985 US Patent No. 4,493,795

Rothbard JB, Fernandez R, Schoolnik GK 1984 Strain-specific and common epitopes of gonococcal pili. J Exp Med 160:208-221

Rothbard JB, Fernandez R, Wang L, Teng NNH, Schoolnik GK 1985 Antibodies to peptides corresponding to a conserved sequence of gonococcal pilins block bacterial adhesion. Proc Natl Acad Sci USA 82:915-919

Tainer JA, Getzoff ED, Alexander H et al 1984 The reactivity of anti-peptide antibodies is a function of the atomic mobility of sites in a protein. Nature (Lond) 312:127-134

Wilson IA, Haft DH, Getzoff ED, Tainer JA, Lerner RA, Brenner S 1985 Identical short peptide sequences in unrelated proteins can have different conformations: a testing ground for theories of immune recognition. Proc Natl Acad Sci USA 82:5255-5259

Influence of local structure on the location of antigenic determinants in tobacco mosaic virus protein

M. H. V. VAN REGENMORTEL*, D. ALTSCHUH*† and A. KLUG†

*Institut de Biologie Moléculaire et Cellulaire du CNRS, 15, rue René Descartes, 67084 Strasbourg, France and †MRC Laboratory of Molecular Biology, Hills Road, Cambridge CB2 2QH, UK

Abstract. Early work on protein antigenicity led to the common belief that proteins possess a finite number of antigenic determinants located in accessible regions of the molecule's surface. This view is now changing. As a result of extensive studies, seven continuous epitopes have been located on tobacco mosaic virus (TMV) protein by measuring the antigenic activity of short peptides with anti-protein antibodies. The structure of the viral protein has been refined in Cambridge, enabling the Strasbourg workers to correlate the position of these epitopes with regions of high segmental mobility in the protein. Surface accessibility is not a sufficient condition for antigenicity, because six short peptides corresponding to accessible regions of the protein possess no antigenic activity.

Recent work in Strasbourg shows that when longer peptides of TMV protein are used, more antigenic determinants are found and these lie in more structured regions of the protein (e.g. helices). In these cases the longer peptide may be folding up in solution to mimic part of the native structure.

1986 Synthetic peptides as antigens. Wiley, Chichester (Ciba Foundation Symposium 119) p 76-92

The accumulated knowledge of the antigenic structure of well-characterized proteins has led to a search for empirical rules that would make it possible to predict the position of their epitopes. Such predictions would be extremely useful, in view of the current attempts to develop synthetic peptide vaccines against viral and other infectious diseases (Van Regenmortel & Neurath 1985).

Most antibodies recognize discontinuous epitopes formed by residues adjacent in space but not in the primary sequence (Atassi & Smith 1978). However, only a small proportion of anti-protein antibodies is able to bind to peptide fragments of the protein in solution. These antibodies recognize continuous epitopes. Recent studies on synthetic vaccines have concentrated on this type of epitope since they can theoretically be reproduced by synthesizing small peptides. Also, in many instances, the only available information on the antigen of interest is its amino acid sequence.

One popular method for predicting antigenicity consists in identifying regions along the polypeptide chain that contain a high proportion of hydrophilic residues (Hopp & Woods 1981, Kyte & Doolittle 1982). In many cases, local maxima in the hydrophilicity plots of proteins correspond to residues which are exposed to the solvent at the surface of the molecule and are also part of epitopes. However, this rule is not absolute, since regions of the protein that are rich in hydrophobic residues are also sometimes implicated in epitopes. The link between hydrophilicity and antigenicity is based on the fact that accessibility is necessary for antigenicity and that accessibility in turn correlates with hydrophilicity.

The surface location of many chain termini in proteins (Thornton & Sibanda 1983) probably explains at least partly why the terminal residues are so often implicated in protein epitopes. It has also been suggested that the higher than average antigenicity of chain termini could be due to the fact that they are less constrained than other sections of the polypeptide chain and that they have a high relative flexibility. Similar suggestions of a link between local disorder of short segments of a protein and antigenicity have been made occasionally in the past (Niman et al 1983). In the case of cytochrome c, for instance, it was observed that one of its six known epitopes is located very close to a particularly mobile amino acid (Moore & Williams 1980).

The importance of the internal dynamics of protein molecules is becoming increasingly recognized (Gurd & Rothgeb 1979, Karplus & McCammon 1983). Recently, two independent groups have reported that the location of continuous epitopes in proteins is correlated with the segmental mobility along the polypeptide chain: peptides corresponding to highly mobile regions in the protein are able to bind to anti-protein antibodies (Westhof et al 1984) and, when used as immunogens, they elicit antibodies which react strongly with the native protein (Tainer et al 1984).

Crystallographic structure of tobacco mosaic virus protein

The structure of the protein disk of tobacco mosaic virus (TMV) was solved by A.C. Bloomer et al (1978) and refined by A. Mondragon (PhD Thesis, University of Cambridge 1984). The refinement method provides the atomic temperature factors, the so-called B values, which represent the mean-square displacement of each atom from a well-determined average position. The two rings of protein subunits of the TMV disk are crystallographically independent and so have been refined independently, yielding very similar B factors, which indicates that these values are significant.

Antigenic structure of tobacco mosaic virus protein

The antigenic structure of the coat protein of TMV (TMVP) has been extensively studied over the last 20 years (Benjamini 1977, Van Regemortel 1982). By 1983, seven continuous epitopes varying in length from five to 10 residues had been identified in TMVP corresponding to residues 1–10, 34–39, 55–61, 62–68, 80–90, 108–112 and 153–158 (Altschuh et al 1983) (Fig. 1).

Most of these studies concentrated on measuring the capacity of natural and synthetic fragments of TMV protein to inhibit the reaction between TMV protein and anti-TMV protein antibodies. Because the peptide competes with

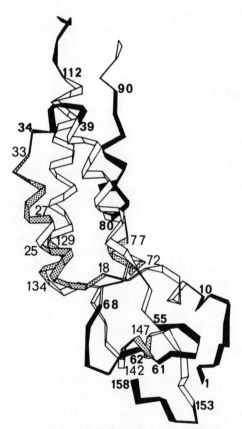

FIG. 1. Drawing of the α-carbon backbone of the TMVP subunit at the present stage of refinement of the protein disk (A ring). All residues are shown except for 94–106, which are omitted because this region of the polypeptide has no specific conformation in the disk. The locations of the seven continuous antigenic determinants are indicated by solid lines. Regions corresponding to short peptides which showed no antigenic activity are stippled.

antibodies able to bind to the protein, it is the reaction of the peptide with anti-protein antibodies which is being measured.

The immunochemical tests used were the ELISA (enzyme-linked immunosorbent assay) and microcomplement fixation test, in which very small amounts of protein and of antiserum are used. Typically in ELISA the antibody dilution is of the order of $1/50\,000$ to $1/200\,000$ and the protein concentration of 100 to $300\,ng/ml$. The high dilution of antiserum used in the assay ensures that these anti-protein antibodies have a good affinity for the protein.

In control experiments in which the competitor in ELISA was the native protein rather than the peptide, the amount necessary to inhibit the reaction was of the same order as that applied to the plate. This indicates that a high proportion of the protein adsorbed to the plastic of the microtitre plates is close to its native state. Also, the fact that large molar excesses of peptide over protein are needed in inhibition experiments indicates that the assay is not detecting antibodies to the denatured protein. Furthermore, the inhibitory activity of the small peptides was verified by complement fixation assays which are performed in solution (Milton & Van Regenmortel 1979, Altschuh et al 1983).

Segmental mobility and the antigenic structure of tobacco mosaic virus protein

When plotted against residue number, B factors provide a graphic image of the degree of mobility existing along the polypeptide chain. The refined coordinates of the viral subunit determined at the MRC Laboratory of Molecular Biology in Cambridge as described above were made available to the Strasbourg Immunochemistry laboratory. When E. Westhof and D. Altschuh in Strasbourg examined the location of the seven epitopes of TMVP in the polypeptide backbone by computer graphics, they noticed that the position of the epitopes agreed closely with the regions of high segmental mobility (i.e. a continuous run of high B values). There is a good correlation between the mobility of short stretches of the main-chain atoms and the location of epitopes (Fig. 2). The side-chain mobility does not correlate so well, presumably because the individual side groups can move even when the backbone is less mobile. Six of the epitopes correspond to the six major peaks in the plot of the backbone temperature factors. The remaining epitope of TMVP (residues 55–61) is located in a region of low mobility; however, the lack of mobility in this epitope could be due to the fact that it corresponds to a region where there are strong intermolecular contacts within the crystal, resulting in a lower apparent mobility than would be observed for an isolated molecule.

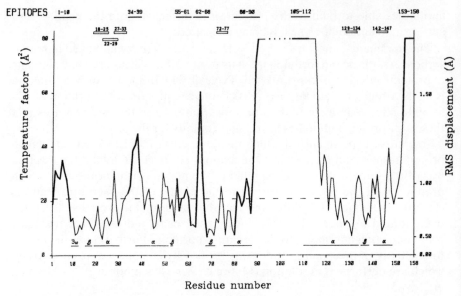

FIG. 2. The mean temperature factor of the main-chain atoms in each residue plotted against residue number for the TMVP disk (adapted from Westhof et al 1984). These temperature factors are from the constrained crystallographic refinement (Jack & Levitt 1978) of the disk of TMVP at 2.8 Å resolution. Temperature factors for the A ring are shown here, although those for the B ring are essentially the same (A. Mondragon & A. C. Bloomer, in preparation). The mean value of the temperature factor (omitting residues for which $B > 80$) is shown by a dashed line. Regions of secondary structure are denoted α, β, 3_{10}. At top, the locations of the seven continuous antigenic determinants are indicated by underlining. Antigenically inactive peptides are indicated by boxes.

Antigenicity and surface accessibility

The weak cross-reactivity between native and denatured proteins implies that most anti-protein antibodies are specific for a folded conformation (Crumpton 1974) and therefore react only with residues accessible in the native antigen. However, surface accessibility is not a sufficient condition for the antigenic reactivity of peptides: the significance of the correlation between antigenicity and mobility was reinforced by the finding that three hexapeptides corresponding to protruding, and therefore accessible, areas of the protein (residues 72–77, 129–134 and 142–147) possessed no antigenic activity. They are all situated outside mobile regions. Recently, three additional short peptides (residues 18–25, 22–29 and 27–33) have been found to be antigenically inactive (Al Moudallal et al 1985). These results are summarized in Fig. 3, which represents the exposed area along the polypeptide chain of TMV protein.

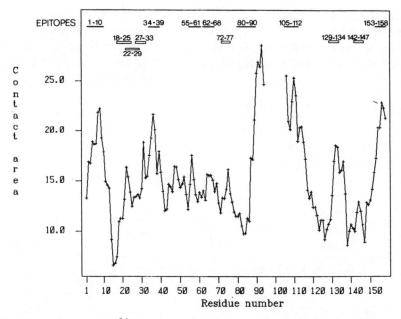

FIG. 3. The contact area (in Å²) for each residue in the protein is plotted against residue number for a probe with radius 1.5 Å. The value plotted is the running average of the contact area for seven residues. At top, the locations of the seven continuous antigenic determinants are indicated by underlining. Antigenically inactive peptides are indicated by boxes.

The value plotted for each residue is the contact surface (Lee & Richards 1971) averaged over seven residues, which is the average length of the peptides used to test for antigenicity. This plot shows that the correlation between the location of epitopes and the area of contact surface is not as good as that with segmental mobility. The correlation between antigenicity and mobility is thus not solely based on the fact that flexible regions in proteins tend to be situated predominantly at the surface on the molecule, nor do all the epitopes found correspond to the most protruding regions of the surface.

Antigenic activity of longer peptides

It should be stressed that the seven continuous epitopes of TMVP discussed above do not represent the total antigenic activity of the molecule. In a recent study using long synthetic peptides, three additional antigenic regions of 14–20 residues were discovered (Al Moudallal et al 1985). These new regions are structured in the protein: two of them (residues 19–32 and 115–134) correspond to two helices of TMV protein. The third (residues 134–146) contains a region with a β-bend at the end of an α-helix. The importance of structure for the activity of these peptides has been shown for one of the helices, where none of three short peptides, spanning between them the whole length of the helix, possesses antigenic activity (Table 1). The presence of antigenicity only in

TABLE 1 Antigenic reactivity of synthetic TMVP peptides

	Peptide (length)			
Anti-TMVP antisera	19–32 (14)	18–25 (8)	22–29 (8)	27–33 (7)
HA 5	0.42	0.08	0.19	0.08
HA 9	1.26	0.08	0.26	0.08
HA 12	1.25	0.08	0.12	0.08
LA 30	0.33	0.08	0.20	0.07
JU 18	0.98	0.08	0.16	0.07
JI 19	1.56	0.07	0.16	0.07
Mouse antiserum (M 7)	0.08	0.08	0.19	0.08

Data from Al Moudallal et al (1985): antigenic activity of synthetic TMVP peptides measured in ELISA by direct binding. Microtitre wells were coated with 1 μM of peptide. The following antisera diluted 1/500 were then incubated in the wells for 2 h: HA 5, HA 9 and HA 12 (three bleedings of one rabbit); LA 30, JU 18 and JI 19 (three bleedings from different rabbits) and M 7 (mouse antiserum). Anti-globulin conjugates were used to reveal positive reactions. The lack of activity of the short peptides was confirmed by an ELISA inhibition assay.

the longer peptide is probably linked to the need to stabilize a particular conformation, or to make its probability of occurrence much more likely. Indeed, it is possible that the peptide is not actually helical in solution but that it is 'helix-going' and the final conformation is induced by binding to the antibody. The contact residues involved in antibody binding are impossible to identify when such long peptides are used and probably correspond to residues in successive turns of the α-helix; that is, residues not contiguous in the primary sequence.

These results are perhaps not surprising, since it is well known that longer peptides possess more antigenic activity than short peptides (Crumpton 1974). Long peptides react with more antibodies for several reasons: they may carry several epitopes; they may have a tendency to be structured or to become structured by binding to the antibody; also, non-specific interactions on either side of the antigenic determinant may enhance specific binding (Benjamini 1977). Fig. 4 illustrates the results obtained by measuring the capacity of tryptic peptides of strain U2 of TMV to inhibit the reaction between U2 protein and anti-U2 protein antibodies. The maximum percentage inhibition is approximately proportional to the peptide length. For example, tryptic peptide 1 of U2 (residues 1 to 41) probably carries two flexible epitopes (1–10 and 34–39) and a structured region (helix 20–32).

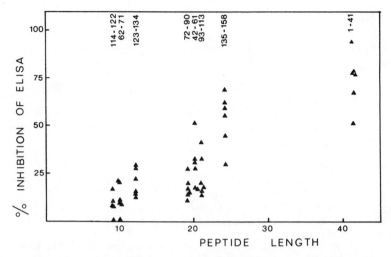

FIG. 4. Influence of peptide length on the maximum percentage inhibition of ELISA (data from D. Altschuh, Thesis, University of Strasbourg 1984). The reaction between the protein of strain U2 of TMV and anti-U2 protein antibodies was inhibited by increasing amounts of tryptic peptides of U2 protein. Each triangle represents the value obtained with a different antiserum. Numbers above each set of points indicate the position in the sequence of the tryptic peptides. Strain U2 of TMV differs from the wild-type by 27% of its amino acid sequence.

Concluding remarks

Since only a small part of the protein surface is made up of linear arrays of residues, most epitopes must be discontinuous (Todd et al 1982). In another study using monoclonal antibodies, several discontinuous epitopes have also been identified in this antigen (Altschuh et al 1985).

Each experimental approach will emphasize a particular aspect of the many types of interactions that constitute the immune response. When short peptides (6–8 residues) are used as probes, it is mostly loops and turns corresponding to mobile segments of the protein that are identified as epitopes. Studies with short peptides are thus biased toward the detection of antigenicity in mobile regions of the protein. When longer peptides are used as probes, regions of the molecule that are more structured are also able to reveal their antigenicity. Monoclonal antibodies usually do not react with peptides but are specific for the tertiary or quaternary structure of the antigen.

Acknowledgement

D. A. thanks the European Molecular Biology Organization for support.

REFERENCES

Al Moudallal Z, Briand JP, Van Regenmortel MHV 1985 A major part of the polypeptide chain of tobacco mosaic virus protein is antigenic. EMBO (Eur Mol Biol Organ) J 4:1231-1235

Altschuh D, Hartman D, Reinbolt J, Van Regenmortel MHV 1983 Immunochemical studies of tobacco mosaic virus. V. Localization of four epitopes in the protein subunit by inhibition tests with synthetic peptides and cleavage peptides from three strains. Mol Immunol 20:271-278

Altschuh D, Al Moudallal Z, Briand JP, Van Regenmortel MHV 1985 Immunochemical studies of tobacco mosaic virus. VI. Attempts to localize viral epitopes with monoclonal antibodies. Mol Immunol 22:329-337

Atassi MZ, Smith JA 1978 A proposal for the nomenclature of antigenic sites in peptides and proteins. Immunochemistry 15:609-610

Benjamini E 1977 Immunochemistry of the tobacco mosaic virus protein. In: Atassi MZ (ed) Immunochemistry of proteins. Plenum Press, New York vol 2:265-310

Bloomer AC, Champness JN, Bricogne G, Staden R, Klug A 1978 Protein disk of tobacco mosaic virus at 2.8 Å resolution showing the interactions within and between subunits. Nature (Lond) 276:362-368

Crumpton MJ 1974 Protein antigens: the molecular bases of antigenicity and immunogenicity. In: Sela M (ed) The antigens. Academic Press, London vol 2:1-78

Gurd FRN, Rothgeb TM 1979 Motions in proteins. Adv Protein Chem 33:73-165

Hopp TP, Woods KR 1981 Prediction of protein antigenic determinants from amino acid sequences. Proc Natl Acad Sci USA 78:3824-3828

Jack A, Levitt M 1978 Refinement of large structures by simultaneous minimization of energy and R factor. Acta Crystallogr Sect A Cryst Phys Diffr Theor Gen Crystallogr 34:931-935

Karplus M, McCammon JA 1983 Dynamics of proteins: elements and function. Annu Rev Biochem 52:263-300

Kyte J, Doolittle RF 1982 A simple method for displaying the hydropathic character of a protein. J Mol Biol 157:105-132

Lee B, Richards FM 1971 The interpretation of protein structures: estimation of static accessibility. J Mol Biol 55:379-400

Milton RC de L, Van Regenmortel MHV 1979 Immunochemical studies of tobacco mosaic virus. III. Demonstration of five antigenic regions in the protein subunit. Mol Immunol 16:179-184

Moore GR, Williams RJP 1980 Comparison of the structures of various eukaryotic ferricytochromes c and ferrocytochromes and their antigenic differences. Eur J Biochem 103:543-550

Niman HL, Houghten RA, Walker LE, Reisfeld RA, Wilson IA, Hogle JM, Lerner RA 1983 Generation of protein-reactive antibodies by short peptides is an event of high frequency: implications for the structural basis of immune response. Proc Natl Acad Sci USA 80:4949-4953

Tainer JA, Getzoff ED, Alexander H, Houghten RA, Olson AJ, Hendrickson WA, Lerner RA 1984 The reactivity of anti-peptide antibodies is a function of the atomic mobility of sites in a protein. Nature (Lond) 312:127-134

Todd PEE, East IJ, Leach SJ 1982 The immunogenicity and antigenicity of proteins. Trends Biochem Sci 7:212-216

Thornton JM, Sibanda BL 1983 Amino and carboxy-terminal regions in globular proteins. J Mol Biol 167:443-460

Van Regenmortel MHV 1982 Serology and immunochemistry of plant viruses. Academic Press, New York

Van Regenmortel MHV, Neurath AR 1985 Immunochemistry of viruses. The basis for serodiagnosis and vaccines. Elsevier Life Sciences, Amsterdam

Westhof E, Altschuh D, Moras D, Bloomer AC, Mondragon A, Klug A, Van Regenmortel MHV 1984 Correlation between segmental mobility and the location of antigenic determinants in proteins. Nature (Lond) 311:123-126

DISCUSSION

Altschuh: I should like to make some additional points not covered in our main paper which Dr Klug presented. Viral antigens present an additional complexity compared to monomeric proteins, because assembly into quaternary structure modifies the antigenic properties of proteins. Antisera against whole virus particles have been generally found to cross-react only weakly with monomeric coat proteins. The new antigenic determinants which appear in viruses can result from the juxtaposition of residues from two adjacent subunits or from a modified conformation of the protein surface (Van Regenmortel 1982). These new antigenic properties seem to play an important role in virus neutralization (Meloen et al 1979, Bachrach et al 1975).

Tobacco mosaic virus is a good model with which to study the influence of quaternary structure on antigenicity because the protein assembles into a helix to form the viral capsid. The C- and N-terminal tryptic peptides of TMV protein bind well to anti-protein antibodies, but only weakly to anti-virus antibodies, although these terminal regions are accessible at the virus surface. This suggests that the epitopes recognized by anti-virus antibodies are mostly discontinuous.

One approach commonly used to localize discontinuous epitopes is to compare the binding of monoclonal antibodies to mutant proteins. If a mutant binds less to the antibody than does the parent protein, it is concluded that the mutation is part of the epitope; but, as I shall illustrate, this is not always true.

By comparing the ability of anti-TMV monoclonal antibodies to bind to mutant viruses containing single or double point mutations, Al Moudallal et al (1982) showed that each antibody has a different reactivity pattern. However, it was not possible to map the antigenic determinants for two reasons. (1) The antigen–antibody interaction was found to be sensitive to conformational changes produced by mutations outside the epitope. For example, substitutions at positions 107 and 20 which are respectively 50 and 20Å away from the virus surface alter the binding of some antibodies. (2) This type of study is limited by the number of mutants available.

Some information on the region recognized by some of these antibodies can however be obtained by also studying their ability to cross-react with TMV strains, and with the isolated protein, and to bind to the N- and C-terminal peptides (Altschuh et al 1985). Half of the antibodies are so specific in conformation that they do not cross-react with the monomeric protein. The others bind to the virus and to the protein but only three of those are able to react with peptides. For example, antibody 22 reacts with the N-terminal tryptic peptide and also with strain HR, which is totally different from the wild-type in the N-terminal region. The residues recognized in strain HR are probably among residues 150, 152 and 153 which are common to these two strains and adjacent in space to the N-terminal region. The fact that mutations at positions 153 and 156 influence the binding of antibody 22 confirms that the epitope is formed by residues from both the C-terminal and N-terminal regions. Antibody 21 has a similar behaviour with peptides and strains, but a different reactivity with point mutants. Antibody 28 reacts with the C-terminal synthetic peptide 149–158, but its binding is not affected by substitutions at positions 153 and 156. The epitope could comprise the accessible residues 149, 150, 152 and 154. A substitution at position 140 which modifies the binding of the antibody is likely to act through a conformational change, since residue 140 is not adjacent to the region 149–154.

These examples, which can be analysed for only a small proportion of the total number of monoclonal antibodies (three out of 18), emphasize the difficulty of mapping the antigenic determinants of viruses. The influence of a mutation located outside the epitope on antibody binding is probably more important in viruses than in monomeric proteins because mutations can change the subunit packing. Because of these conformational effects, only the binding of antibodies to peptides gives clear information on the epitope location. However, the cross-reactivity of anti-virus monoclonal antibodies with peptides is rare, and always weak.

Furthermore, even when the antibody reacts with a peptide, the peptide often represents only part of the epitope. Space-filling models of protein surfaces show that only very small areas of the surface correspond to linear arrays of residues, suggesting that the chances of mimicking a virus-neutralizing epitope with linear peptides are small.

Edmundson: Dr Klug, within the regions of your viral protein that react with antibodies, do you notice any long stretches of hydrophobic residues that might be partially exposed? It is not obvious that there is a correlation between antigenicity and hydrophobicity in TMV.

Klug: No.

Crumpton: Information on the structure of an antigenic determinant that is acquired from studying the relative antigenicities of increasingly smaller fragments of a larger, antigenically active oligopeptide can often be misleading. I am referring, in particular, to a study carried out some time ago by Benjamini et al (1968) on a 20-amino acid fragment of TMV protein. A tripeptide fragment of the oligopeptide, namely Ala-Thr-Arg, had no measurable immunological reactivity. Specific binding activity was, however, 'recovered' on N-octanoylation. My interpretation of these data is that the unsubstituted tripeptide was bound by the antibody combining site, but the strength of interaction was insufficiently high to give a stable complex. However, the octanoate group provided additional non-specific hydrophobic interaction which supplemented the specific interaction to give measurable activity. It seems to me that such effects have implications for the interpretation of your data.

Klug: The Benjamini peptide was, as you suggest, narrowed down, but it occurs in the region of the TMV molecule which is more or less fully disordered, so the set of antibodies is really seeing a chain which is so highly flexible that it goes through all the conformations, and can actually see all the individual residues. (The other antigenic regions are mobile but here the motion is about a well-defined mean conformation.) Presumably, in the case of the peptide, there is recognition of arginine, and perhaps one or two of the other amino acids, but the binding would, as you say, be very weak for a very small peptide.

Crumpton: My point is that non-antigenic peptides do not necessarily tell us as much as we expect about the antigenic structure of the protein. It is always possible that the binding by antibody is not sufficiently stable as to register positively in the competitive tests normally used. Nevertheless, by necessity, our interpretations are always based upon measurable reactivity.

Geysen: The real interest in peptide vaccines came about from the ready access to sequences made possible by direct translation from the genes. To go back now and say that we have to determine mobility, say, as being the only true predictor of which regions are likely to be useful, takes us a step backwards. In many cases we shall have the actual sequence, and we may never have the X-ray crystal structure for the useful antigens. So what is the real value of being able to demonstrate a valid correlation with mobility in regions that might be the best candidates for a vaccine?

Altschuh: The value lies in the explanation of the results that we are getting.

Geysen: That may not help us to determine how to make peptide vaccines.

Lerner: Obviously there are two agendas: one is to understand the chemistry, irrespective of whether one ever achieves a vaccine, and the other is to make better vaccines. One can't say that there's no point in doing this.

Geysen: I said that this approach is taking a step backwards on the road to getting vaccines, which is something different!

Nussenzweig: There is not a complete deadlock here, in fact, because you can look at natural immunity to the pathogen as a guideline. It is now possible to find the sequence of the epitopes of the natural immunogens; and if a sequence is immunodominant, that sequence should be chosen for a vaccine, if the antibodies have a neutralizing effect. We shall discuss an example later on (see p 150-159).

Geysen: We have published a table of the frequencies of the amino acids as they occur in immunogenic epitopes (restricted to continuous epitopes), determined by examining anti-protein responses to various antigens (see Table 2 in Geysen et al 1985). You could use these frequencies in an algorithm for predicting epitopes.

Klug: Such algorithms are likely to have weak predictive power; at least, those for protein folding have.

Geysen: Ours is not an algorithm for protein folding, but an algorithm for the frequency at which each amino acid is likely to occur in an epitope, and it turns out that the highest frequencies are for hydrophobic amino acids such as valine.

Skehel: Isn't that based on three-dimensional structure information?

Geysen: No; it's purely based on looking at an antibody response to the whole antigen and asking which regions are expressed by the immune response; that is, to which sequences can you show an antibody response.

Klug: If you are working on a protein which you want to develop for a vaccine, and it has a known three-dimensional structure, would you pay attention to it, or would you use your prediction based on all the other proteins?

Geysen: We do not think that three-dimensional structure will identify epitopes, because in several cases where we have tried to map the contact residues we have found that invariably one of these has no exposure at the surface, as determined from the X-ray crystal structure. I don't know how to interpret that other than by saying that antibody binding induced a significant conformational change. We have seen the need for a complete side-chain to be rotated out for binding to occur.

Klug: That is very possible, because in solution, parts of the protein are moving about. A residue on the edge of a mobile region could be rotated out, perhaps with some help from the antibody. There is also the case reported in influenza virus where there is a hidden site. But, in general, is it not true that antibodies are raised against residues which are on the surface?

Geysen: Not by our earlier assessment (Geysen et al 1985). We have now determined contact residues which are completely buried.

Sela: The results presented by Dr Klug are very relevant to any efforts to make synthetic vaccines, because they have shown that those areas of a protein that have the highest flexibility are very good candidates for the synthesis of peptides for vaccines.

Ada: This work is an attempt to discover whether there are any rules that are important for this. So far, we seem not to have found any hard-and-fast rules.

Lerner: One ought to distinguish between work on anti-protein antibodies, and on anti-peptide antibodies. When you start with an anti-protein antibody, you make an antibody which can cause a free peptide to adopt some structure. Doing it the other way round, you are asking the sequence in the protein to adopt a structure. We should always consider which way the experiment is being done.

Corradin: When we talk about cross-reactivity we should be careful to determine the difference in the binding constant between the native protein and the denatured peptide; there may be a 10^4 or 10^5 difference. For example, Dr Altschuh showed that some larger peptides inhibited the interaction better than smaller peptides, but if they inhibit at a concentration 100- or 1000-fold higher than that of TMV protein, it is difficult to say that this is not due to contamination by the native protein.

Altschuh: With TMV protein, a large molar excess of peptides over native protein (around 1000) is needed to inhibit the reaction between the protein and anti-protein antibodies, which means that peptides do not mimic epitopes on the native protein very well. In other words, even antibodies reacting with peptides are partly specific for a conformation. The only exception is the C-terminal region of TMV protein which is totally disordered. The maximum percentage inhibition is reached with smaller amounts of C-terminal peptide and is higher than for other peptides of equal length (six residues). This is consistent with the view that peptides have a higher antigenic activity with anti-protein antibodies if the corresponding region in the protein is mobile and mimics a peptide in solution.

On the question of purity, all tryptic and synthetic peptides were checked by amino acid analysis and recently also by high pressure liquid chromatography.

Klug: You can put the peptides in rank order according to the degree of inhibition, if you want to attempt to be quantitative. There is a rough relation between the rank orders of *B* values and the degrees of inhibition, but the amount of data is not sufficient for a proper correlation.

Williams: If we confine discussion to short peptides taken from proteins in the first instance, rather than getting confused by taking longer stretches which may have several different antigenic sites, several groups have shown that the antigenic short peptides are from rather exposed, mobile pieces of proteins and on the whole don't belong to pieces of a helix or pieces of a sheet (see references in Williams & Moore 1985). If this is so, the next step towards understanding is to ask whether there are general rules about the amino acids in these sequences. Rules may not be highly specific, but if they are quite good—for example, that the amino acids are largely hydrophilic—then we could attempt to put together the information obtained from the different proteins studied, in order to derive antigenicity indices, if such exist. For example, it seems often to be the case that the N-terminus is disordered in solution and antigenic: in cytochrome *c*, the N-terminus is not 'seeable' in the structure, so presumably it is disordered even in the crystal. I do not know how disordered the termini are in TMV protein, however. Do mobile N-terminal sequences have a limited set of amino acids?

Klug: The last three residues in the C-terminus can't be seen, so they are probably totally disordered.

Williams: These disordered regions do look to be more antigenic than other sequence regions. So there is some lead to a systematic approach. The question is whether we can rationalize this in terms of composition.

Klug: You have to measure the antigenicity quantitatively.

Ada: And you also have to agree on the antibody preparations to be used.

Williams: Paterson (1985) has studied amino acid substitution in cytochrome *c*, and has shown by the use of synthetic sequences that antigenicity can be in a particular small region, and this is in the mobile N-terminus.

V. Nussenzweig: When one immunizes with the total TMV protein, is it known what proportion of antibodies are directed against the more rigid, α-helical structure, as compared to the rest? Which structure is the most immunogenic, in other words?

Altschuh: The proportion of antibodies directed against each type of structure is not known. We are testing antigenicity, not immunogenicity. But Anderer & Schlumberger (1965) showed that antibodies obtained by immunization with peptides corresponding to the C-terminal region precipitate the virus and neutralize its infectivity.

Ada: It is rather more difficult to determine immunogenicity than antigenicity.

V. Nussenzweig: Another problem is establishing the rules for choosing the immunogenic areas of a polypeptide. In the case of the malaria parasites, many protein antigens contain repetitive sequences of amino acids such as glycine, alanine, proline, asparagine and glutamine. These are strongly immunodominant, although other regions of the antigen molecule may contain sequences which are much more hydrophilic. In other words, hydrophilicity of a sequence does not guarantee immunogenicity.

Ada: Perhaps we can reflect on Bob Williams' comments and see whether we can reach some general agreement about them, and whether we think the data support what seems to be a general principle there.

Lerner: In our myohaemerythrin work, we wished to put limits on the degree of disorder, and that is not easy to do, in solution at least. But this molecule contains an iron atom, so in every study on antigen–antibody union we always confirmed that the iron was not released. Thus we knew, within those constraints, that the protein was not so altered or disordered as to release the bound iron ligand. So we did not ignore the problem of the degree of disorder.

Williams: Cytochrome *c* is said to be one of the least immunogenic of proteins, and its fold is very stable, much more so than lysozyme. So it is interesting also to look at the stability of folds, and look for correlations with antigenicity. There is a potential connection to mobility, of course.

Corradin: Cytochrome *c* is not immunogenic if you use the horse or beef protein, but if you use tuna or *Candida* or pigeon cytochrome *c*, then it is.

Ada: It's a question of how hard you try. You can make almost anything immunogenic. One must do comparable studies.

Lachmann: As I understand it, these experiments are all done with antisera raised against the protein, so you are looking at the immunodominant determinants. It would be interesting to know how these antigenic analyses would turn out if you did a second 'cascade' immunization by inhibiting the antibody response to the immunodominant determinants by the passive administration of the antibodies raised in the first immunization. Perhaps you would produce antibodies where the rules are entirely different!

Ada: If we are to get practical results from this approach we want to know what happens in primary immunization.

Lachmann: Not necessarily; you may want to make a particular antibody. Take immunoglobulin, for example, where something is known about the order in which antibodies are made. If you wanted to make antibodies to the Fd fragment (because these had some desired biological effect), you would be unlikely to learn how to do this by primary immunization with the whole Ig molecule, because the anti-Fc response competes against anti-Fd. However, if you give anti-Fc antibodies together with whole Ig, antibodies to Fd are readily made (Taussig & Lachmann 1972). If we are trying to establish rules, we should be clear whether we are establishing the rules of immunodominance or the rules of immunogenicity, because they are not the same.

Rothbard: Or establishing the rules for antibodies against peptides to cross-react with intact proteins. Both your paper, Dr Klug, and John Tainer's paper, which have proposed that the cross-reaction of anti-peptide antibodies with proteins is correlated with flexibility, have confused this issue with the natural immunogenicity of the proteins (Tainer et al 1984, Westhof et al 1984).

Klug: Perhaps if we abandon the word 'rules', we shall get further. That is a strong word. It may be more appropriate to talk about indications or pointers or suggestions.

Stanworth: Another issue might be the way in which the antigen is presented. If it is presented in complete Freund's adjuvant, you are emulsifying the protein and essentially administering it in denatured form. This is sometimes not recognized.

REFERENCES

Al Moudallal Z, Briand JP, Van Regenmortel MHV 1982 Monoclonal antibodies as probes of the antigenic structure of tobacco mosaic virus. EMBO (Eur Mol Biol Organ) J 1:1005-1010

Altschuh D, Al Moudallal Z, Briand JP, Van Regenmortel MHV 1985 Immunochemical studies of tobacco mosaic virus. VI. Attempts to localize viral epitopes with monoclonal antibodies. Mol Immunol. 22:329-337

Anderer FA, Schlumberger HD 1965 Properties of different artificial antigens immunologically related to tobacco mosaic virus. Biochim Biophys Acta 97:503-509

Bachrach HL, Moore DM, McKercher PD, Polatnick J 1975 Immune and antibody responses to an isolated capsid protein of foot-and-mouth disease virus. J Immunol 115:1636-1641

Benjamini E, Shimizu M, Young JD, Leung CY 1968 Immunochemical studies on the tobacco mosaic virus protein, Parts VI and VII. Biochemistry 7:1253-1260, 1261-1264

Geysen HM, Mason TJ, Rodda SJ, Meloen RH, Barteling SJ 1985 Amino acid composition of antigenic determinants: implications for antigen processing by the immune system of animals.

In: Lerner RA et al (eds) Vaccines 85. Cold Spring Harbor Laboratory, Cold Spring Harbor, NY, p 133-137

Meloen RH, Rowlands DJ, Brown F 1979 Comparison of the antibodies elicited by the individual structural polypeptides of foot-and-mouth disease and polio viruses. J Gen Virol 45:761-763

Paterson Y 1985 Delineation and conformational analysis of two synthetic peptide models of antigenic sites on rodent cytochrome c. Biochemistry 24:1048-1055

Tainer JA, Getzoff, ED, Alexander H et al 1984 The reactivity of antipeptide antibodies is a function of the atomic mobility of sites in a protein. Nature (Lond) 312:127-134

Taussig MJ, Lachmann PJ 1972 Studies on antigenic competition. II. Abolition of antigenic competition by antibody against or tolerance to the dominant antigen: a model for antigenic competition. Immunology 22:185-197

Van Regenmortel MHV 1982 Serology and immunochemistry of plant viruses. Academic Press, New York

Westhof E, Altschuh D, Moras D et al 1984 Correlation between segmental mobility and the location of antigenic determinants in proteins. Nature (Lond) 311:123-126

Williams RJP, Moore GR 1985 Protein antigenicity, organization and mobility. Trends Biochem Sci 10:96-97

The importance of conformation and of equilibria in the interaction of globular proteins and their fragments with antibodies

MICHAEL J. CRUMPTON

Imperial Cancer Research Fund, Lincoln's Inn Fields, London WC2A 3PX, UK

Abstract. Oligopeptide fragments of globular proteins often inhibit the interaction of anti-bodies with native protein. Although such fragments appear to possess in aqueous solution an unfolded conformation it is apparent, in those cases where the protein's three-dimensional structure is known, that the antibody-bound fragment possesses a folded conformation mimicking that of the corresponding portion of the whole protein. The probable explanation of this dichotomy is that the fragment has various conformations in equilibrium including a small proportion of molecules whose shape is recognized and stabilized by the antibody. A related situation can exist in the interaction of antibody(ies) with the whole protein. Thus, antibodies against an altered form of the protein can induce the native antigen to adopt the conformation of the altered form. In this case, it appears that localized regions of the protein's surface are flexible, adopting various conformations in equilibrium, one of which is stabilized (selected) by interaction with the appropriate antibody. In both instances interaction with antibody perturbs an equilibrium, leading to the selection of a particular conformation. Such dynamic effects have profound implications on the choice of peptides as synthetic vaccines.

1986 Synthetic peptides as antigens. Wiley, Chichester (Ciba Foundation Symposium 119) p 93-106

My contribution is concerned with the importance of conformation and of equilibria in the interaction of globular proteins and their peptide fragments with antibodies raised against the native protein. These parameters and their interrelationship will be explored by making use of two studies that were carried out in my laboratory about 15 years ago using sperm whale metmyoglobin as a model globular protein. In spite of their age, I believe the interpretations of the results are still valid. If so, they provide valuable insights into the conformation of relatively short peptides (up to 14 amino acid residues) in aqueous solution and into the flexibility of globular proteins. The results also serve to illustrate the profound changes in conformation that can be induced in a fairly rigid globular protein by antibodies directed against epitopes with varying conformations in equilibrium with one another. These insights in turn have significant implications for the use of synthetic peptides as antigens and especially as vaccines.

Peptide conformation

It is now well-established that peptide fragments of globular proteins, corresponding to regions in the whole protein of folded conformation, often react with antibodies directed against the native protein (Crumpton 1974, Benjamin et al 1984). This principle relies upon the observations that both natural and synthetic peptides can inhibit the reaction of the native protein with homologous polyclonal antisera and/or monoclonal antibodies. Under these circumstances, it is reasonable to assume that the peptide when bound by the antibody combining site possesses the same conformation as the corresponding region of the native protein, although this asumption discounts the possibility that the antibodies can select and stabilize alternative localized, including unfolded, conformations of the protein (see below). In these studies myoglobin and haemoglobin represent valuable experimental model proteins because the presence of haem in the immune precipitate provides a marker of the protein's native conformation; albeit, a rather gross marker which will not reveal subtle localized changes in shape. Although the conformation of the peptide when bound by antibody can be predicted, the conformational state of the free peptide and the molecular bases of its recognition and interaction with antibody are less well-established.

The problem of peptide conformation in relation to the reactivity of the peptide with antibody against the whole protein was first explored in the late 1960s by using two chymotryptic fragments (namely, B1 and Cla; Crumpton & Wilkinson 1965) of sperm whale myoglobin (Crumpton & Small 1967). These peptides were of similar size and corresponded essentially to helical and non-helical portions of the protein; as well, a similar proportion of each peptide was exposed on the surface of the protein. As judged from the X-ray crystallographic structure of sperm whale metmyoglobin (see Fig. 1), peptide B1, which comprised 14 amino acid residues (56 to 69 inclusive), has 12 consecutive helical residues; whereas Cla, which contained 13 residues (77 to 89 inclusive), has eight consecutive non-helical residues followed by four helical residues. Both peptides also contained 'corners' between either successive helical, or helical and non-helical segments of metmyoglobin. As shown in Table 1, each peptide inhibited the precipitation of metmyoglobin or apomyoglobin, using pools of serum collected from several individual rabbits immu-

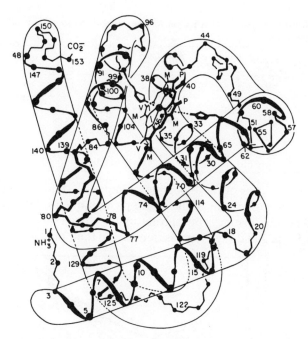

FIG. 1. A two-dimensional representation of the conformation of a molecule of crystalline sperm whale metmyoglobin. The amino acid residues are numbered from the N- to the C-termini.

nized with metmyoglobin. Most importantly, peptide B1 inhibited the precipitation of metmyoglobin but not apomyoglobin by antiserum WF. As apomyoglobin is more unfolded (flexible) than metmyoglobin (Crumpton & Polson 1965), this result argues strongly in support of the view that the conformation of peptide B1 in the immune complex resembles that of the corresponding region of metmyoglobin. In contrast, peptide Cla failed to react with antiserum WF, although it inhibited the precipitation of apomyoglobin by antiserum WH.

TABLE 1 Capacities of peptides to inhibit immunoprecipitation of metmyoglobin and/or apomyoglobin

| Peptide | Maximum inhibition (%) | | |
| | Antiserum WF | | Antiserum WH |
	Apomyoglobin	Metmyoglobin	Apomyoglobin
B1	0	8	0
Cla	0	n.t.[a]	9

[a]n.t., not tested.

TABLE 2 Optical rotatory dispersion parameters for aqueous solutions of peptides B1 and Cla at various temperatures

Dispersion parameter	Peptide B1		Peptide Cla			
	7 °C	55 °C	11 °C	33 °C	48 °C	63 °C
λ_0	221	228	216	218	222	222
$-a_0$	464	404	620	586	561	548
$-b_0$	52	89	47	70	80	85
$[m']_{233}$ at 25 °C		-2610			-1920	

If the conformations of these peptides in aqueous solution resemble those of the corresponding regions of the native protein, then solutions of the peptides should possess distinct optical rotatory dispersion properties. However, as shown in Table 2 and Fig. 2, measurements of their optical rotatory disper-

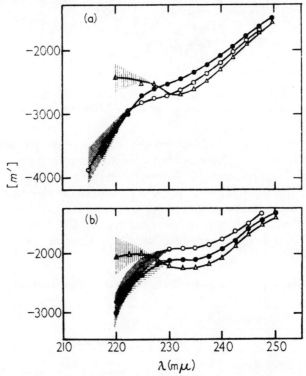

FIG. 2. Optical rotatory dispersion curves of aqueous solutions of (a) peptide B1 and (b) peptide Cla at 25 °C (○) and 75 °C (△), and of solutions of B1 and Cla which had been heated at 75 °C and then cooled to 10 °C and 33 °C, respectively (●). The width of the curves below 230 nm (mμ) indicates the reproducibility of the measurements.

sion parameters and of their optical rotatory dispersion curves failed to reveal any significant differences. In other words, no evidence for any difference in their conformations was obtained. Furthermore, both the dispersion parameters and the shapes of the curves indicated that both peptides possessed conformations which resembled that of a random coil (i.e. unfolded) and which incorporated very little ($< 5\%$) helical structure. Although no evidence for any non-random conformation (e.g. 'corners') was obtained, if such a conformation contributed to the dispersion properties then it was common to both peptides.

Similar but more elegant studies have been executed more recently using improved instrumentation, the more compelling technique of circular dichroism and peptide synthesis to prepare more suitable pairs of peptides for comparison (for example, see Paterson 1985). The results of these studies have endorsed the initially derived conclusions; namely, that oligopeptides comprising up to about 20 amino acid residues and corresponding to a helical region in the native protein possess an unfolded conformation in aqueous solution. Thus, for example, the C-terminal, 22-amino acid peptide of sperm whale myoglobin that comprises 16 consecutive residues of the H helix of myoglobin is essentially non-helical ($< 5\%$ α-helix) in aqueous solution at pH 7.2 (Epand & Scheraga 1968).

The above conclusion is superficially at variance with the capacities of peptides B1 and Cla to inhibit the precipitation of metmyoglobin or apomyoglobin by antisera against metmyoglobin. *A priori*, this apparent dichotomy can be resolved in a number of ways, two of which appear more probable. Firstly, the antibodies could have combined with a limited region of unchanged conformation, such as the corners, which would not necessarily have been revealed by optical rotatory dispersion. The alternative explanation is not mutually exclusive but is more satisfying. It is based upon the proposition that each peptide possesses a variety of conformations in continuous interchange including, in the case of peptide B1, a small fraction of molecules with a helical conformation. In this case, the homologous antibodies could have reacted with those molecules whose conformations resembled that of the corresponding region in metmyoglobin, thereby stabilizing this conformation and perturbing the equilibrium in favour of the native structure. It is envisaged that antibody selects a complementary structure rather than *inducing* a complementary structure subsequent to the initial interaction. Although these mechanisms differ fundamentally and cannot be distinguished at the present time, their consequences are the same. Some support for this explanation comes from the observation that the S-peptide of ribonuclease, which in aqueous solution has a random conformation (Scatturin et al 1967), acquires a helical conformation when bound by the rest of the molecule to form ribonuclease S (Wyckoff et al 1967). This explanation has also been promoted by Sachs et al (1972) who proposed a mathematical model which predicted that at any one moment in time the relative amount of peptide with a native conformation will be too small to be detectable by conventional techniques. There is, however, an absolute requirement to demonstrate experimentally that this explanation is indeed correct. This will, undoubtedly, be achieved by X-ray crystallographic analyses of the structures of relevant antibody–peptide complexes.

The above deductions have significant implications for the use of peptides as immunogens. Most importantly, peptides corresponding to helical (folded) regions of a protein are very unlikely to give rise to antibodies which will react with the native protein, unless the corresponding region of the protein is itself flexible; that is, exists in a variety of conformations, one of which resembles that of the unfolded peptide sufficiently to permit a stable interaction with antibody (see below).

Perturbation of protein conformation

A variety of effects induced on proteins by antisera have been variously interpreted as indicative of conformational changes in the antigen. These interpretations have been principally identified with antibody-induced changes in enzyme activity, especially of mutant penicillinases and β-galactosidase (Celada & Strom 1972), and the promotion of dissociation of proteins comprising non-covalently bonded subunits, such as class I major histocompatibility antigens and actomyosin (Peterson et al 1974, Mazander & Groschel-Stewart 1985). One of the most dramatic examples is the release of haem from sperm whale metmyoglobin induced by antisera against apomyoglobin (Crumpton 1966, 1972). Thus, rabbit antisera against sperm whale apomyoglobin invariably (from 25 different rabbits) formed precipitates with metmyoglobin that contained no haem (see Fig. 3), whereas Fab fragments of purified antibodies caused a slow decrease in the Soret band absorption of metmyoglobin, indicative of the release and subsequent aggregation of haem (Table 3).

The choice of explanation of this phenomenon is influenced by various considerations, especially by the fact that some distortion of the conformation of metmyoglobin, as revealed by X-ray crystallographic analysis (see Fig. 1), is essential for the release of haem, because the dimensions of the mouth of the haem pocket are less than those of the haem group. The most satisfying explanation depends upon the current generally accepted view that localized regions of a globular protein show high segmental motility; that is, undergo small rapid and reversible fluctuations in motility (Moore & Williams 1980, Westhof et al 1984). In this case, recognition and combination of a localized transient shape with antibody will result in the freezing of this conformation. Furthermore, stabilization of particular localized conformations by their speci-

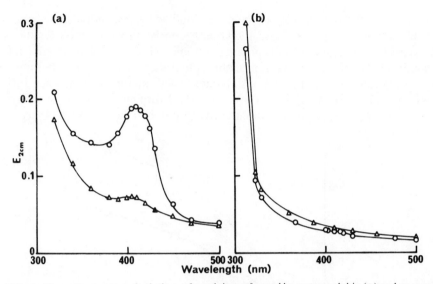

FIG. 3. Absorption spectra of solutions of precipitates formed by metmyoglobin (○) and apomyo-globin (△) with (a) an antiserum to metmyoglobin and (b) an antiserum to apomyoglobin.

fic antibodies may well promote more extensive conformational changes else-where in the molecule. This explanation permits anti-(metmyoglobin) and anti-(apomyoglobin) sera to be made up of populations of antibodies which recognize (and thus stabilize) different conformations of the same portion of the myoglobin molecule. As a result, metmyoglobin bound to metmyoglobin antibodies can possess a different conformation from that of metmyoglobin bound to apomyoglobin antibodies. As the release of haem from metmyoglo-bin is associated with an unfolding of the protein, this model also predicts

TABLE 3 Release of haem from sperm whale metmyoglobin induced by Fab fragments of anti-(apomyoglobin) serum

Time (min)[a]	$E^{2\,cm}_{410\,nm}$	
	Anti-Apo[b]	Anti-Met[b]
1	0.498	0.499
10	0.478	0.497
20	0.470	—
75	0.447	—
190	0.418	0.494
23 h	0.320	0.490

[a]Time after mixing metmyoglobin with Fab fragments.
[b]Fab fragments of antisera against apomyoglobin and metmyoglobin, respectively.

that anti-(apomyoglobin) sera contain antibodies against unfolded segments of the polypeptide chain. This prediction is consistent with the observations that anti-(apomyoglobin) sera contain antibodies which react with apomyoglobin unfolded by treatment with citraconic anhydride (see Fig. 4). Furthermore, it appears that these antibodies also combine with metmyoglobin, since anti-(apomyoglobin) serum that had been adsorbed with citraconylated apomyoglobin formed less precipitate with metmyoglobin than the unadsorbed serum.

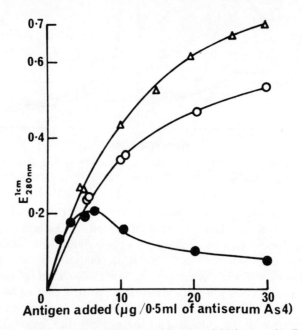

FIG. 4. Amounts of precipitate formed by an anti-(apomyoglobin) serum (As4) with increasing amounts of sperm whale metmyoglobin (○), apomyoglobin (△) and citraconylated apomyoglobin (●).

The antibody-induced release of haem from metmyoglobin, which is a fairly rigid protein, may be used as evidence in support of metmyoglobin showing segmental motility. A cogent question is: how extensive is this motility? For metmyoglobin, the answer to this question must be that it is not very extensive, for the following reason. In spite of containing 21 peptide bonds which are sensitive to breakage by trypsin, native sperm whale metmyoglobin in aqueous solution is completely resistant to degradation by trypsin.

If the phenomenon of segmental motility is widespread among globular proteins, it suggests that antibodies raised against a synthetic peptide whose conformation when attached to the carrier bears little apparent relationship to the corresponding region of the whole protein may nevertheless still react with the whole protein, provided this region of the protein shows high segmental motility. In other words, synthetic peptides corresponding to regions of high motility (i.e. 'corners' of the folded chain; Westhof et al 1984) are most likely to stimulate the production of antibodies which react with the native protein. In contrast, synthetic peptides representing folded regions of low motility are very unlikely to give rise to antibodies reactive with the native protein.

REFERENCES

Benjamin DC, Berzofsky JA, East IJ et al 1984 The antigenic structure of proteins: a reappraisal. Annu Rev Immunol 2:67-101

Celada F, Strom R 1972 Antibody induced conformational changes in proteins. Q Rev Biophys 5:395-425

Crumpton MJ 1966 Conformational changes in sperm-whale metmyoglobin due to combination with antibodies to apomyoglobin. Biochem J 100:223-232

Crumpton MJ 1972 Conformational changes in protein antigens induced by specific antibodies: sperm-whale myoglobin. In: Jaenicke R, Helmreich E (eds) Protein–protein interactions. Springer-Verlag, Heidelberg, p 395-408

Crumpton MJ 1974 Protein antigens: the molecular bases of antigenicity and immunogenicity. In: Sela M (ed) The antigens. Academic Press, New York, vol 2:1-78

Crumpton MJ, Polson A 1965 A comparison of the conformation of sperm whale metmyoglobin with that of apomyoglobin. J Mol Biol 11:722-729

Crumpton MJ, Small PA 1967 Conformation of immunologically-active fragments of sperm whale myoglobin in aqueous solution. J Mol Biol 26:143-146

Crumpton MJ, Wilkinson JM 1965 The immunological activity of some of the chymotryptic peptides of sperm whale myoglobin. Biochem J 94:545-556

Epand RM, Scheraga HA 1968 The influence of long-range interactions on the structure of myoglobin. Biochemistry 7:2864-2872

Mazander KD, Groschel-Stewart U 1985 Dissociation of actomyosin complex by monovalent fragments of polyclonal antibodies to myosin. FEBS (Fed Eur Biochem Soc) Lett 182:287-290

Moore GR, Williams RJP 1980 Comparison of the structure of various eukaryotic ferricyto-chromes c and ferrocytochromes and their antigenic differences. Eur J Biochem 103:543-550

Paterson Y 1985 Delineation and conformational analysis of two synthetic peptide models of antigenic sites on rodent cytochrome c. Biochemistry 24:1048-1055

Peterson PA, Rask L, Lindblom JB 1974 Highly purified papain-solubilized HL-A antigens contain β_2-microglobulin. Proc Natl Acad Sci USA 71:35-39

Sachs DH, Schechter AN, Eastlake A, Anfinsen CB 1972 An immunologic approach to the conformational equilibria of polypeptides. Proc Natl Acad Sci USA 69:3790-3794

Scatturin A, Tamburro AM, Rocchi R, Scoffone E 1967 The conformation of bovine pancreatic ribonuclease S-peptide. Chem Commun 1273-1276

Westhof E, Altschuh D, Moras D et al 1984 Correlation between segmental mobility and the location of antigenic determinants in proteins. Nature (London) 311:123-126

Wyckoff HW, Hardman KD, Allewell NM, Inagami R, Johnson LN, Richards Fm 1967 The structure of ribonuclease-S at 3.5 Å resolution. J Biol Chem 242:3984-3988

DISCUSSION

Lerner: There are now answers to the question of what are the antigenic proteins in viruses. Poliovirus and rhinoviruses are both close to being solved. One of the antigenic determinants seems to be a highly flexible loop that extends out from the surface. So if we look at viruses as geometric objects with lumps sticking out from their surfaces, these projections or loops are probably the main antigenic determinants. The next question is whether, if antibody is bound to those determinants, this disrupts the much more ordered array of surface structure.

Crumpton: Given the B cell repertoire and the fact that a motile area, at a single moment in time, will present a variety of conformational states, does this mean that a larger spectrum of B cells will recognize a motile region than a fixed region? If so, this corresponds to saying that a motile area is more immunogenic than a less motile one, because a greater proportion of the B cell repertoire will recognize it.

Lerner: I can answer that with another question. After all, the immune system is a contingency plan, with antibody to everything, and to nothing. Could one build 10^{11} perfect binders—perfectly shaped binding pockets—within the confines of the amount of genetic material available? My guess is that mobility gives one a lot of room that one wouldn't otherwise have. Rather than saying that the repertoire must be expanded, by virtue of all of the structures and all their conformations, I would say that it is rather the other way round. The limited repertoire that you have goes a longer way.

Klug: Mobility also extends to IgG molecules. The antibody binding site is not an old-fashioned 'lock' to fit a 'key'; it may be mobile. Unfortunately, not enough antibody molecules have been solved to a high enough resolution with reliable B factors for us to study, but a preliminary look shows that some sites are equally mobile. One would expect the hypervariable regions of the Ig molecule to be rather mobile. Thus, in the case of TMV protein injected into an animal which has never seen tobacco mosaic virus before, the antibodies don't know what is going to hit them ultimately, so there must be adaptation on both sides.

Williams: I would like to present some data derived from study of the cytochrome *c* molecule by myself and my colleagues, Dr G.R. Moore and Dr G. Williams. From our data we can draw a mobility map (Fig. 1) showing that for example some of the aromatic rings are turning over rapidly, flipping at a rate of something like 10^5 times a second, while others are flipping slowly, at say 10 times a second. We can describe much of the mobility of other side-chains of this molecule, too. While the inside has many regions of restricted mobility, on much of the outside surface of the cytochrome *c* molecule many of the side-chains, especially lysines, are twirling around in solution. They don't have fixed

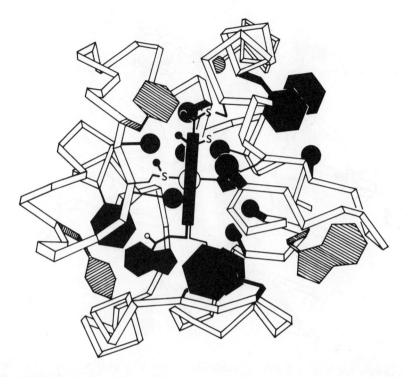

FIG. 1 (*Williams*). A side-chain mobility map of cytochrome *c*, derived from NMR studies. The filled-in side-chains are very rigid and are largely on the side of the haem group away from the methionine. The most mobile surface groups are hatched. Of the main chain, all methods indicate that the termini, especially the N-terminus, and the part of the chain on the methionine side, are most mobile.

conformations. (The fact that some crystallographic studies represent them as fixed is because the lysine groups are drawn, to enable one to recognize the amino acid; but they are not actually seen.)

One might expect that tryptophan residues would be rigid, but on the surface of proteins they are not always so. We can actually measure their time constants for motion. So one must not imagine that even the hydrophobic surface of the protein is grossly confined to any particular structure. Inside the protein, too, the rigidity may be confined to certain regions only. On one side of the porphyrin ring in cytochrome *c* the rigidity of side-chains is such that leucines and valines cannot twist around, but on the other side, where the sulphur of methionine 80 is bound, several side-chains are moving rapidly, and thus this 'side' of the haem is different in mobility from the other 'side'. We suspect that

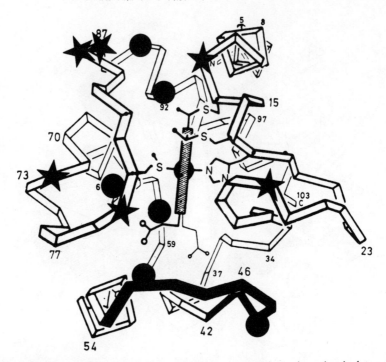

FIG. 2 (*Williams*). Ribbon diagram of cytochrome *c* showing the main antigenic determinants (circles) suggested by the work of Margoliash and co-workers (Urbanski & Margoliash 1977, Jemmerson & Margoliash 1979). The main antigenic region proposed by Atassi (1981) is shown by the solid ribbon. The lysine residues of cytochrome *c* responsible for the binding of its redox partners are shown by stars. Probably they all have very high mobility in their side-chains. (Reproduced from Williams & Moore 1985 by permission of *Trends in Biochemical Sciences*.)

the internal side-chain mobility generally is related to segmental mobility. This mobility may be very important for the opening of a groove to the haem iron, for the attack of reagents on the iron. By NMR we can test for this segmental mobility, not only by the internal motions but by the reactivity of the interior. One method is to use hydrogen exchange and another is to use access for a binding molecule. When we examined the binding of cytochrome *c* with cyanide and repeated the structure study, we saw what had changed, and we can deduce what had to move to allow access for cyanide. Cyanide breaks the methionine–iron bond and binds to the iron. While it only slightly perturbs the protein structure, it does so most in the regions on the methionine side of the haem, opening this segment out a little. The major regions of this mobility also correlate with the antigenic regions around amino acids 40–50 and 55–65 (Fig. 2).

We deduced from these studies that certain loops of proteins are more mobile than others and will expose quite hydrophobic parts of the protein for part of the time. It is these regions, we proposed, rather than the actual surface present for most of the time, which give rise to antigenicity. The most apparent parts of the protein surface, such as the lysines and glutamates, are used in protein–protein organization within the organism, giving rise to only weak binding and little antigenicity.

Finally, I don't believe that complete disordering is necessary to antigenic determinants. If there is a helix in a protein, as seen by crystallography, then in solution the helix may be antigenic, since it could rotate to make new hydrophobic groups exposed. The main thrust of this description is that there will not be a rule such as 'antigenic regions keep the same conformation when bound to antibody as that seen in the intact protein'.

Klug: Reverting to Mike Crumpton's paper, the question of equilibria seems fairly simple. You need only a factor of 10:1 for one particular conformation to dominate. For example, in the NMR experiment that Dr Lerner discussed, that is all that is needed to give a dominant signal. And 10:1 corresponds to a relatively small difference of energy to achieve, of the order of 2 kcal. Moreover, as long as you have a metastable structure there for a sufficient part of the time, the antibody can select it. In the case of TMV that I described, where there is a long helix showing antigenic activity but the short constituent peptides do not, probably the result is telling us that the long peptide is sufficiently helical for enough of the time for antibody to fix this conformation. We don't, however, know how to measure the fractional times spent in each conformation.

Williams: There is a peculiar point in Dr Crumpton's work. If an antibody is required to remove haem from myoglobin, that costs a factor of about 10^{10} against the binding constant for haem in the protein. Thus it is enormously difficult for an antibody to bind to the apoprotein when presented with the holoprotein.

Klug: That may have been done by more than one antibody at a time. It wasn't done with a single monoclonal antibody.

Ada: Do you know how many molecules of antibody bind to the antigen molecule?

Crumpton: Only in the sense that if you extrapolate the precipitin curve to antibody excess, it corresponds to a maximum of about three moles of IgG bound per mole of antigen.

Lerner: It wasn't helped along by the sodium azide in the solution, was it?

Crumpton: No! It might be helped by the albumin in the serum, in that this should act as a sink for the free haem. However, this doesn't appear to be a valid explanation. Thus, purified immunoglobulin was as effective in displacing the haem as the whole antiserum; also, in the experiment using Fab fragments, the addition of albumin did not increase the rate of decrease in Soret-band absorption.

Anders: Do any of the many monoclonal antibodies made against myoglobin have the same effect?

Crumpton: No.

REFERENCES

Atassi MZ 1981 Immune recognition by cytochrome C. I. Investigation by synthesis whether antigenic sites of polymeric cytochrome coincide with locations of sequence differences between the immunizing and host cytochromes. Mol Immunol 18:1021-1025

Jemmerson R, Margoliash E 1979 Topographic antigenic determinants on cytochrome *c*. Immunoadsorbent separation of the rabbit antibody populations directed against horse cytochrome *c*. J Biol Chem 254:12706-12716

Urbanski GJ, Margoliash E 1977 Topographic determinants on cytochrome *c*. I. The complete antigenic structures of rabbit, mouse, and guanaco cytochromes *c* in rabbits and mice. J Immunol 118:1170-1180

Williams RJP, Moore GR 1985 Protein antigenicity, organization and mobility. Trends Biochem Sci 10:96-97

Three-dimensional analyses of the binding of synthetic chemotactic and opioid peptides in the Mcg light chain dimer

ALLEN B. EDMUNDSON and KATHRYN R. ELY

Department of Biology, University of Utah, Salt Lake City, Utah 84112, USA

Abstract. Synthetic peptides with chemotactic or opioid activity were bound to crystals of a light chain dimer and their three-dimensional structures and modes of binding were determined by X-ray analysis. The chemotactic series consisted of di- and tripeptides initiated with *N*-formylmethionine or *N*-formylnorleucine residues. Opioid peptides included the enkephalins and casomorphins ranging in length from four to seven residues. The binding region of the protein proved to be malleable in adjusting to the surface contours of the peptides. Aromatic contact residues, as well as polypeptide segments of hypervariable loops, moved to improve the complementarity with the ligands. The peptides were even more flexible and tended to conform fairly closely to the space and geometry available for occupancy in the binding sites. Binding interactions were not confined to the interior of the cavity. In both the chemotactic and opioid series, the carboxyl tails of the peptides encroached upon the outer surfaces of the rim and contributed to the binding energies for the protein–ligand complexes. The peptide bond in *N*-formylmethionyltryptophan was found to be in the energetically unfavourable *cis* configuration. There was also evidence for less severe distortions in peptide bond geometry when *N*-formyltripeptides were bound to the dimer.

1986 Synthetic peptides as antigens. Wiley, Chichester (Ciba Foundation Symposium 119) p 107-129

The immunoglobulin light chain dimer to be discussed in this article was isolated in large quantities (100 g) from the urine of a patient (Mcg) with amyloidosis. Such proteins tend to have greater affinity for tissue components than light chains obtained from myeloma patients without accompanying amyloidosis (see Bertram et al 1980). The Mcg dimer possesses a large and malleable binding region which may be responsible for this tissue affinity. The binding region is located along the interface of the two 'variable' (V) domains of the dimer and is structurally divided into a conical main cavity and a deep pocket. The main cavity consists of constituents from the three 'hypervariable' loops of each monomer. Of the 21 side-chains lining the cavity, 12 are aromatic (eight tyrosines and four phenylalanines). It is not surprising that the dimer binds a wide variety of aromatic and hydrophobic aliphatic compounds (Edmundson et al 1974, 1984). Although the four aromatic residues constituting the floor of the main cavity are in van der Waals contact in the native structure, they can be reversibly displaced to allow ligands with appropriate chemical structures to enter the deep pocket. In some cases, forced entry into the pocket by over-sized ligands (e.g., bis(dinitrophenyl)lysine) presages overt damage or even dissolution of the crystals used in the binding studies. The ellipsoidal pocket is much smaller than the main cavity and is lined by glutamine 40, proline 46 and tyrosine 89 from each monomer.

In the binding of fluorescein, lucigenin and 6-carboxytetramethylrhodamine, the relative orientations of the two ring moieties in each compound were influenced by interactions with protein constituents. Moreover, the conformations of the binding site components were adjusted to approximate the contours of the ligands. To explore the process of mutual conformational adjustments more thoroughly, we expanded the binding studies to include very flexible ligands like peptides. We reasoned that the geometric and dynamic properties of the Mcg dimer would be favourable for the binding of hydrophobic peptides but we were initially perplexed over the selection of potential ligands. Our earlier studies (Edmundson et al 1974) indicated that randomly chosen hydrophobic dipeptides did not bind, and we decided to limit the present screening to peptides with well-characterized biological activities.

Even primitive immune systems were probably challenged with bacterial antigens, some of which had amino acid sequences beginning with N-formylmethionine residues. We hoped that a contemporary hydrophobic binding site would retain vestiges of a structure which could recognize peptides with similar N-terminal sequences. There were many commercially available N-formylated chemotactic peptides for binding trials, and their properties had been correlated with the structural requirements for binding to specific high affinity receptors on neutrophils (Schiffmann et al 1975, Showell et al 1976, Williams et al 1977, Freer et al 1982). The binding studies of the chemotactic peptides in the Mcg dimer were successful beyond expectation, and the results will be discussed here.

There are other groups of hydrophobic peptides with activities mediated through receptors. We had found that morphine and methadone could be bound to the Mcg dimer (Edmundson et al 1974) and wondered if opioid peptides (enkephalins and casomorphins) would mimic the properties of the drugs. Again, suitable peptides were available in a variety of lengths and sequences. These variations were reflected in different binding patterns, which will be described after consideration of the chemotactic peptides.

Brief description of the experimental procedure

The Mcg dimer was crystallized in 1.6–1.9 M-ammonium sulphate, buffered at pH 6.2 with 0.19 M-phosphate. A single barrel-shaped crystal, 0.4–0.5 mm wide in the middle and 1.0–1.2 mm long, was suspended in 0.4 ml of the crystallizing medium. Many peptides were sparingly soluble in this medium, but usually dissolved in quantities (>0.5 mM) sufficient for detection by X-ray analysis. In most experiments a peptide was added to the solution over a crystal to the point of saturation. After a soaking period of at least two weeks at 12 °C the crystal was mounted in a thin-walled capillary and exposed to Cu Kα X-irradiation with an automated Nicolet P21 diffractometer. Diffraction data were first collected to 6.5 Å resolution and compared with the data for the 'native' (unliganded) protein by difference Fourier analysis. If the peptide was found to be present in the binding region in significant amounts, the data collection was extended to 2.7 Å resolution. The results of the difference Fourier analyses were displayed in terms of three-dimensional 'cage' electron density with an Evans & Sutherland computer graphics system. Skeletal models of the peptide constituents were interactively fitted to this cage density. Models of the native binding region components were simultaneously displayed with the fitted peptides to study the protein–ligand interactions. Space-filling van der Waals surface representations of the protein and ligand were calculated with Connolly's (1983) algorithm. With these representations displayed on the graphics screen, forbidden contacts between protein and ligand could be identified and corrected to reflect the conformational changes in the native protein.

Binding of N-formylated chemotactic peptides

General requirements for binding

N-formylation of a peptide in the chemotactic series proved necessary for significant binding. Comparisons of binding properties were based on acceptance of N-For-Met-Leu-Phe as the prototype chemotactic peptide (see Showell et al 1976). The derivatized peptide Boc-Met-Leu-Phe (where Boc = *t*-butoxycarbonyl) and the parent compound Met-Leu-Phe were bound to the Mcg dimer, but in quantities barely above background levels. Dipeptides with sequences identical to those in various chemotactic peptides failed to bind in significant quantities (e.g., Met-Leu, Leu-Phe, Phe-Leu and Phe-Met).

The N-formyl peptides N-For-Met-Leu-Phe, N-For-Met-Phe-Met, N-For-Met-Met-Met and N-For-Met-Trp bound with relative occupancies of 1.0,

1.0, 0.88 and 0.92. *N*-For-Met-Ala and *N*-For-Met-Leu-Phe-Lys did not bind. An *N*-formylated eosinophilic tetrapeptide, *N*-For-Val-Gly-Ser-Glu (Snyderman & Goetzl 1981), showed some binding activity (relative occupancy 0.17), but a similar non-formylated peptide, Ala-Gly-Ser-Glu, did not. In summary, an *N*-formyl tripeptide was of optimum size for binding, but an *N*-formyl dipeptide could be accommodated if the second amino acid side-chain was large.

Methionine in position 1 could be replaced with norleucine, as in *N*-For-Nle-Leu-Phe (relative occupancy 0.75). In repeated tests with the norleucyl peptide, however, the occupancies were always lower than those for the methionyl derivative.

Structures of bound N-formylated tripeptides

The three-dimensional structures and the orientations of the *N*-formyl tripeptides were very similar when these were bound to the Mcg dimer. A skeletal model of the prototype *N*-For-Met-Leu-Phe ligand is shown in Fig. 1 in the orientation in which it was interactively fitted to the cage electron density in the difference Fourier map. In both nuclear magnetic resonance (NMR) solution studies (Becker et al 1979) and X-ray analyses of single crystals (Eggleston et al 1984), *N*-formylated chemotactic peptides adopted an extended

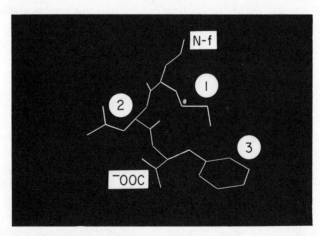

FIG. 1. Skeletal model of the chemotactic tripeptide *N*-For-Met-Leu-Phe displayed in the wedge-shaped conformation it adopted when bound to the Mcg dimer. The *N*-formyl and α-carboxyl groups are labelled N-f and COO⁻ and the three side-chains are represented by numbers (1: methionine; 2: leucine; 3: phenylalanine). This model was fitted by interactive computer graphics to three-dimensional 'cage' electron density in a difference Fourier map at 2.7 Å resolution.

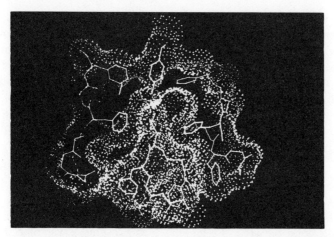

FIG. 2. Top, cut-away view of a van der Waals surface dot representation (Connolly 1983) of the binding of N-For-Met-Phe-Met in the main cavity of the Mcg dimer. Before this photograph was taken, the skeletal models of the peptide and protein were co-displayed with the surface dots on the graphics screen. As in Fig. 1, this photograph emphasizes that the chemotactic peptide assumed a wedge shape conforming closely to the contours of the binding cavity.

conformation similar to that of segments in a β-pleated sheet. Note that the bound N-formyl tripeptide is not fully extended, but has assumed a wedge shape with its side-chains swept back toward the entrance of the main binding cavity of the Mcg dimer. This shape conforms closely to the space available for binding in the main cavity (see Fig. 2).

Just as the peptide has adjusted to the binding site, the protein constituents have also moved to improve the complementarity with the ligand. Among these conformational adjustments were rotations and translations of aromatic side-chains and local expansion of the cavity by movements of the first, second and third hypervariable loops.

The N-formyl group of the tripeptide was within hydrogen-bonding distance of the phenolic hydroxyl groups of two tyrosine residues on the floor of the main cavity (tyrosine 38 from each monomer). In the difference map there was continuous electron density to one of these hydroxyl groups, direct evidence for a specific and relatively linear hydrogen bond in an otherwise hydrophobic environment. Formation of this hydrogen bond was of prime importance in orienting each of the N-formyl peptides in the cavity. Peptides with a free α-amino group or with a different derivatizing group could not sterically make such a hydrogen bond and would therefore be unsuitable for binding.

The methionyl or norleucyl side-chain in position 1 in each peptide occupied a distinctive pocket in which it was anchored by contact with tyrosine 93 of monomer 2. The subsite for residue 2 was more spacious, and therefore more permissive of movements and variations in size of the ligand constituent. Although the α-carboxyl group of a tripeptide was technically located inside the boundary of the cavity, the third side-chain was outside and impinging on components of the rim. While a bulky hydrophobic residue like methionine could readily be accommodated in this subsite, an aromatic residue like phenylalanine was preferable for maximizing interactions.

Distortions of peptide bond geometry during binding

Initially, we assumed that all peptide bonds in the ligands and protein were in the energetically more favourable *trans* configurations. However, it was not possible to achieve fully satisfactory fits to the electron density when the peptide bond between methionine 1 and residue 2 was placed in either the *cis* or *trans* configuration. The ligand appeared to be under torsional strain and it is possible that the peptide bond had partial *cis* character. In the *N*-formyl tripeptides, complete isomerization from the *trans* to the *cis* configuration was probably prevented by distal interactions involving the third residue. The dipeptide *N*-For-Met-Trp was not subject to such restrictions, as discussed in the following section.

Presence of a cis peptide bond in bound N-For-Met-Trp

N-For-Met-Trp was found in two overlapping subsites with approximately equal occupancies. The deep subsite was very similar to that of an *N*-For-Met tripeptide, but the peptide bond between methionine and tryptophan could only be fitted to the electron density in the *cis* configuration (see Fig. 3). In the outer subsite, in which the tryptophan side-chain occupied the same general space as phenylalanine 3 in a tripeptide, the peptide bond was in the expected *trans* configuration. Especially in sites in which the requirements for binding are strict, it appears that the alteration of peptide bond geometry can be considered a distinct possibility for the enhancement of protein–ligand interactions.

Binding of opioid peptides

Selection of opioid peptides for binding trials

Methionine- (Met-) and leucine- (Leu-) enkephalins are endogenous opioid peptides originally detected in brain homogenates (Hughes et al 1975). The

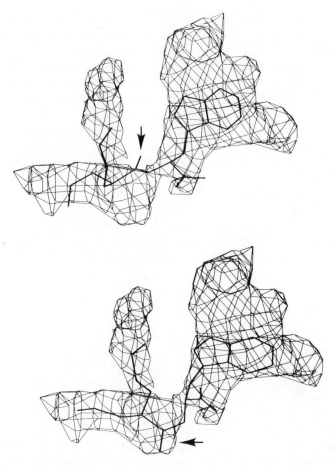

FIG. 3. Binding of *N*-For-Met-Trp in the deeper subsite of the Mcg dimer. The cage electron density in a 2.7 Å difference Fourier map was co-displayed with the skeletal model of the fitted peptide. The cage density was too extensive for a single ligand molecule but was appropriate for two molecules binding in different (but overlapping) subsites. Only the fitting of a model to the deeper subsite is shown. *Upper panel*: the peptide bond between methionine and tryptophan was built in the energetically favourable *trans* configuration. Note that the carbonyl group (arrow) was outside the electron density envelope, an indication that this configuration was very unlikely. *Lower panel*: the peptide bond was constructed in the *cis* configuration and the carbonyl group could be placed in the cage density with confidence.

enkephalins interact with at least two classes of receptors, δ and μ, with generally higher affinity for the former (Lord et al 1977, Chang et al 1979). Morphine binds strongly to μ receptors, a preference shared by β-casomorphins (Brantl et al 1981). These peptides were first isolated from enzymic digests of the milk protein β-casein.

The naturally occurring enkephalins are pentapeptides with the general sequence Tyr-Gly-Gly-Phe-(Met or Leu). Hundreds of analogues have been synthesized and tested for binding to receptors. Amino-terminal tyrosine is necessary, but not sufficient for binding. Residues 4 and 5 are also important. In some analogues, D-amino acids have been inserted into positions 2 and 5 and proline has been placed in position 4, mainly to deter rapid enzymic hydrolysis of the peptides *in vivo* and secondarily to improve the binding to receptors. In binding experiments with the Mcg dimer, we have screened [Met^5]- and [Leu^5]enkephalins, a heptapeptide extension of [Met^5]enkephalin (Arg-6, Phe-7), and various analogues, including peptides with D-amino acids in positions 2 and 5. Di-, tri- and tetrapeptides together representing the sequence of an enkephalin were also subjected to binding trials.

β-Casomorphin(1–7) has the sequence Tyr-Pro-Phe-Pro-Gly-Pro-Ile. In assays for binding to receptors, both the (1–4) and (1–5) fragments were more potent than the heptapeptide, and the (1–3) fragment was inactive (Brantl et al 1981). The (1–4), (1–5) and (1–7) peptides were all tested for binding in the Mcg dimer.

General binding characteristics of the opioid peptides

As in δ receptors, the presence of N-terminal tyrosine was essential for the binding of enkephalins to the Mcg dimer. For example, the following compo-nents of enkephalins minus tyrosine all failed to bind in measurable quantities: Gly-Gly-Phe-Met, Gly-Gly-Phe, Phe-Met and Phe-Leu. In further analogy with receptors, N-terminal tyrosine was not sufficient for binding since Tyr-Gly-Gly and Tyr-Gly did not form complexes with the protein. A brominated derivative, 3,5-dibromo[Leu^5]enkephalin, showed no binding activity but this compound was practically insoluble in the buffered ammonium sulphate used in the soaking procedure. As expected, cyclo(Leu-Gly-), a morphine-tolerance peptide, and Tyr-Arg, an analgesic, also did not bind.

The remaining peptides, all with the minimum requirements for receptor binding, exhibited a variety of binding patterns in the Mcg dimer. Collectively, these ligands occupied subsites along most of the interface between the two V domains, including the main cavity and deep pocket. Moreover, the C-terminal portions of some of the ligands interacted with protein constituents outside the boundaries of the cavity. These binding patterns will now be dis-cussed in more detail.

Binding of [Met]- and [Leu]enkephalins

[Met]enkephalin occupied two overlapping sites with a preference of about 1.3 to 1.0 for the deeper site. In the deeper site the N-terminal tyrosine residue

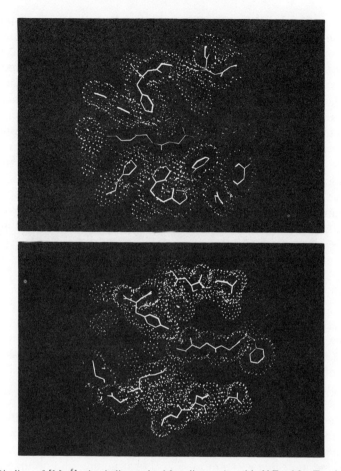

FIG. 4. Binding of [Met⁵]enkephalin to the Mcg dimer. As with *N*-For-Met-Trp (see Fig. 3), [Met⁵]enkephalin was bound in two overlapping subsites. *Upper panel*: surface dot representation and skeletal model of [Met⁵]enkephalin in the deeper subsite (cut-away side view of the binding region). Note that the peptide is almost fully extended, with its N-terminal tyrosine residue anchored in the deep binding pocket on the left and its carboxyl portion in the main cavity on the right. *Lower panel*: cut-away side view of the [Met⁵]enkephalin molecule bound in the outer subsite. The empty deep pocket appears on the left and the phenyl ring of residue 4 of the peptide is outside the main cavity on the far right. The peptide backbone of the last two residues is bent sharply upward to interact with constituents of the outer rim of the main cavity.

penetrated into the pocket, and the remainder of the peptide trailed in a completely extended conformation in the main cavity (see Fig. 4). The peptide bond involving the carbonyl group of tyrosine bridged the junction between the main cavity and pocket.

In the second subsite, N-terminal tyrosine was stacked between phenylalanine 99, monomer 2, and the floor of the cavity near phenylalanine 101, monomer 2. At the position of glycine 3 the ligand exited the cavity and turned abruptly upward to interact with rim constituents of monomer 1 (Fig. 4.). [Leu]enkephalin did not enter the deep pocket, but was bound in a subsite very similar to the outer site for [Met]enkephalin. These differences in the binding patterns of [Met]- and [Leu]enkephalins were surprising, and therefore open to question. However, the initial observations were confirmed when the experiments were repeated.

In single crystals of [Leu]enkephalin in N,N-dimethylformamide and water, the peptide assumed four different conformations (Karle et al 1983). These conformers, with extended peptide backbones, were aligned side-by-side to form an antiparallel β-pleated sheet in the crystal lattice. When bound in the Mcg dimer, these extremely flexible enkephalin molecules did not adopt an extended conformation unless their amino ends reached the deep pocket.

Binding sites for the remaining enkephalins

The heptapeptide, (Arg-6, Phe-7)[Met^5]enkephalin, displayed a similar pattern to the deep-seated molecule of [Met]enkephalin. Amino-terminal tyrosine was situated in the pocket and the rest of the peptide extended to the entrance of the main cavity and beyond. The Arg-6 and Phe-7 side-chains flattened out against the external surface of the cavity.

Peptides with D-amino acids in positions 2 and 5 were not always predictable in their binding behaviour. For example, Tyr-D-Ala-Gly-Phe-D-Leu occupied two subsites. The innermost ligand molecule assumed an extended conformation very similar to that of the deep-seated [Met]enkephalin. The second ligand molecule was almost helical in structure, and occupied a more external position. Tyr-D-Met-Gly-Phe-Pro(NH$_2$) was also highly convoluted. While less convoluted, Tyr-D-Ala-Gly-Phe-Met was primarily an external binder which entered the cavity only with its tyrosine residue. In contrast to these peptides, Tyr-D-Ser-Gly-Phe-Leu-Thr mimicked the binding behaviour of [Leu]enkephalin with, of course, additional external interactions involving C-terminal threonine.

Binding of casomorphins

The N-terminal portions of the (1–4) and (1–5) β-casomorphins were confined to the main cavity, but the (1–7) derivative spanned the cavity and the tyrosine side-chain penetrated into the pocket (see Fig. 5). The presence of proline

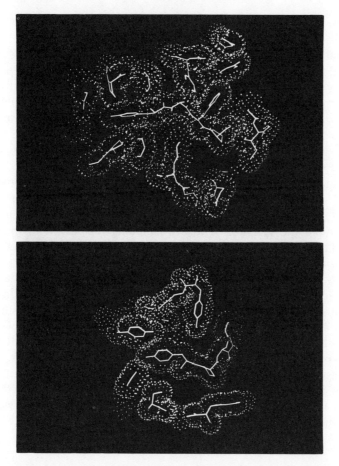

FIG. 5. *Upper panel*: binding pattern of β-casomorphin(1–7). This peptide spanned nearly the entire length of the binding region, with its N-terminal tyrosine in the deep pocket on the left and its carboxyl end outside the main cavity on the right. *Lower panel*: cut-away view of β-casomorphin(1–4) in its binding site. The N-terminal part of the peptide is inside the main cavity on the left and the carboxyl region bends upward to impinge on the outer rim on the right.

residues resulted in compact conformations of the peptides, but their carboxyl regions still protruded from the cavity. Inside the cavity the structures of the bound casomorphins were quite similar, but externally their structures were different. Peptide bonds involving proline are more easily isomerized to the *cis* configuration than other bonds, but there were no indications of *cis* configurations in the bound casomorphins.

Summary of the general binding properties of the opioid peptides

N-terminal tyrosine was essential for binding in all enkephalins and casomorphins, and four residues appeared to be the minimum number in a productive ligand. As many as four residues of a bound ligand were found to interact with external flat or convex surfaces of the binding region. The internal or concave parts of the binding region accommodated from one to five residues of various opioid peptides. The proportion of the peptide entering the cavity seemed to be dependent on its length and its sequence, including the presence or absence of D-amino acids.

The Met-enkephalin pentapeptide, its [Arg-6, Phe-7] heptapeptide extension, and the casomorphin heptapeptide penetrated the floor of the main cavity to the deep pocket. This penetration involved conformational changes in and around the junction of the two binding regions. With the tyrosine side-chain rather rigidly held in the deep pocket, the remainder of each ligand assumed an almost fully extended conformation.

[Leu]enkephalin and its analogues generally penetrated less deeply and showed a tendency to bend sharply around glycine 3 to participate in external interactions with rim constituents of the cavity. The external surfaces of monomer 1 components seemed to be favoured for interactions with about two-thirds of the ligands. Peptides with D-amino acids adopted conformations that were particularly complementary with the monomer 1 surfaces. It should be emphasized that the surface binding interactions were influenced by the local packing of protein molecules and the distribution of solvent in the crystal lattice. In general, the external interactions of the opioid peptides were more variable than those in the more protected internal environment.

Acknowledgements

This investigation was supported by grant CA 19616, awarded by the National Cancer Institute, Department of Health and Human Services. We gratefully acknowledge the graphics work and photography of Barbara Staker and Brad Nelson, and the unstinting aid of Maurine Vaughan in the preparation of the manuscript for publication. Our colleague James Herron has been extremely helpful in modifying and implementing computer programs.

REFERENCES

Becker EL, Bleich HE, Day AR et al 1979 Nuclear magnetic resonance conformational studies on the chemotactic tripeptide formyl-L-methionyl-L-leucyl-L-phenylalanine. A small β sheet. Biochemistry 18:4656-4668

Bertram J, Gualtieri RJ, Osserman EF 1980 Amyloid-related Bence Jones proteins bind dinitrophenyl L-lysine (DNP). In: Glenner GG et al (eds) Amyloid and amyloidosis. Excerpta Medica, Amsterdam, p 351-360

Brantl V, Teschemacher H, Bläsig J, Henschen A, Lottspeich F 1981 Opioid activities of β-casomorphins. Life Sci 28:1903-1909

Chang K-J, Cooper BR, Hazum E, Cuatrecasas P 1979 Multiple opiate receptors: different regional distribution in the brain and differential binding of opiates and opioid peptides. Mol Pharmacol 16:91-104

Connolly ML 1983 Solvent-accessible surfaces of proteins and nucleic acids. Science (Wash DC) 221:709-713

Edmundson AB, Ely KR, Girling RL et al 1974 Binding of 2,4-dinitrophenyl compounds and other small molecules to a crystalline λ-type Bence-Jones dimer. Biochemistry 13:3816-3827

Edmundson AB, Ely KR, Herron JN 1984 A search for site-filling ligands in the Mcg Bence-Jones dimer: crystal binding studies of fluorescent compounds. Mol Immunol 21:561-576

Eggleston DS, Jeffs PW, Chodosh DF, Heald SL 1984 Conformational influences of N^2-methylation in chemotactic peptides. Abstr Am Crystallogr Assoc Annu Meet, Lexington, Kentucky, PB4:36

Freer RJ, Day AR, Muthukumaraswamy N 1982 Formyl peptide chemoattractants: a model of the receptor on rabbit neutrophils. Biochemistry 21:257-263

Hughes JW, Smith T, Kosterlitz HW et al 1975 Identification of two related pentapeptides from the brain with potent opiate agonist activity. Nature (Lond) 255:577-579

Karle IL, Karle J, Mastropaolo D et al 1983 [Leu^5]enkephalin: four cocrystallizing conformers with extended backbones that form an antiparallel β-sheet. Acta Crystallogr Sect B Struct Crystallogr Cryst Chem 39:625-637

Lord J, Waterfield AA, Hughes J, Kosterlitz HW 1977 Endogenous opioid peptides: multiple agonists and receptors. Nature (Lond) 267:495-499

Schiffmann E, Corcoran BA, Wahl SM 1975 N-formylmethionyl peptides as chemoattractants for leucocytes. Proc Natl Acad Sci USA 72:1059-1062

Showell HJ, Freer RJ, Zigmond SH et al 1976 The structure–function relations of synthetic peptides as chemotactic factors and inducers of lysosomal enzyme secretion for neutrophils. J Exp Med 143:1156-1169

Snyderman R, Goetzl EJ 1981 Molecular and cellular mechanisms of leucocyte chemotaxis. Science (Wash DC) 213:830-837

Williams LT, Snyderman R, Pike MC, Lefkowitz RJ 1977 Specific receptor sites for chemotactic peptides on human polymorphonuclear leucocytes. Proc Natl Acad Sci USA 74:1204-1208

DISCUSSION

Lerner: Is one implication of this work that if you knew the structure of the endorphin receptor, for example, it would combine with the peptide in a very similar way to the dimer?

Edmundson: I wouldn't say that, because the binding site of the Mcg dimer dealt with the opioid peptides in different ways. Maybe the difference between binding in the Mcg dimer and high affinity binding lies in the specificity of a receptor, as compared to a generalized hydrophobic binding site of the right size and shape. I would be surprised if the size and shape of a receptor were not similar, but I would also be very surprised if the detailed kinds of binding were identical to those in the dimer.

Ada: Can you have binding where the cleft isn't filled at all?

Edmundson: We have peptides in which only the tyrosine residue enters the cavity and the rest of the peptide is binding on the outside. Therefore, entry into the cavity isn't essential for peptide binding.

Crumpton: And is the number of contacts between the tyrosine and the binding site about 70, in this instance?

Edmundson: No; that number is obtained only when it goes into the deep pocket.

Stanworth: Do I understand that only Bence-Jones proteins from amyloid patients show this binding?

Edmundson: We think so. Bertram et al (1980) found that the light chain dimers from seven patients with amyloidosis bound DNP-lysine like the Mcg dimer. Six proteins from patients with multiple myeloma, but without amyloidosis, failed to bind this hapten-like compound.

Stanworth: So this binding might not be relevant to ligand-binding to the Fab regions of antibodies?

Edmundson: I don't know that, but I wouldn't say it was *not* relevant. It is at least a good model!

Anders: To my knowledge, there is no evidence that any ligand is bound in amyloid deposits involving immunoglobulin light chains. With the appropriate light chains, amyloid fibrils can be generated *in vitro* in the absence of any ligand.

Edmundson: You can generate fibrils with some light chains that aren't even amyloidogenic, but they must first be treated with pepsin. All amyloid deposits contain some intact light chain molecules. I think the light chains accumulate in organs because of their affinity for tissue components, as mediated through their binding sites. We don't know what these components are.

Rothbard: With the smaller ligands that do not fill the combining site, do you see any changes where you could conclude that the antibody has compacted the site rather than expanded it?

Edmundson: Our only experiment on compaction involved the use of high hydrostatic pressures. When Jim Herron subjected liganded dimers to pressures of about 2.5–3 kbar, which is about half the pressure normally required for a protein to unravel, the affinity for one ligand (bis[1-anilinonaphthalene-8-sulphonate]) increased 300-fold.

Rothbard: Is this due to the restraints of the crystal lattice, or is it that to compact a binding site is energetically less favourable than to expand it?

Edmundson: It's difficult to do, because of external crystal-packing interactions with other protein molecules. But you can put the dimer under pressure in solution and it compacts and increases the affinity. What surprised us was the fact that on decompression of the solution to atmospheric pressure, the dimer retained an affinity for the ligand ten times higher than the starting value.

Crumpton: What happens in solution? Are the peptides bound with the same relative affinities as you see in the crystal? Furthermore, is it possible to make a complex in solution and crystallize it? If so, does it have the same structure as when you diffuse the ligand into the crystal? I am wondering whether the flexibility of the site in solution is greater than that in the crystal.

Edmundson: We suspect that it is. There are ligands which you can test in solution, and some you can't; for instance, bis(DNP)lysine binds both in the crystal and in solution. In the crystal only one molecule is bound because the second potential site is blocked by crystal-packing interactions. In solution there are two nominally identical sites available for binding, and two molecules of ligand can be bound in one dimer. You cannot co-crystallize the dimer with two ligands in the cavity, however, because the second ligand would interfere with the known crystal packing of the native dimer.

Williams: This work illustrates what antigenic and other forms of specificity really are about. The first ideas historically on specificity were of a die fitting into its mould—an exact fitting between two objects. Then followed the concept of a lock and a key, which is different in that as you insert the key into the lock, you make small twisting movements of the key to get it into the lock—induced fit—which show that the dynamics of the system are needed to make a final fit. The die going into the mould causes an almost infinite problem in the speed of fitting, if it's a perfect fit; you cannot force the die into the mould at all easily. Putting a round peg in a round hole is actually very difficult if they are very closely the same size. How far can one go with the principle of increasing dynamics to increase speed—what do you lose and what do you gain? You can go to the extreme of the model of a hand going into a glove, where both are mobile initially and where mobility remains even when the fit is perfect. When the fingers of the hand are in the glove they can twist around. Specificity has something to do with shape at one extreme, but time also needs to be described to analyse access and also to allow subsequent action rather than a static combination. Unless you have mobility, a tight fitting requirement could so seriously jeopardize rate that no reaction would ever occur. The realities of reaction mean that some specificity must be thrown away in order to allow combination and consequential action.

Edmundson: In recent experiments with very high affinity antibodies (anti-fluorescein monoclonals), we think that the last little bit of conformational adjustment is still based on flexibility, even though the association constant is $10^{10}\,M^{-1}$.

Stevens: If this model does relate to antigen–antibody binding, where the antibody is concave and the antigen is convex, how would you characterize anti-idiotype binding to antibody?

Edmundson: I don't see that there has to be a concave surface on the antibody. The Kol myeloma protein is convex in shape, and the potential binding site is filled. There are many sites that one could imagine simply as slight invaginations, or even a flat surface. Any antibody combining site that interacts with large molecules could easily be flat or slightly concave. We have been thinking about DNA-binding monoclonals; there is no way in which DNA will insert end-on into a cavity. We think that the binding site is a groove. It's just that, in our dimer, there is a cavity, and we want to see how far we can push this model.

Lerner: Is this system peculiar to the antibody molecule? If you picked out some other crystal with a deep pocket, could you achieve the same binding? I would not see this as specific to antibody binding; other pockets might do just as well. Have you tried to diffuse similar ligands into crystals of other proteins?

Edmundson: We haven't gone to other proteins.

Crumpton: In the past, immunochemists have imagined the antibody combining site as a collection of subsites, one of which contributes preferentially to the affinity and specificity of interaction. The group occupying this subsite represents the immunodominant group. You have given us, in terms of the deep tyrosine binding, a very good demonstration of such an immunodominant group.

Edmundson: We found this with the fluorescein series too. As we increased the size of a ligand by two phenyl rings at a time, each ligand occupied a different subsite in the cavity, and progressively had more contacts as we made them bigger (e.g. fluorescein, lucigenin and dimers of 6-carboxy-tetramethylrhodamine). The immunodominant group in fluorescein is clearly the three-membered ring.

Geysen: We have characterized monoclonal antibodies and some polyclonal antibodies for their reactions with single amino acids. This is quite easy to do; you get signal-to-background ratios of from 4:1 to as high as 8:1. It is clear that of all the monoclonal antibodies examined, only one of about five amino acids ever reacts, and it does so with very clear signals. These are single amino acids, each on the end of a long polyacrylic acid polymer. You can change the link between the amino acid and the support, so this has very little to do with the interaction. It seems that you observe sufficient binding in the outer part of the antibody cavity, which is very specific for a given amino acid and differs enormously between monoclonal antibodies.

Edmundson: We have a similar case with the leucine 110 side-chain that goes into the binding site of an adjacent dimer in the crystal lattice. This side-chain fits very well in the cavity; yet it's not the primary determinant in the binding process. All the other closely packed protein surfaces around the cavity make the major contribution to binding.

Geysen: A number of our monoclonal antibodies show reactions with single leucine residues attached to our solid support.

Ada: Presumably a single amino acid wouldn't distort the binding site of the antibody?

Edmundson: By itself a side-chain might not distort, but you could get distortion due to more distal interactions with other parts of the molecule. We had multi-site attachment in all cases. In Dr Geysen's example, you would have to assume that the multi-site attachment is in and around the binding site, but the specificity would centre on a single amino acid.

Lerner: Take trypsin: no one would say that the enzyme 'sees' lysine alone, but this residue gets into the pocket and the enzyme makes additional contacts with the rest of the protein substrate.

Edmundson: We have hybridized other light chains with our Mcg protein and have crystallized them. One molecule (Weir) with the same C gene as Mcg has 36 differences in the variable domain. The Weir dimer doesn't bind DNP at all. When we hybridize this molecule with the Mcg protein, the hybrid binds DNP compounds just as Mcg does. The crystal of the hybrid structure is almost identical with the Mcg dimer except for the substitutions. However, the binding site on the Mcg portion of the binding cavity is not hindered by the second chain. The Weir protein has serine substituted for tyrosine in position 34, and Tyr-34 is the primary contact residue for DNP. Serine is sufficiently small and is on the other side of the cavity, and therefore does not interfere with the capacity of Mcg to bind DNP; it collaborates with Mcg in forming a binding site compatible with the binding of such compounds.

Ada: What is the maximum flexibility of the binding site in one of your hybrid molecules? To what extent does it change?

Edmundson: We are thinking in terms of 1–2 Å of translation of a polypeptide loop or side-chain, and relatively free rotation about the α–β bonds of the aromatic rings. In many cases in the binding site the ring orientations appear to be relatively fixed in the crystal structure of the native protein. They change when the ligands move in.

Klug: I gather that the tyrosine at the bottom of the cavity moved over by about 1 Å. That tyrosine in the unliganded structure might be mobile, but not necessarily through a distance as large as that. But the tyrosine moves from one place to another.

Edmundson: Yes; that seems to be true.

Ada: Is the flexibility of the binding site actually so great? We have been discussing segmental flexibility of proteins with parts that are more motile than others being more important. Are these differences so critical, if the flexibility of the binding site of the antibody is great enough to accommodate different molecules?

Edmundson: It's not quite like that. Many compounds that look promising don't bind. What is significant is that an appropriate ligand can move rings that are in van der Waals contact out of the way, 17 Å from the entrance, and force its way into the deep pocket.

Ada: I am wondering whether the flexibility of the binding site of the antibody is great enough to decrease the importance of flexibility in the ligand.

Edmundson: I don't think so. I would add that our model is very useful for looking at cross-reactivity, and may indicate the mechanism involved. In such cases you don't have to have a binding site tailor-made, but just a site which is complementary in shape and in its chemical properties. Even in high affinity systems, we think that final adjustments are probably made before the binding is finished; there is some kind of mutual adjustment.

Klug: There is no contradiction between high affinity and mobility. The key and the lock, as Bob Williams said, can both be slightly wobbly. The final object that is made can nevertheless be a pretty tight and highly specific structure, depending on how many groups are interacting.

Williams: The best example must be oxygen binding onto haemoglobin, because for oxygen to reach the iron, some groups have to move. The oxygen molecules cannot see the iron directly. Interestingly, site flexibility is shown by different substrates. Oxygen binds nicely; carbon monoxide also binds but with a slightly different structure. It has the same problem of getting to the iron, but it binds with a slightly different final stereochemistry. CO is actually pushed out again, if you wish to say so, by the structural requirements. Of course, if equilibrium is not reached, the rate of the process, getting to the site, can also be part of the selectivity. Competition in transient states is not the same as that at equilibrium.

Anders: High affinity interactions might be favoured by mobility in the antigen. We haven't yet referred to the fact that somatic mutation in the variable regions of lymphocyte Ig receptors is probably very critical to the eventual generation of high affinity antibody responses. This may bias the immune response towards epitopes that are capable of flexibility.

Lerner: Not exactly; because diversity is a sharpening mechanism under selection, so you are driving the system to higher and higher affinity.

Anders: Antigen is driving the system and somatic mutations are occurring which are selected by antigen.

Ada: The antigen doesn't change, though.

Anders: The antibody is changing, due to somatic mutations that will alter affinity. If there is also the capacity for the epitope to change conformation, antigen selection of somatic mutants is more likely to generate high affinity antibody responses.

Lerner: Do you know that you are driving towards a higher affinity antibody?

Anders: Not yet for somatic mutations in hybridomas making antibodies to influenza haemagglutinin (Clarke et al 1985), but in the secondary response to arsonate, somatic mutation generates higher affinity antibodies (Manser et al 1985).

Klug: Are you saying that the descendants of the cells involved in the primary response are no longer highly represented in the secondary and later responses?

Anders: No; the descendants of those cells *are* represented in the secondary response, but the antibodies they produce may be changed in affinity and fine specificity.

McConnell: You can recall particular clones present in the primary response on subsequent immunization. The original specificity can still be elicited.

Skehel: At limiting antigen concentration they would be different. That's the basis of the high affinity secondary immune response.

McConnell: In limiting conditions of antigen one selects clones which were not present before. B cells of higher affinity are selected. However, the original clone, possibly of lower affinity, may still be present.

Anders: The highest affinity antibodies in a secondary immune response, from the results on influenza haemagglutinin (Clarke et al 1985), have probably accumulated quite a number of somatic mutations in the complementarity-determining regions.

Klug: One advantage of flexibility in the antigenic determinant is that the antibody can make a rough-and-ready interaction in a quick response, if that is required in a given situation. Then the system can adapt itself later, by selecting rare descendants of cells which have hardly reacted, or not reacted at all.

Lerner: This is a good point, because in some instances the earliest immune response is the 19S antibody, which is very ready and very rough. Later on the response switches to 7S Ig and the affinity sharpens up. It is an interesting idea that you need to get a response started, and since an individual cannot own all the collection of perfectly shaped antibodies, the whole cascade is started with any old binder.

Ada: Of course, there are avidity effects as well.

Lerner: Yes, even if it's a different class of Ig.

V. Nussenzweig: The idea of mimicking a peptide antigen with a rigid structure would not be so good, in view of Allen Edmundson's results, because a rigid structure would be recognized by fewer antibody combining sites with sufficient energy. No 'adaptation' would be possible to trigger a response.

Edmundson: I think that is so. It would be difficult to decide what your site should look like, since binding is multi-point and since it changes from peptide to peptide. Even with the same peptide, the binding pattern can change, if we allow the soaking period to extend to two months or so. The ligand and protein have plenty of time to equilibrate. In some cases the ligands actually change sites over a period of time, as they alter the binding region.

Lerner: I don't think Dr Nussenzweig's point necessarily follows. Something we think is important for our science would be to build these shapes out of non-peptide chemicals. Consider the fact that the opioid receptor sees endorphins and alkaloids; if you knew the rules, you could build the peptide mimic out of an alkaloid, and the receptor would see them both with good affinity. Theoretically, I can keep changing the structure chemically and checking it against the opioid receptor. Every time I make a chemical change and do not lose the affinity of binding, I am permitted to make the next change. If I did this long enough, always checking against the proper receptor, I might drive up the affinity of binding.

V. Nussenzweig: That is a different question. I am concerned about the repertoire of B cells, and the number that will be triggered by an epitope. For greater immunogenicity, you want to get many cells going. The question is whether this is better achieved with a rigid or flexible epitope. Can you make a shape which would be as immunogenic as the peptide epitope for the random population of B cells? That seems unlikely, in view of Dr Edmundson's results.

Lerner: I don't think so. If you immunize with the opiate alkaloid, would that antibody see endorphin, for example? That is the experiment.

Edmundson: We have been able to bind morphine and methadone to the dimer.

Rothbard: Have you ever seen a crystal containing more than one conformation? In other words, did you get an average structure of your ligand?

Edmundson: If this happened, we might see an ill-defined structure in the difference electron density maps.

Rothbard: Did you ever see *cis-trans* isomerization in a peptide bond in any of your antigens?

Edmundson: We would not pick that up without doing a complete structural analysis.

Ada: Do your large peptides by themselves crystallize? I am wondering about the extent to which the shape bound by the antibody is different from the shape in free solution or as a crystal.

Edmundson: Some did; [Leu]enkephalin, for instance. It had four different conformers, all of which were extended (Karle et al 1983). There was an infinite β-pleated sheet in the crystal, with four conformers arranged in antiparallel fashion. But each shape was different from the ones we obtained in the bound forms. When the tyrosine of the peptide went to the deep pocket and the remainder was firmly held in the cavity, the peptide adopted an extended structure.

Ada: Can we try to formulate any general principles or guidelines for peptide-based vaccines, at this stage?

Stevens: We have discussed the fit of a given antibody to a particular epitope and how we can obtain stronger binding. Is there a rule that one should prepare a peptide immunogen containing more than one epitope, to increase the overall strength of binding of antibodies to the target antigen, in addition to increasing the binding avidity of antibody to single epitopes, or will that depend on the individual target antigen of the disease state being tackled? That is to say, if in a region of a protein you find one epitope and another epitope in a distant region, could you put those in one long carrier chain, or inject them as two separate carrier–peptide conjugates, and obtain stronger binding of the resulting antibodies for neutralizing or eliminating the protein?

Edmundson: Are you asking whether we should build a discontinuous determinant?

Stevens: Not necessarily. I am asking whether one wants an immunogen that, following an immune response, evokes antibodies with two separate specificities such that they each bind to different parts of the molecule; so that as well as increasing the strength of binding at one site, you also have more than one site of the protein being bound by antibody simultaneously.

Geysen: I think the answer is yes, with some qualifications. If you think of two protein molecules, the native molecule seen in solution, with a given biological activity, and a conformationally different molecule with no biological activity, you could calculate an energy difference for the two different states. If you were to use a single antibody to stabilize the conformationally altered protein, with subsequent loss of biological activity, then in its binding it has to provide the total energy for the conformational change. If you use two antibody molecules simultaneously binding at different parts of the same protein molecule, both of which bind to (effectively) the altered version, they share the energy penalty for the conformational change. With three antibodies binding simultaneously, there is an even smaller effect on the affinity of each of the antibodies. Perhaps a polyclonal response often gives good protection (neutralization) because that is what is happening: each of the binding antibodies stabilizes to a small extent a conformational change which is transmitted and allows another antibody molecule to bind, and so on. It is a cascade event. That may explain why examples of synergism between antibody molecules have been found; that is, individual monoclonal antibodies don't bind with high affinity but two antibodies (which don't bind on an overlapping site) both bind at higher affinity. So the question is whether the best vaccine consists of multiple epitopes which are not overlapping but all contribute to the same eventual conformational change of the protein molecule, causing loss of activity. Is that what you have in mind?

Stevens: Yes; I wanted to know if it is generally better to seek synergistic antibody action than single-site antibody binding.

Klug: Logically, the longer the peptide you make, the more chance you have of a multiple reaction with antibodies; so the longer the better, surely.

Geysen: Yes; but you may have to tailor one epitope to the other, because one antibody may produce a conformational change in the antigen molecule in one direction and the other antibody, which binds at a distant place on the antigen, could produce a conformational change in the other direction, so the two antibodies are antagonistic to the binding of one another. Thus it is necessary for two epitopes to be tailored so that they complement each other, and lead to a synergistic antibody response resulting in the loss of biological activity, as measured in a suitable test or animal system.

Evan: If you take Dr Klug's argument to its logical conclusion, you may run into problems. Many people are now immunizing with bacterially expressed proteins which are large chunks of gene products of interest. Very often polyclonal or monoclonal antibodies raised against these proteins don't react with the native gene product. This is the reason why smaller synthetic peptides are being used more now.

Klug: The larger peptides fold up wrongly, then?

Evan: Either that, or they have immunodominant sites which are not reflected by sites on the intact protein.

Crumpton: The reason for the problem that you describe is that these proteins actually lack flexibility. This seems to me to be a key ingredient.

Evan: Perhaps. Certainly, if they are too big, they might well fold up the wrong way initially.

Lerner: We ought to say more about neutralization at some point; there are very few sites on viruses which, when hit, lead to neutralization.

Ada: We have discussed antibodies to structures such as peptides which do not bind to the native protein; the situation is not very different to what we find when we immunize with a viral particle. Most of the antibody formed has no neutralizing activity.

REFERENCES

Bertram J, Gualtieri RJ, Osserman EF 1980 Amyloid-related Bence Jones proteins bind dinitrophenyl L-lysine (DNP). In: Glenner GG et al (eds) Amyloid and amyloidosis. Excerpta Medica, Amsterdam, p 351-360

Clarke SH, Huppi K, Ruezinsky D, Staudt L, Gerhard W, Weigert M 1985 Inter- and intraclonal diversity in the antibody response to influenza hemagglutinin. J Exp Med 161:687-704

Karle IL, Karle J, Mastropaolo D, Camerman A, Camerman N 1983 [Leu^5]enkephalin: four cocrystallizing conformers with extended backbones that form an antiparallel β-sheet. Acta Crystallogr Sect B Struct Crystallogr Cryst Chem 39:625-637

Manser T, Wysocki LJ, Gridley T, Near RI, Gefter ML 1985 The molecular evolution of the immune response. Immunol Today 6:94-101

The delineation of peptides able to mimic assembled epitopes

H. MARIO GEYSEN, STUART J. RODDA and TOM J. MASON

Department of Molecular Immunology, Commonwealth Serum Laboratories, 45 Poplar Road, Parkville, Victoria 3052, Australia

Abstract. Present methods allow a detailed study of the immune system's recognition of sequential epitopes. The results so far suggest that peptides homologous with these epitopes may not fulfil the early promise of synthetic vaccines. A procedure is described which now allows the study and evaluation of assembled epitopes.

Using a monoclonal antibody which had been shown both to strongly neutralize foot-and-mouth disease virus, and to bind to a discontinuous epitope, peptides mimicking this epitope were determined *a priori*. An iterative procedure based on the progressive identification of amino acids in a random mixture of antibody-binding octapeptides was used. Strongly binding peptides consisted of the two elements W-Q-M (Trp-Gln-Met) and H-S (His-Ser) separated by a spacer. It was also shown that element W-Q-M was best composed of D-isomers, and the element H-S of L-isomers. Comparison of the sequence of these peptides with that of the immunologically important coat protein of the virus leads to the prediction that the epitope recognized by this monoclonal antibody consists of the residues occurring at positions 29–30, 54–55 and 88.

Application of this general approach will answer questions about the nature of discontinuous epitopes and the stereochemical requirements for antigen–antibody interactions, as well as defining useful peptide immunogens.

1986 Synthetic peptides as antigens. Wiley, Chichester (Ciba Foundation Symposium 119) p 130-149

Recombinant DNA technology now makes it possible to deduce, from the determined nucleotide sequences, reliable amino acid sequences of biologically important proteins. The early prospect of synthetic peptide vaccines was suggested, even though our understanding both of the relationship between the amino acid sequence and the tertiary structure of a protein, and of the way in which the immune system interacts with protein antigens, was limited (Lerner 1983). This led to the formulation of predictive algorithms aimed at identifying suitable candidate peptides for evaluation as vaccines against a variety of pathogens (Hopp & Woods 1983, Westhof et al 1984). We, however, chose to apply the much-used solid-phase methods of peptide synthesis to systematically identify immunogenic sequential epitopes, as well as to investigate the basis for antigen–antibody interactions.

Sequential epitopes as peptide immunogens

Overlapping sets of peptides based on the sequences of several protein antigens were synthesized and subsequently tested for reactivity with antisera raised against the respective whole antigen. Antisera shown to contain peptide-reactive populations of antibodies were absorbed with excess antigen and retested for reactivity with the corresponding set of peptides. Sequential epitopes accessible to antibodies correspond to those peptides initially reactive, but for which no reaction could be demonstrated after absorption (Geysen et al 1984). Fig. 1(a & b) shows the identification of a surface or antibody-accessible sequential epitope of a model antigen, sperm whale myoglobin (swMb).

Significant differences were obtained in the responses of individual members of the same species to identical antigen preparations. The individual immune responses to the small (153 residues), well-defined antigen swMb, were determined for members of the same species and compared with the differences observed between species. Different responses obtained from two rabbits are shown in Fig. 1(a & c), and Fig. 2 shows the range of responses of members of the same species for rabbits, rats and chickens. It is clearly seen that the three species tested respond very differently to the same antigen, and that no peptide corresponds to a 'universally' recognized epitope.

It was also found that the antibodies reactive with the peptide L-K-T-E-A-E (peptide 49) could be absorbed from a rabbit serum by swMb (Fig. 1b), whereas chicken antibodies to the same peptide were not. Fig. 3 shows the reactivity patterns for rabbit and chicken antibodies when each was reacted with the set of peptides comprising all single amino acid substitutions of the sequence L-K-T-E-A-E. From the observed patterns, the principal residues contributing directly to antibody binding (contact residues) were determined to be L-§-T-#-A-§ for the rabbit antibodies, and #-#-T-E-A-# for the chicken antibodies (§ represents a residue for which limited replacement is allowed, and # a freely replaceable residue). At this resolution of a single amino acid, recognition of the peptide by antibodies from the two species is clearly different and may account for their different reactivity with native swMb.

These specific examples emphasize the difficulties which arose in a number of viral systems for which we attempted to define sequential surface epitopes suitable for evaluation as synthetic vaccines, and are summarized as follows:

1. Only a small number of sequential epitopes are exposed at the surface of protein antigens, as identified by testing peptides for their reaction with anti-whole protein sera.

INDIVIDUAL VARIATION

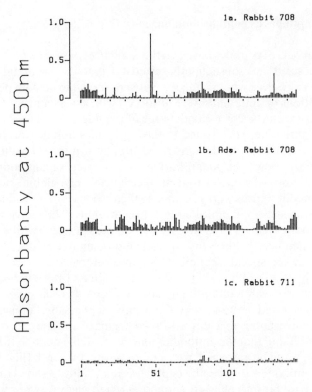

FIG. 1. The variation in the immune response between individuals of the same species. The figure shows the results of scanning the antisera from two rabbits which had been immunized with sperm whale myoglobin. The horizontal axes represent the overlapping heptapeptides which can be synthesized from the sperm whale myoglobin (swMb) sequence. Each peptide is numbered according to the position in the swMb sequence of its N-terminal residue. The vertical bars represent the absorbance of the substrate solution after an enzyme-linked immunosorbent assay (ELISA) on peptides. Fig 1b gives the response after the antiserum from Rabbit 708 had been adsorbed with swMb. Note that the peaks at peptides 47 and 48 have been lost after adsorption, whereas the peak at peptide 132 remains.

2. Within the same species, individual animals do not necessarily respond to the same small number of sequential epitopes.

3. Different species may not recognize any common sequential epitopes.

4. Different species responding to a common sequential epitope may produce binding antibodies with very different fine specificities.

SPECIES VARIATION

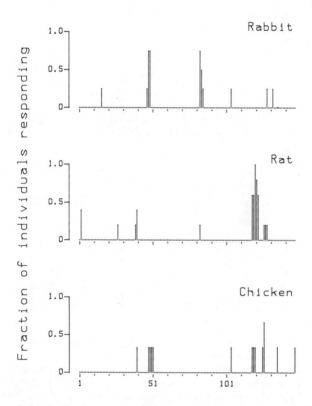

FIG. 2. The variation in the immune response among different species. The horizontal axes are the same as in Fig. 1. The vertical axes represent the fraction of animals whose antisera reacted with the peptide to a highly significant level. Sera from four rabbits, five rats and three chickens were tested.

In addition, we have shown that the immune response to small peptide immunogens, while generating a greater antibody diversity than the corresponding folded protein antigen, is of lesser diversity than would have been predicted from the stochastic model applied to that response. This is consistent with the hypothesis that the immune repertoire of animals is less than the potential repertoire. Differences observed between responding animals of the same species, and those between species, may reflect their individual expressed repertoires.

Taken altogether, the evidence suggests that the realization of effective

SPECIES VARIATION

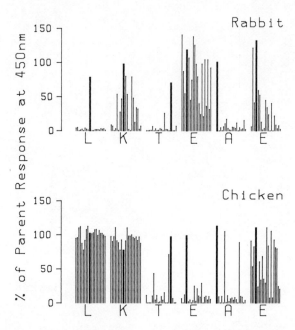

FIG. 3. Replacement Set analysis of antibodies binding to the peptide L-K-T-E-A-E. Vertical axes represent the absorbancy of an ELISA on a peptide given as a percentage of the mean absorbancy of the parent hexapeptide L-K-T-E-A-E. The peptides are hexapeptides related to L-K-T-E-A-E by the replacement of each residue by each of the 20 genetically coded amino acids, one at a time. The residue which has been substituted is identified below each block of bars. The replacement residues within each block are in the alphabetical order of their single-letter codes. For instance, the left-most bar represents A-K-T-E-A-E, and the right-most bar represents L-K-T-E-A-Y. The thicker bars represent the parent sequence L-K-T-E-A-E.

vaccines based on synthetic peptides corresponding to sequential epitopes presents a number of problems:

1. Identification of potentially useful sequential epitopes shoud be made using antisera raised in members of the target species only. If the very different responses to the same antigen observed between some species reflects 'holes' in the immune repertoire of these species, then peptide immunogens based on the sequential epitopes for one species may be totally non-immunogenic in another. This could necessitate the identification of several sets of peptides, to allow formulation of vaccines effective in different species.

2. The specificity of the immune response to small peptides has been found

to discriminate between antigens differing by as little as one amino acid (Alexander et al 1983, Rowlands et al 1983, Geysen et al 1985). This narrow specificity may enable an infectious microorganism to 'escape' with a sufficiently high frequency to negate the effect of the vaccination.

3. The number of sequential epitopes that can be identified is too small to provide for a vaccine consisting of a 'cocktail' of peptides. This will be necessary to ensure protection against a microorganism differing by only a single amino acid in the corresponding epitope on the relevant protein.

Antigens mimicking assembled epitopes

The above summary presents a pessimistic view of the potential of synthetic peptides as immunogens. Two lines of experimental evidence suggest that assembled (that is, discontinuous) epitopes determine a very significant component of the immune response to an antigen. The first is the observed low frequency with which monoclonal antibodies react with short peptides homologous with the sequence of the inducing antigen (Berzofsky et al 1982, Benjamin et al 1984), and the second is the inability of small peptides to absorb from antiserum substantial fractions of antibodies reactive with the native antigen (Lando et al 1982). We suggest that the present inability to delineate synthetic mimics for assembled epitopes limits the further development of peptide vaccines.

Studies of competition between monoclonal antibodies to the same antigen suggest that the immune response is to overlapping epitopes, a cluster of such epitopes defining an immunogenic domain (Webster et al 1979, Underwood 1982, Lafon et al 1983). A polyclonal response to a large antigen probably represents a redundant response to each immunogenic domain. However, this redundancy may ensure that escape from an induced immune response requires more than a single amino acid change in any domain, an event which is observed with sufficient frequency to limit the usefulness of a monospecific response (typically 10^{-5} per amino acid). Protein folding (tertiary structure) limits the number of continuous stretches of amino acids exposed or at least accessible to the immune response. A peptide vaccine which induces sufficient redundancy in the immune response is unlikely to be based on immunogens restricted to continuous epitopes.

Delineation of assembled epitopes

The amino acids directly contributing to antibody binding may be deduced by reacting monoclonal antibodies with sequence-related protein antigens.

This assumes that amino acid changes correlating with loss of antibody binding act at the binding interface and not at a distance as a result of a conformational change extending into the binding site. Predicting the three-dimensional configuration of the binding interface then relies on the availability of the X-ray crystal structure of the relevant antigen, and on the further assumption that antibody binding occurs with no local conformational change in the antigen.

Even assuming that the structures of immunogenic domains of the antigen have been correctly deduced, there remains the problem of synthesizing the equivalent molecular arrangements. Peptide vaccines consisting of immunogens derived from this strategy are, at best, a matter of speculation at present.

We now show that the sequence of a peptide able to bind to the antigen-combining site of a monoclonal antibody can be deduced *a priori*, even though that monoclonal antibody recognizes a discontinuous epitope. Starting with a weakly binding peptide, more strongly binding peptides are progressively identified. We further show that the binding conformation of the more completely defined peptides can be deduced. Generalization of this procedure should lead to the ready synthesis of peptides able to mimic assembled epitopes, which then may elicit an antibody response cross-reactive with the antigen that induced the defining antibody.

Monoclonal antibody #15 recognizes a discontinuous viral epitope

Monoclonal antibodies raised against foot-and-mouth disease virus (FMDV), type A_{10}, were characterized in terms of their reactivity with the viral subunit and the immunologically important coat protein VP1, isolated from the homologous virus (Meloen & Barteling 1983). In radioimmunoassays, a preparation of MAb #15 (isotype IgG2) gave a lower titre with the subunit than with intact homologous virus, a hundred-fold lower titre with trypsin-treated homologous virus, and failed to react with isolated VP1. MAb #15 neutralized type A_{10} virus in a micro-neutralization test. No reaction was observed when MAb #15 was titrated against type O_1 whole virus. These results show that MAb #15 recognizes a serotype-specific, neutralizing epitope, whose conformational integrity is optimum on the whole virus. There is considerable evidence that of the four capsid proteins, VP1, as folded in the intact virus, carries the major virus-neutralizing epitopes. This suggests that the epitope for MAb #15 is also on this protein (Wild et al 1969, Bachrach et al 1975, Kaaden et al 1977).

On the basis of the published sequence of the VP1 protein, type A_{10} (Booth-royd et al 1982), we synthesized complete sets of overlapping peptides (hexapeptides to nonapeptides), as has been described for type O_1 virus (Geysen et al 1984). In an enzyme-linked immunosorbent assay (ELISA), anti-whole virus sera reacted with a number of these peptides (Geysen et al, unpublished results). However, MAb #15 failed to react with any of the synthesized peptides. This was interpreted to indicate that this antibody recognized a discontinuous epitope on the whole virion, and a search was begun for a binding peptide without making any assumptions about its amino acid sequence.

Deducing the starting point for a binding peptide

The specificity of antibody binding to hexapeptides has been investigated by reacting monoclonal or polyclonal antibodies with sets of peptides in which each peptide is related to a known antibody-binding sequence by the replacement, one at a time, of the amino acid residue at each position within that sequence with all 19 other common amino acids. Essential residues within the peptide are identified as those for which replacement by dissimilar residues results in a loss of antibody-binding activity (Geysen et al 1984, 1985). This systematic replacement technique showed that a minimum condition for detectable binding to an antibody was that three amino acid residues within the sequence of the peptide should have both the correct identity and position. In all tests, at least two of these three amino acids were found to be adjacent to one another. By reacting any antibody with a set of hexapeptides representing the complete set of combinations of at least these three amino acids at various relative spacings, we should then identify partial sequences able to bind to antibody. This would require the synthesis and testing of about 24 000 (3×20^3) peptides, an impractical task.

A realistic compromise is to synthesize peptide mixtures representing all 400 possible adjacent pairings of the 20 commonly occurring L-α-amino acids. Each of these 400 peptide mixtures then consists of many individual octapeptides with the general formula: acetyl-*-*-D_1-D_2-*-*-*-*-S_s, where D_1 and D_2 represent the positions of the defined amino acids within each peptide in a peptide mixture. An asterisk represents an undefined position with respect to amino acid composition and is filled at random by one of the 20 amino acids. S_s represents the solid support on which the synthesis was carried out. Ideally, each solid support has, coupled to its surface, a large number of peptides (in total, greater than $10 \, nmol/S_s$) comprising all combinations of amino acids for the six undefined positions, but of known composition at the third and fourth positions (D_1 and D_2). The third amino acid necessary for significant antibody binding is then present in at least a proportion (about 5%) of the peptides. Amino acids (D_1 and D_2) important for antibody binding are determined by reacting this set of peptides with a designated monoclonal antibody in a suitable test. From the initial identification of the optimal antibody-binding octapeptide mixture, two further sets of peptides are synthesized with the general formulae acetyl-*-D_3-A_1-A_2-*-*-*-*-S_s and acetyl-*-*-A_1-A_2-D_4-*-*-*-S_s. In these formulae, A_1 and A_2 represent the amino acids present in the initial optimal antibody-binding peptide mixture, and D_3 and D_4 represent positions within these octapeptides where each of the 20 amino acids is incorporated one at a time. In this manner, non-defined positions in the original reacting octapeptide mixture are progressively defined as the amino acid giving the maximum antibody binding activity. Table 1 summarizes the iterative procedure used to delineate the more strongly antibody-binding peptides.

Improving spatial relationships

To allow for the possibility that the internal spacing between the determined amino acids may require independent optimization, peptides were synthesized in which a glycine or a β-alanine residue was incorporated between adjacent

TABLE 1 Iterative procedure used to delineate the strongly antibody-binding hexapeptides

Level of definition	Relative activity
Initial optimal antibody-binding peptide acetyl-*-*-M-K-*-*-*-*-S_s	
Second level of definition acetyl-*-*-M-K-*-*-*-*-S_s acetyl-*-W-M-K-*-*-*-*-S_s acetyl-*-*-M-K-H-*-*-*-S_s	 1.00 2.50 2.85
Optimization from all single-residue replacements acetyl-*-W-M-K-H-*-*-*-S_s acetyl-*-Q-M-K-H-*-*-*-S_s acetyl-*-W-M-R-H-*-*-*-S_s	 1.00 2.13 1.61
Third level of definition acetyl-*-Q-M-R-H-*-*-*-S_s acetyl-W-Q-M-R-H-*-*-*-S_s acetyl-*-Q-M-R-H-S-*-*-S_s	 1.00
Optimization from all single-residue replacements acetyl-W-Q-M-R-H-S-*-*-S_s acetyl-W-Q-M-G-H-S-*-*-S_s	 1.00 2.09
Final level of definition of hexapeptide acetyl-W-Q-M-G-H-S-S_s	

The identity of the preferred amino acids was determined either by an extension strategy of the intermediate optimum sequence, or by evaluating the effect on antibody binding of all single residue replacements within this sequence. The antibody-binding activity of each 'improved' peptide is shown relative to the intermediate optimum sequence.

residues in each of the five positions, one at a time. The results suggest that the peptide-binding site of MAb #15 accommodates the two elements, W-Q-M (Trp-Gln-Met) and H-S (His-Ser) and that the orientation of the bound peptide is as shown in Fig. 4 (upper). This was confirmed by showing that peptides with up to three β-alanine residues inserted between these two elements bound to the antibody. It is also consistent with the demonstration that peptides in which the order of these elements was reversed bound equally well to the antibody (Fig. 4, lower).

Stereochemistry of individual residues

Peptides based on the sequence W-Q-M-G-H-S were synthesized in which each amino acid was replaced one at a time with the D-optical isomer, all

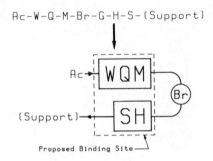

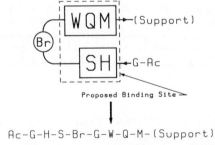

FIG. 4. Peptides predicted to bind MAb #15 in an equivalent configuration. The upper diagram shows the predicted geometry of the peptide W-Q-M-β-G-H-S on binding to MAb #15. The direction of the main-chain peptide bonds is given by the arrowheads on the chain. The peptide bridge (Br) linking the elements (W-Q-M and H-S) comprises the β-alanine and glycine residues. The lower diagram shows how the peptide of sequence G-H-S-β-G-W-Q-M can form an equivalent configuration and preserve the main-chain direction. Retained in this peptide is the glycine next to histidine at the N-terminus.

combinations of two amino acids were replaced with the D-optical isomer, and likewise all combinations of three, four and five. The optimum antibody-binding peptide was determined to be w-q-m-G-H-S, where the lower case letters indicate those residues incorporated as the D-optical isomer.

Peptides based on the sequence W-Q-M-G-H-S specifically bind MAb #15

In order to confirm the specificity of the antibody-binding reaction of the determined group of related peptides for MAb #15, the titre of MAb #15 for a number of the peptides was compared with the titres of a monoclonal antibody to sperm whale myoglobin or hepatitis A (Table 2). The specificity

TABLE 2 Specificity of MAb #15 for W-Q-M-G-H-S-related peptides

Peptide	Titre		
	MAb #15	Anti-hepatitis	Anti-myoglobin
Ac-*-*-M-K-*-*-S$_s$	<2000	<200	<200
Ac-*-W-M-K-*-*-S$_s$	14 000	<200	1600
Ac-*-*-M-K-H-*-S$_s$	17 000	<200	<200
Ac-*-W-M-K-H-*-S$_s$	36 000	<200	800
Ac-W-Q-M-R-H-S-S$_s$	100 000	<200	<200
Ac-W-Q-M-G-H-S-S$_s$	120 000	<200	<200
Ac-w-q-m-G-H-S-S$_s$	135 000	<200	<200
Ac-W-Q-M-β-G-H-S-S$_s$	>256 000	<200	<200

Antibody titres for each MAb were determined by ELISA and correspond to the reciprocal dilution of the ascites fluid giving an extinction of three times the test background. Values were corrected for non-specific absorption as determined by reacting each dilution of ascites fluid with unrelated peptide controls (Ac-G-D-L-G-S-I-S$_s$ and Ac-G-D-L-Q-V-L-S$_s$). MAbs tested were: MAb #15, anti-FMDV, type A$_{10}$, as described in the text (titre against the whole virus, 1.3×10^6); anti-hepatitis A, site of reaction unknown (titre against hepatitis A virus, 10^6); and anti-myoglobin (sperm whale), site of reaction also unknown (titre against sperm whale myoglobin, $>10^6$). Lower case indicates those amino acids incorporated as the D-optical isomer. β, β-alanine. Ac, acetyl.

of the antibody-binding reaction is clearly for MAb #15, the antibody used to determine the sequence of those peptides.

Relationship between virus epitope and deduced peptide

The possibility cannot be excluded that the antibody-binding peptide deduced by the use of this iterative procedure may consist of amino acids which

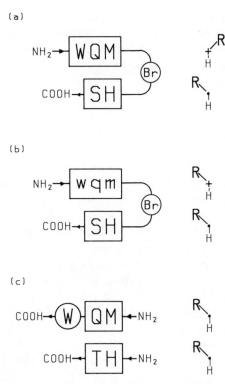

FIG. 5. D-Optical isomers compensate for reversed side-chain orientation. The diagrams represent the postulated antibody-binding conformations. The right-hand side of the figure shows the orientation about the α-carbons of the residues as seen when looking towards the bridge (Br). Lower-case letters represent the D-optical isomers of the amino acids. Fig. 5a represents an antiparallel arrangement of the main-chain directions of the two elements (W-Q-M and H-S) and their side-chain orientations, as found in the mimotope made up entirely from L-isomers. Fig. 5b is similar, except that the element W-Q-M consists of the D-isomers, as found in the optimum antibody-binding peptide. Note the change in side-chain orientation. Fig. 5c represents a parallel arrangement of the main-chain directions of the two elements and their side-chain orientation, as predicted to occur in the discontinuous epitope of the virus. Tryptophan (W) is shown separated from M-Q because they are not contiguous in VP1. Threonine replaces serine, as discussed in the text. Note that the mimotope shown in (a) cannot duplicate the side-chain orientation shown in (b) and (c).

are different from those constituting the epitope on the virus. It is likely that the only criterion which requires to be satisfied is that complementarity between the antigen-combining site of the antibody and the molecular surface of the binding peptide is maintained in regard to both shape and charge. It follows from this that the deduced antibody-binding peptide is best considered to be a 'mimotope' of the epitope which induced the antibody, rather than an accurate model of that epitope. A mimotope is defined as a molecule able to bind to the antigen-combining site of an antibody molecule, not necessarily identical with the epitope inducing the antibody, but an acceptable mimic of the essential features of the epitope.

Predicted virus epitope

The closest homology between either mimotope element (W-Q-M and H-S) and capsid protein VP1 of FMDV, type A_{10} occurred with the pair M-Q at position 54–55 of the VP1 sequence. The reverse order of this pair to Q-M as determined is consistent with the preference for the D-optical isomers. No direct match for the element H-S is found. However, assuming that serine is a conservative replacement for threonine, the pair H-T at position 29–30 satisfies the observed preference both for H and S as the L-optical isomers, and for the inclusion of spacers between the two elements in the strongly binding mimotopes. Tryptophan (W) occurs only once, at position 88. With the assumption that in this example the residues determined for the binding peptide are the same as those making up the antibody-inducing epitope, we predict that this site of virus neutralization is an assembled epitope consisting of the residues occurring at positions 29–30, 54–55 and 88.

Concluding comments

We have described a procedure that delineates the sequence and the binding conformation of peptides mimicking an assembled epitope. This was achieved without the need for either the sequence of the protein carrying this epitope, or the three-dimensional structure of the virus particle itself. We anticipate that the extensive 'mapping' (used here to describe the method as outlined) of the antigen-combining site of antibodies will answer important questions about the nature of assembled epitopes. We also anticipate that it will provide a direct method for defining potentially useful peptide immunogens to be used in vaccines. The choice of vaccine candidates can then be made, taking into account any particular properties of these peptides which may favour their immunogenicity or stability within the target animal. The important question which still remains to be answered is whether or not a significant proportion of the antibodies present in antisera raised against the mimotope are those which share valued characteristics, such as virus neutralization, with the original monoclonal antibody.

Acknowledgements

We thank Peter Schoofs, John Hussey, Philip Clayton and Marisa Cachia for their enthusiastic and skilled assistance. We also thank Dr R. Meloen of the Central Veterinary Institute, Lelystad, The Netherlands for the anti-FMDV monoclonal antibody.

REFERENCES

Alexander H, Johnson DA, Rosen J et al 1983 Mimicking the alloantigenicity of proteins with chemically synthesized peptides differing in single amino acids. Nature (Lond) 306:697-699

Bachrach HL, Moore DM, McKercher PD, Polatnick J 1975 Immune and antibody responses to an isolated caspid protein of foot-and-mouth disease virus. J Immunol 115:1636-1641

Benjamin DC, Berzofsky JA, East IJ et al 1984 The antigenic structure of proteins: a reappraisal. Annu Rev Immunol 2:67-101

Berzofsky JA, Buckenmeyer GK, Hicks G, Gurd FR, Feldmann RJ, Minna J 1982 Topographic antigenic determinants recognized by monoclonal antibodies to sperm whale myoglobin. J Biol Chem 257:3189-3198

Boothroyd J, Harris TJ, Rowlands DJ, Lowe PA 1982 The nucleotide sequence of cDNA coding for the structural proteins of foot-and-mouth disease virus. Gene (Amst) 17:153-161

Geysen HM, Meloen RH, Barteling SJ 1984 Use of peptide synthesis to probe viral antigens for epitopes to a resolution of a single amino acid. Proc Natl Acad Sci USA 81:3998-4002

Geysen HM, Barteling SJ, Meloen RH 1985 Small peptides induce antibodies with a sequence and structural requirement for binding antigen comparable to antibodies raised against the native protein. Proc Natl Acad Sci USA 82:178-182

Hopp TP, Woods KR 1983 A computer program for predicting protein antigenic determinants. Mol Immunol 20:483-489

Kaaden OR, Adam KH, Strohmaier K 1977 Induction of neutralizing antibodies and immunity in vaccinated guinea pigs by cyanogen bromide-peptides of VP_3 of foot-and-mouth disease virus. J Gen Virol 34:397-400

Lafon M, Wiktor TJ, Macfarlan RI 1983 Antigenic sites on the CVS rabies virus glycoprotein: analysis with monoclonal antibodies. J Gen Virol 64: 843-851

Lando G, Berzofsky JA, Reichlin M 1982 Antigenic structure of sperm whale myoglobin. 1. Partition of specificities between antibodies reactive with peptides and native protein. J Immunol 129:206-211

Lerner RA 1983 Synthetic vaccines. Sci Am 248(2):48-56

Meloen RH, Barteling SJ 1983 Further study of the neutralizing antigenic determinants of FMDV types O_1 and A_{10} with the aid of monoclonal antibodies. Report of the Research Group of the Standing Technical Committee of the European Commission for the Control of FMDV, 20–23 September

Rowlands DJ, Clarke BE, Carroll AR et al 1983 Chemical basis of antigenic variation in foot-and-mouth disease virus. Nature (Lond) 306:694-697

Underwood PA 1982 Mapping of antigenic changes in the haemagglutinin of Hong Kong influenza (H3N2) strains using a large panel of monoclonal antibodies. J Gen Virol 62:153-169

Webster RG, Kendal AP, Gerhard W 1979 Analysis of antigenic drift in recently isolated influenza A (H1N1) viruses using monoclonal antibody preparations. Virology 96:258-264

Westhof E, Altschuh D, Moras D et al 1984 Correlation between segmental mobility and the location of antigenic determinants in proteins. Nature (Lond) 311:123-126

Wild TF, Burroughs JN, Brown F 1969 Surface structure of foot-and-mouth disease virus. J Gen Virol 4:313-320

DISCUSSION

Stanworth: How practical is this new method of peptide synthesis, in relation to conventional solid-phase methods? Is it technically easier, or more demanding?

Geysen: We use technicians with no chemistry training, and it takes them about a week to learn the synthetic procedure. There is a lot of help from the computer; the total synthesis is designed by computer software. It tells the technician what to weigh out, how to make up the solutions, and where to put them. The results are all read directly from the ELISA reader into the computer, building up a data base that already occupies 75 floppy discs, of the peptides synthesized so far. We have software written for designing all types of peptide synthesis. The kind of analysis and the presentation of results is also software-driven.

Stanworth: Do you need to coat the pins on which the peptides are synthesized with extra polymer?

Geysen: The pins are moulded and are sent away for radiation-grafting. We graft a polymer of acrylic acid onto the pins. We currently use hexamethylene diamine as the first step in the reaction, coupling that to the polyacrylic acid, and then we have a fairly conventional solid-phase format. The polymer is partially blocked. It is a soluble polymer, so the assay is a part solid-phase, part solution-phase assay. The pin has the soluble polymer bound to it with a peptide hanging on the end. The polymer is about 40000 monomers per unit. We find no influence of the type of polymer link on the kind of assay result. In all cases where we have identified a peptide and subsequently synthesized it by conventional means in large quantities (as opposed to the 40 nmol synthesized per pin, synthesized in a way that is dependent on the specificity of the immune system to select out the correct peptides), and coupled it back after purification to the pins, we see no difference from the peptide originally synthesized in the less precise manner.

Crumpton: If you don't couple it back to the pin, what then?

Geysen: It is more difficult to show a reaction. We work with short peptides, and we believe that you can't have a short peptide binding simultaneously to a plate, say, and to an antibody. If you radiolabel the peptide and use it in solution phase, it also reacts.

Lerner: We have just done a joint study with Mario Geysen; his group did the experiment their way and we did it our way, and the agreement was exellent.

Rothbard: Have you completed the circle by immunizing with the peptides synthesized by your method?

McConnell: And do you know if the peptide induces neutralizing antibody? You use a non-neutralizing monoclonal antibody to select the peptide in the first place.

Geysen: In all tests so far where we have used a peptide corresponding to a sequential epitope, the anti-peptide response has reacted well with the whole protein antigen. With the mimotope, the prediction is that it is folded when bound to the antibody and, as shown in Table 2 (p 140), the hexapeptide W-Q-M-G-H-S has a high specificity for this antibody. The longer peptide, however, with the inserted β-alanine, gave a much higher titre when reacted with the monoclonal, of over one million, which was greater than the titre when reacted with the virus. This indicated that the greater conformational flexibility of the longer insert was important to binding. The mimotope peptide synthesized as the hexapeptide (with only the glycine residues in the bridge) induced an immune response which did not recognize FMDV. We suggest that the folded conformations, which might have been expected to induce antibodies reactive with the virus, were almost excluded energetically from the conformations in equilibrium of the linear peptide in solution. So if each conformation produced an antibody response, the number of antibodies recognizing the folded form would be very low, or excluded alogether. We are now in the process of synthesizing a cyclized version of the peptide with β-alanine–glycine bridges on both sides. When this is used as the immunogen we hope to induce a response to which the overlap with virus-reactive antibodies is much higher.

McConnell: The difficulty in your system is that you are using the 'end-point' of the immune system, namely antibody formation, to predict the structure of an immunogen. Efficient production of neutralizing antibody requires a considerable number of different stages. Although you consider the immune system as a black box, it really is in effect a series of black boxes whose functions range from the initial pick-up of antigen and presentation, through T cell help and T cell suppression, and finally antibody formation. Furthermore, the immune system is not symmetrical, in as much as the determinants seen by the T cell are not necessarily identical to the determinants seen by the B cell. Yet it is the B cell specificity which you are trying to influence by your approach.

In a system where you have T cell help, how do you predict the epitope which the T cell is going to see so that the B cells make the correct specificity?

Geysen: We haven't addressed the question of T cell responses; we are about to use all our sets of peptides to map T cell receptors. If it is absolutely necessary that a peptide immunogen has T cell help, we won't see it. As I said,

s where we have gone back into animals, we have not had a
e fact that we failed the first time with the mimotope was almost
:cause the energetics of folding the two elements, W-Q-M and
H-S, about a glycine were unfavourable. By constraining the mimotope in the folded form we exclude the linear conformations. I shall be surprised if we don't elicit a response which overlaps with the virus epitope.

Alkan: In this beautiful design, I am afraid that you are ignoring antigen processing, as has been said. One thing you *can* predict is that the D isomers will not be immunogenic, probably because they cannot be processed by accessory cells; therefore they will stay in the body for a long time.

Geysen: Work at the Scripps Institute shows that they are very antigenic, though. We would like to make stable immunogens with the D optical isomers of amino acids.

Alkan: The D isomers are perfect antigens; that is, one can obtain antibodies against them. But they will not be immunogenic, in the sense that they do not induce T cell help. In other words, they need a carrier to be immunogenic.

Sela: The nomenclature needs explaining here. Antigenicity means the capacity to react with specific antibodies, whereas immunogenicity is a property of the whole molecule. If one talks about whether one peptide within an immunogen expresses itself better than another in terms of immune response, I prefer to use the term 'immunopotent'. It is true that we once said that polymers of D-amino acids are not antigenic. This was wrong! We showed later that they are similar to some of the immunologically paralysing polysaccharides, namely that if you inject sufficiently small quantities of the polymer built exclusively of D-amino acids, good antibody responses are obtained. When it comes to the antigenic determinants, the D peptides are infinitely more immunopotent than the L peptides.

Geysen: There is no reason why the D-amino acids should be more antigenic, or immunogenic, or whatever you like to call it, than the L versions. We are talking about the response to a molecule. The only reason we use D-amino acids is to change the direction of the main chain. In terms of antibody binding, the side-chain interactions dominate over the main-chain interactions. Another possibility is to synthesize mimotopes using all L-amino acids, but to synthesize two chains parallel to one another.

Sela: I would not like to use peptides of D-amino acids for human vaccination.

Ada: This is a first approach, and is different to what has been done in the past. Dr Geysen is trying to make a molecule which is a perfect fit to an antibody which neutralizes viral infectivity. When you come to test that molecule as an immunogen, there might be other factors. You may have to add some PPD or other molecule, as a carrier. We just don't know, yet.

Lachmann: What Dr Geysen is doing is something which the immune system does all the time. If one looks at the immune system in the way that Niels Jerne (1972, 1974) does, all antibody specificities are actually generated by the variable regions of immunoglobulin molecules, and immunoglobulins are therefore the 'primary' molecules to which they are directed. All the environmental antigens which we encounter are the cross-reactions which happen to fit the same binding site. Just as NIP and DNP and nickel ions are not actually the true structures to which antibody specificity is generated, but happen to fit the combining site, so presumably are the less than totally physiological peptides that Mario Geysen makes. Since there is no difficulty in raising antibodies to NIP, DNP or nickel ions if they are bound to suitable carriers, I can similarly see no difficulty in raising antibodies to other structures that fit antibody combining sites, providing that they too are bound to appropriate carriers. After all, Michison's (1967) 'accurate sample' hypothesis tells us that for B cells, selection is by the capacity of antigen to fit at high affinity with the receptor.

Geysen: As Gordon Ada pointed out when he first heard of our work, we are actually making anti-idiotypes, and there is a great similarity between the two processes. Both start by taking an antibody. In one case we fit the antigen-combining site by selecting from chemically synthesized peptides. To make an anti-idiotype, you select from a set of molecules produced by the immune response.

Lachmann: In the Jernian view, all antibodies are anti-idiotypes.

Geysen: And it is possible to make anti-idiotypes to antibodies that recognize polysaccharide antigens. We were not surprised that when we took monoclonal antibodies to blood group antigens, we found signals from our initial set of peptides. We feel that it's just a matter of extending the selected pair of amino acids and we will make a mimic of a polysaccharide antigen. We are trying to produce a set of amino acids with greater numbers of hydroxyl groups in the side-chains, because we think that if we are going to make a mimotope for an epitope that is polysaccharide, we may need to use polyhydroxy side-chain amino acids and increase the repertoire in our molecular Lego set! That is, the number of building blocks is not big enough.

Williams: Can you say why you bother to go back and look at the sequence of a protein at all? You concluded that there was virtually no connection to sequence; and there might well not be, from your logic.

Geysen: We were interested in any relationship which could be observed. In fact, the correlation wasn't too bad, because a Q-M was found in exactly the main-chain direction that was predicted from the mimotope. As you say, there is no need to go back to the sequence. In fact, we get more than one 'starting signal'; that is, the initial reactive octapeptide containing a defined pair of amino acids. So, if we work from different starting points, do we converge to the same sequence or do we diverge to different sequences? If they diverge, then there is a large collection of molecules which are adequate mimics. If most converge, there isn't such a great number.

Williams: You have to be careful that you don't deduce too much about the nature of the antigenicity of the original protein from this procedure. This type of search may or may not link up with our earlier discussion of antigenicity, since it is a random search for the best solution, which may not lead to a sequence which was in the original protein at all.

Liu: I wonder if you have selected any mutant that has an amino acid substitution in the mimotopes? This kind of result might help to determine whether your mimotopes are viral antigenic sites or just compounds that can combine with virus-neutralizing monoclonal antibodies.

Geysen: We are now trying to do that for influenza virus. Foot-and-mouth disease virus was not a good choice because we can't continue to work on it in Australia. With influenza virus we shall do those more comprehensive studies. We have monoclonal antibodies and a set of viral mutants with known sequences, selected in the presence of the monoclonal. We intend to map the monoclonal antibody to see what the relationships are, and to test back with anti-mimotope serum, to see whether the response to the mimotope would select out the same mutants and whether it shows the same sort of selectivity for the mutants.

Humphrey: I imagine that in the long run you would like to produce clonal expansion of antibody-forming cells which make something resembling the original monoclonal antibody, with all its properties. Let us assume that the animal to be immunized possesses a clone, or can generate a clone, with these properties. The problem will be to present the antigen or peptide on a carrier which will stimulate the right clones. I take it that at this stage you don't particularly want to stimulate T cells which also recognize the same epitopes; you would need quite different carriers for that.

Ada: I don't think we are concerned with carriers yet; but that would be a question for the future.

Humphrey: If only you knew the right choice of carrier, though! Peter Lachmann would say that you should use PPD.

Brown: Have you studied a biological system where you can measure an effect of one of these mimotopes?

Geysen: Not yet! The first delineation of a mimotope was only completed at the beginning of 1985, and in fact we now use a modified procedure, different from that described. In the eight months it took to develop the process we had to solve the problems of obtaining approximately equimolar amino acid incorporation at the mixture positions, and to form an understanding for the analysis of the data from the starting set of 400 peptide mixtures, as well as to test the procedures for the insertion of spacers into the correct position for optimum binding. We now use three sets of 400 peptide mixtures, $D_1 - D_2$, $D_1 - P - D_2$, and D_1 spaced from D_2 by o-aminobenzoic acid. This gives reactive pairings with different spatial relationships imposed on the defined amino acids. We expect that the results from these will allow us to more quickly and accurately define the mosaic or pattern of the important amino acids as they bind to the antibody. We have mapped four antigen-combining sites to reasonable completion, one polyclonal serum and three monoclonal sera. One monoclonal was against lysozyme and one to myoglobin; the polyclonal was an anti-peptide serum. We are now identifying mimotopes to blood group antigens, rabies antigens, malaria antigens, and two monoclonals against transformed cell antigens from two human cancers; also influenza and hepatitis virus. We are able to work towards about 20 mimotopes simultaneously, and at present it takes about six weeks to complete the steps for the identification of a mimotope.

Anders: I was intrigued to see how good a match you got when you went back to the original structure in FMDV. Have you done this with the other mimotopes that you have synthesized? It might tell us something about inherent biases of the immune system.

Geysen: We predicted the spatial relationship of the important residues for a monoclonal antibody to myoglobin. When we looked at the structure, we found exactly those side-chains (H,E,L,F) present across two main chains. That may be coincidence; we haven't verified that the monoclonal binds with that point. That was the prediction from the initial assessment of the reactive octapeptides, and, when we looked at the molecule, we saw that those residues occur sufficiently close together to be the epitope.

Crumpton: Are the side-chains adjacent to one another in the folded structure?

Geysen: Yes.

Heusser: One way of determining whether you were able to optimally mimic the epitope of the native antigen would be to measure the corresponding binding affinities. Have you measured and compared the affinity obtained with your epitope and with the native antigen?

Geysen: No; because we cannot import either anti-FMDV sera, or the virus itself.

REFERENCES

Jerne NK 1972 What precedes clonal selection? In: Ontogeny of acquired immunity. Elsevier/ Excerpta Medica/North-Holland, Amsterdam (Ciba Found Symp) p 1-15

Jerne NK 1974 Towards a network theory of the immune system. Ann Immunol (Paris) 125c:373-389

Mitchison NA 1967 Antigen recognition responsible for the induction *in-vitro* of the secondary response. Cold Spring Harbor Symp Quant Biol 32:431-439

Experimental basis for the development of a synthetic vaccine against *Plasmodium falciparum* malaria sporozoites

VICTOR NUSSENZWEIG and RUTH NUSSENZWEIG

Department of Pathology, Kaplan Cancer Center and Department of Clinical and Molecular Parasitology, New York University Medical Center, New York, NY 10016, USA

Abstract. Malaria continues to cause extensive morbidity and mortality in man. The exact number of individuals affected is not known. Estimates vary from 200 to 400 million, and more than one million die each year. Protective immunity against malaria can be obtained by vaccination with irradiated sporozoites. The protective antigens are polypeptides (circumsporozoite [CS] proteins) which cover the surface membrane of the parasite. CS proteins contain species-specific immunodominant epitopes, formed by tandem repeated sequences of amino acids. The dominant epitope of *Plasmodium falciparum* is represented in the synthetic peptide asparagine-alanine-asparagine-proline repeated in tandem three times; that is, (NANP)$_3$. Monoclonal antibodies and most or all polyclonal human antibodies to *P. falciparum* sporozoites react with (NANP)$_3$. Polyclonal antibodies raised against the synthetic peptide (NANP)$_3$ react with the surface of the parasite and neutralize its infectivity. Since (NANP)$_3$ repeats are present worldwide in CS proteins from *P. falciparum*, this epitope is a logical target for vaccine development.

1986 Synthetic peptides as antigens. Wiley, Chichester (Ciba Foundation Symposium 119) p 150-163

When inoculated into the mammalian host, sporozoites develop exclusively inside hepatocytes. Sporozoites are detected inside these cells within a few minutes after intravenous injection and fewer than 100 sporozoites are sufficient to infect a susceptible host. Therefore it is likely that the invasion is a specific event and that hepatocytes contain a high avidity recognition system for surface molecules of the parasite.

Malaria remains one of the most important infectious diseases of man. An urgent need for malaria vaccines arises from the difficulties in controlling the *Anopheles* mosquito vector and from the alarming increase in the incidence and distribution of multiple-drug-resistant strains of *Plasmodium falciparum*, a species which causes extensive morbidity and most of the mortality associated with the disease.

The development of vaccines is complicated by the fact that the protective antigens are specific for each of the main developmental stages of the development of the parasite in the human host: the sporozoites, which are present in the salivary glands of the *Anopheles* mosquito, and are injected during the bite; the blood stages, which develop in red cells and cause the clinical disease; and the gametocytes, which are infectious for *Anopheles* mosquitoes. An effective vaccine against sporozoites would be most advantageous because it would block infection and prevent disease and transmission. Even if sterile immunity is not achieved in all individuals, the decrease in sporozoite load may diminish the severity of the disease.

Circumsporozoite proteins as targets for vaccine development

Protective immunity against sporozoites has been achieved by inoculation of irradiated parasites into rodents, monkeys and humans (reviewed in Cochrane et al 1980, Nussenzweig & Nussenzweig 1984). Mice could be also vaccinated with viable sporozoites if curative chemoprophylactic regimens were started soon after the various challenges to prevent the development of the blood stages (Orjih & Nussenzweig 1982).

This immunization did not require adjuvants. Although the protection obtained under these conditions was brief, lasting approximately three months, immunity could be boosted by the repeated bite of infected mosquitoes. Using this procedure, mice remained resistant to *Plasmodium berghei* challenge for more than one year. In endemic areas the repeated bites of mosquitoes and periodic injection of malaria sporozoites probably has a similar effect, namely, to increase resistance to infection. The immunity is stage-specific, and in most instances species-specific (Nussenzweig et al 1969). Incubation of sporozoites with the sera of vaccinated and protected animals results in the formation of a tail-like precipitate (circumsporozoite or CSP reaction) (Vandenberg et al 1969, Cochrane et al 1976). The target antigens of these reactions have been identified by monoclonal antibodies (Yoshida et al 1980). They consist of single polypeptides (circumsporozoite or CS proteins) which cover the entire surface membrane of the parasite and which are shed when cross-linked by antibodies (Potocnjak et al 1980).

In every experimental model of rodent, monkey and human malarias, monoclonal antibodies directed against CS proteins neutralized parasite infectivity. For example, in one group of experiments (Table 1) mice received intravenous injections of a purified monoclonal antibody to the CS protein (Pb44) of *Plasmodium berghei* (a malaria parasite of rodents) and a few minutes later were challenged with sporozoites. Most animals which received as little as 10 μg of antibody were protected. When infection occurred, the prepatent period was prolonged (Potocnjak et al 1980). The effect of the

TABLE 1 Resistance of mice to infection with 10³ P. berghei sporozoites after treatment with monoclonal antibodies to the CS protein, Pb44

Dose of antibodies (µg/mouse)	Number infected / Number injected	Prepatent period (days ± SE)
300	0/5	—
100	0/5	—
50	1/5	7.0
25	1/5	6.0
10	0/5	—
None	5/5	5.2 ± 0.4

antibody was also species- and stage-specific. It did not neutralize sporozoites from another species of rodent malaria, nor affected the blood stages of *P. berghei*.

The CS polypeptides are probably involved in the initial interactions between the parasite and the host's target cells—that is, the hepatocytes. Fab fragments of monoclonal antibodies to CS proteins neutralize parasite infectivity *in vitro* and *in vivo* and prevent the parasites' attachment to target cells (Potocnjak et al 1980, Hollingdale et al 1982, 1984). In addition, there is a close temporal correlation between the acquisition of infectivity and the appearance of CS protein on the membrane of the parasite. Immature sporozoites (found in the mid-gut of *Anopheles* mosquitoes) bear little or no CS protein on the surface membranes (Aikawa et al 1981) and are not infective (Vandenberg 1975). All these observations suggest that CS proteins or selected domains of the polypeptide are logical candidates for vaccine development.

Properties of circumsporozoite proteins

CS proteins of different plasmodial species have similar structural, biosynthetic and immunological properties (Santoro et al 1983). They are one of the major biosynthetic products of sporozoites (Yoshida et al 1981). About 10% of the [³⁵S]methionine incorporated into proteins by salivary gland sporozoites is found in CS proteins. Biosynthetic studies revealed two precursors of the CS protein with a higher M_r and isoelectric point. Although the biosynthetic pathways are still obscure, it appears that the membrane form of CS protein is generated by sequential removal of two small basic peptides from the precursors.

CS proteins have a strikingly immunodominant epitope, and this epitope is present multiple times in a single molecule (Zavala et al 1983). All monoclonal antibodies against sporozoites are directed against this epitope. Preincubation of crude extracts of sporozoites with these monoclonal antibodies inhibits between 70 and 100% of the subsequent binding of the CS proteins to anti-sporozoite antibodies found in human or animal sera.

The structural basis for these properties has been elucidated by cloning and sequencing the CS genes. Only one copy of the CS genes is present per haploid genome and the DNA sequence is uninterrupted. The central area of CS polypeptides is formed by tandem repeated sequences of amino acids: GQPQAQGDGANA in *Plasmodium knowlesi* (Godson et al 1983, Ozaki et al 1983), $_G^PGAAAAGGGGN$ in the Gombak strain of *P. cynomolgi* (Enea et al 1984a) and NANP in the human malaria parasite, *P. falciparum* (Enea et al 1984b, Dame et al 1984).

Structure of the immunodominant epitope of the CS protein of P. falciparum

In *P. falciparum* the immunodominant epitope is defined by only three consecutive repeats (NANP)$_3$. This conclusion is based on a series of experiments which showed that (NANP)$_3$ was recognized by polyclonal and monoclonal antibodies to sporozoites and, conversely, that antibodies to (NANP)$_3$ reacted with sporozoites and prevented their entry into hepatocytes *in vitro* (Zavala et al 1985a, Young et al 1985, Ballou et al 1985).

Previous studies with monoclonal antibodies had shown that they bound to the repeat-containing domain of the CS protein of *P. falciparum*. To determine the structure of the epitope a series of synthetic peptides, (NANP)$_2$, (NANP)$_3$, (NANP)$_4$, (NANP)$_5$, was synthesized and used to inhibit the binding of the antibodies to extracts of *P. falciparum* sporozoites. The results (Fig. 1) showed that (NANP)$_3$, (NANP)$_4$ and (NANP)$_5$ strongly inhibited the binding of one of the antibodies to the antigen with almost equal efficiency on a molar basis. In contrast, (NANP)$_2$ was a poor inhibitor. Similar findings were obtained with several other monoclonal antibodies.

(NANP)$_3$ was then used as the antigen in an immunoradiometric assay (IRMA) to detect anti-sporozoite antibodies in the sera of humans living in an endemic area—The Gambia, West Africa. In agreement with previous epidemiological studies showing that the immune response of humans to sporozoites is age-dependent (Nardin et al 1979), it was found that the percentage of positive sera detected by the IRMA increased with age, ranging from 22% in children one to 14 years old, to 84% in adults older than 34 years. Among many individuals older than 20 years of age, serum titres reached as high as 1/640. The levels of antibodies to (NANP)$_3$ in the serum of a human volunteer (G.Z.) vaccinated with X-irradiated *P. falciparum* sporozoites and protected against malaria infection were also measured. This serum had the

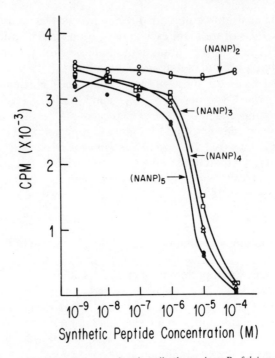

FIG. 1. Inhibition of binding of a monoclonal antibody against *P. falciparum* sporozoites by synthetic peptides. Monoclonal antibody 2A10 at a concentration of 50 ng/ml was incubated with increasing concentrations of peptide. After one hour at room temperature, 30 μl of the mixtures were placed in wells of plates coated with *P. falciparum* sporozoite extracts. After incubation for one hour, the wells were extensively washed with phosphate-buffered saline (PBS) containing 1% of bovine serum albumin (BSA) and 0.05% Tween-20. Then 30 μl of ^{125}I-labelled affinity-purified goat anti-mouse immunoglobulin were placed in each well. After one hour, the wells were washed three times with PBS-BSA, dried and counted in a gamma counter.

highest reactivity measured, and the titre reached 1/4096. Additional observations showed that most or all antibodies to sporozoites present in the human sera were directed against (NANP)$_3$. Indeed, in these sera a highly significant correlation was found between the anti-peptide and anti-sporozoite antibody titres. Moreover, the reactivity of the antibodies with sporozoites was abolished or strongly inhibited when the reaction was carried out in the presence of the (NANP)$_3$ peptide.

Groups of rabbits were then immunized with conjugates prepared by coupling (NANP)$_3$ to tetanus toxoid with glutaraldehyde. The sera were assayed by an IRMA, using (NANP)$_3$ immobilized on the bottom of plastic wells as antigen. All samples from immunized animals were positive (Fig. 2) and the positive reactions were totally inhibited by the synthetic peptide.

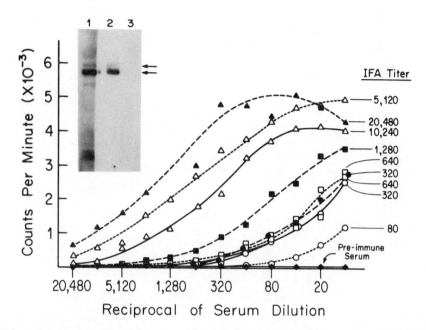

FIG. 2. Immunoassays on sera from rabbits injected with (NANP)₃–tetanus toxoid. Rabbits were injected in one hind foot pad and opposite thigh intramuscularly with 1 mg (▲,△) or 0.1 mg (■,□) of the conjugate with Freund's incomplete adjuvant. Three other rabbits were injected intramuscularly twice, two weeks apart, with 1 mg of conjugate (●,○). Animals were bled four weeks after initial immunization.

The results of the immunoradiometric assay of each serum sample using (NANP)₃ as antigen are plotted. The corresponding indirect immunofluorescence assay (IFA) titres using glutaraldehyde-fixed sporozoites as antigen are shown on the right. The insert shows the results of Western blotting of *P. falciparum* sporozoite extracts revealed by a rabbit antiserum against *P. falciparum* sporozoites (Track 1), against (NANP)₃–tetanus toxoid (Track 2), and normal rabbit serum control (Track 3). The bands indicated by arrows correspond to the precursor (67 000 M_r) and membrane forms (58 000 M_r) of the CS protein, as previously determined using monoclonal antibodies. (Reproduced from Zavala et al 1985a, by permission of *Science*. © The American Association for the Advancement of Science 1985.)

As also shown in Fig. 2, the antibodies to (NANP)₃ reacted in a Western blot with the *P. falciparum* CS protein and its precursors, and with the surface of glutaraldehyde-fixed sporozoites of *P. falciparum*, as determined by indirect immunofluorescence assay (IFA). The sera with highest IFA and IRMA titres gave strong circumsporozoite reactions (titres of 1/50 to 1/100) when incubated with viable parasites.

A highly significant positive correlation was found between the IRMA and the IFA titres, suggesting that most antibodies to (NANP)₃ recognized the CS protein. This question was further examined in the experiment depicted

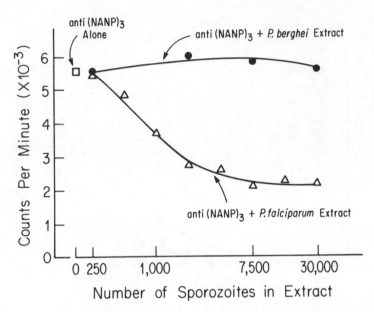

FIG. 3. Inhibition of binding of polyclonal anti-(NANP)$_3$ antibodies by *P. falciparum* sporozoite extracts. Serum was obtained from a rabbit immunized with (NANP)$_3$-tetanus toxoid incorporated in incomplete Freund's adjuvant. Samples of serum diluted 1/1000 in PBS-BSA were incubated with increasing amounts of extracts of sporozoites of *P. falciparum* or, as a control, with extracts of sporozoites of *P. berghei*. After one hour at room temperature, 30 µl of the mixtures were placed in (NANP)$_3$-coated wells. Incubation proceeded for one hour, then the wells were washed with PBS-BSA containing 0.5% Tween-20 and incubated with 30 µl of ^{125}I-labelled affinity-purified goat anti-rabbit immunoglobulin. After one hour the wells were washed with PBS-BSA–Tween-20, dried and counted in a gamma counter. (Reproduced from Zavala et al 1985a, by permission of *Science*. © The American Association for the Advancement of Science 1985.)

in Fig. 3, in which the IRMA of an anti-peptide antiserum was performed after it had been preincubated with increasing amounts of a *P. falciparum* sporozoite extract. As shown, about 70% of the reactivity of the antibody to (NANP)$_3$ was inhibited by the extract. Extracts of sporozoites of the rodent parasite *P. berghei* had no effect.

Immunoglobulin was isolated from the serum of one of these rabbits and tested for its ability to neutralize the infectivity of *P. falciparum* sporozoites *in vitro*. The results showed that the immune IgG inhibited parasite invasion in a dose-dependent fashion. A strong effect was observed with total IgG concentrations as low as 2 µg/ml. When the antibodies to (NANP)$_3$ were removed by absorption with peptide bound to Sepharose beads, the inhibitory effect was abolished (Zavala et al 1985a).

In short, these results strongly suggest that the synthetic peptide (NANP)$_3$

represents the dominant epitope of the domain of the CS protein containing the NANP repeats. Earlier studies involving the CS protein of *P. knowlesi* (Gysin et al 1984) have shown that antibodies to the respective repeats also recognize an uninterrupted sequence of amino acids. Perhaps the repeat domains contain sequential and not configurational epitopes in all CS proteins, since monoclonal and polyclonal antibodies to the repeats of CS proteins of several species react with the denatured antigen heated at 100 °C for 30 minutes or treated with 6 M-urea and 1% β-mercaptoethanol.

In *P. falciparum*, the repeat region contains a very large number of prolines and asparagines, residues frequently found in β-turns. Indeed, the Chou and Fasman algorithm predicts the presence of multiple NANP β-turns in this region. This simple type of secondary structure is formed by a few consecutive amino acid residues, and for this reason its configuration is likely to be adopted by a synthetic peptide. In agreement with this idea, as mentioned above, most of the antibodies to (NANP)$_3$ react with the CS protein.

Rationale for the development of a synthetic malaria vaccine

In view of the difficulties of obtaining large amounts of antigen from the various stages of the development of the parasite, only genetically engineered or synthetic vaccines against malaria are now being contemplated. In the case of *P. falciparum*, synthetic vaccines containing (NANP)$_3$ are attractive candidates for further development. Most of the antibodies to (NANP)$_3$ raised in experimental animals recognize the native CS protein and neutralize the parasite infectivity. Antibodies in the serum of a volunteer vaccinated with X-irradiated sporozoites and protected against malaria infection were mainly or exclusively directed against (NANP)$_3$. The peptide reacted well with the sera from randomly selected individuals living where malaria is endemic. (NANP)$_3$ is repeated many times in each CS molecule, and the CS molecule covers uniformly the surface membrane of sporozoites; therefore the parasite should be particularly vulnerable to attack by anti-(NANP)$_3$ antibodies. Last, but not least, (NANP)$_3$ is present in strains of *P. falciparum* from all over the world (Zavala et al 1985b).

One potential problem of all synthetic vaccines consisting of a peptide conjugated to a carrier protein is that they may not boost the naturally acquired immunity to the pathogen and, more important, that these vaccines will only expand the anti-peptide B memory cells but not prime anti-peptide T cells. That is, if upon vaccination the cellular interactions involved in the processing of the peptide–carrier conjugate lead exclusively to T-cell recognition of the carrier, then the acquired immunity of adults to the pathogen may not be boosted by the vaccine and, more important, a secondary immune response may not be set in motion in vaccinated individuals by the encounter with the pathogen. In this case, the production of antibodies to the peptide would depend exclusively on the effectiveness of the primary immunization or of the secondary response upon revaccination.

Because of the economic and logistic problems involved in delivering vaccines to the underdeveloped areas of the world where they are most needed, it is desirable that a high degree of protective immunity be achieved by a single dose of the immunoprophylactic agent. This is a challenging proposition, particularly in the case of a malaria vaccine, which should ideally contain a mixture of antigens from the various stages of development of the parasite in the human host; that is, the sporozoites, blood stages and gametocytes (reviewed in Ravetch et al 1985). The recent advances in malaria research, immunology and biotechnology permit some measure of optimism that this can be achieved, perhaps in the near future.

Acknowledgements

The work here described was supported by grants from the Agency for International Development DPE-0453-A-00-5012-00, the UNDP/World Bank/WHO Programme for Research and Training in Tropical Medicine, the National Institutes of Health, and the MacArthur Foundation. We thank Mr Roger Rose for editorial assistance.

REFERENCES

Aikawa M, Yoshida N, Nussenzweig RS, Nussenzweig V 1981 The protective antigen of rodent malarial sporozoites (*Plasmodium berghei*) is a differentiation antigen. J Immunol 126:2494-2495

Ballou WR, Rothbard J, Wirtz RA et al 1985 Immunogenicity of synthetic peptides from circumsporozoite protein of *Plasmodium falciparum*. Science (Wash DC) 228:996-999

Cochrane AH, Aikawa M, Jeng M, Nussenzweig RS 1976 Antibody-induced ultrastructural changes of malaria sporozoites. J Immunol 116:859-867

Cochrane AH, Nussenzweig RS, Nardin EH 1980 Immunization against sporozoites. In: Kreier JP (ed) Malaria, vol 3. Academic Press, New York, p 163-202

Dame JB, Williams JL, McCutchan TF et al 1984 Structure of the gene encoding the immunodominant surface antigen on the sporozoite of the human malaria parasite *Plasmodium falciparum*. Science (Wash DC) 225:593-599

Enea V, Arnot D, Schmidt EC, Cochrane A, Gwadz R, Nussenzweig RS 1984a Circumsporozoite genes of *Plasmodium cynomolgi* (Gombak): cDNA cloning and expression of the repetitive circumsporozoite epitope. Proc Natl Acad Sci USA 81:7520-7524

Enea V, Ellis J, Zavala F et al 1984b DNA cloning of *Plasmodium falciparum* circumsporozoite gene: amino acid sequence of repetitive epitope. Science (Wash DC) 225:628-630

Godson GH, Ellis J, Svec P, Schlesinger DH, Nussenzweig V 1983 Identification and chemical synthesis of a tandemly repeated immunogenic region of *Plasmodium knowlesi* circumsporozoite protein. Nature (Lond) 306:29-33

Gysin J, Barnwell J, Schlesinger DH, Nussenzweig V, Nussenzweig RS 1984 Neutralization of the infectivity of sporozoites of *Plasmodium knowlesi* by antibodies to a synthetic peptide. J Exp Med 160:935-940

Hollingdale ML, Zavala F, Nussenzweig RS, Nussenzweig V 1982 Antibodies to the protective antigen of *Plasmodium berghei* sporozoites prevent entry into cultured cells. J Immunol 128:1929-1930

Hollingdale MR, Nardin EH, Tharavanij S, Schwartz AL, Nussenzweig RS 1984 Inhibition of entry of *Plasmodium falciparum* and *P. vivax* sporozoites into cultured cells: an *in vitro* assay of protective antibodies. J Immunol 132:909-913

Nardin EH, Nussenzweig RS, McGregor IA, Bryan J 1979 Antisporozoite antibodies: their frequent occurrence in individuals living in an area of hyperendemic malaria. Science (Wash DC) 206:597-599

Nussenzweig RS, Nussenzweig V 1984 Development of sporozoite vaccines. Philos Trans R Soc Lond B Biol Sci 307:117-128

Nussenzweig RS, Vandenberg JP, Most H, Orton C 1969 Specificity of protective immunity produced by X-irradiated *Plasmodium berghei* sporozoites. Nature (Lond) 227:488-489

Orjih AV, Nussenzweig RS 1982 Comparative studies on the immunogenicity of infective and attenuated sporozoites of *Plasmodium berghei*. Trans R Soc Trop Med Hyg 76:57-61

Ozaki LS, Svec P, Nussenzweig RS, Nussenzweig V, Godson GN 1983 Structure of the *Plasmodium knowlesi* gene coding for the circumsporozoite protein. Cell 34:815-822

Potocnjak P, Yoshida N, Nussenzweig RS, Nussenzweig V 1980 Monovalent fragments (Fab) of monoclonal antibodies to sporozoite surface antigen (Pb44) protect mice against malaria infection. J Exp Med 151:1504-1513

Ravetch JV, Young J, Poste G 1985 Molecular genetic strategies for the development of antimalarial vaccines. Biotechnology 3:729-740

Santoro F, Cochrane AH, Nussenzweig V et al 1983 Structural similarities between the protective antigens of sporozoites from different species of malaria. J Biol Chem 258:3341-3345

Vandenberg JP 1975 Development of infectivity by the *Plasmodium berghei* sporozoite. J Parasitol 61:43-50

Vandenberg JP, Nussenzweig RS, Most H 1969 Protective immunity produced by injections of X-irradiated sporozoites of *Plasmodium berghei*. V. *In vitro* effects of immune serum on sporozoites. Military Med 134 (Suppl):1183-1190

Yoshida N, Nussenzweig RS, Potocnjak P, Aikawa M, Nussenzweig V 1980 Hybridoma produces protective antibodies directed against the sporozoite stage of malaria parasites. Science (Wash DC) 207:71-73

Yoshida N, Potocnjak P, Nussenzweig V, Nussenzweig RS 1981 Biosynthesis of Pb44, the protective antigen of sporozoites of *Plasmodium berghei*. J Exp Med 154:1225-1236

Young JF, Hockmeyer WT, Gross M et al 1985 Expression of *Plasmodium falciparum* circumsporozoite proteins in *Escherichia coli* for potential use in a human malaria vaccine. Science (Wash DC) 228:958-962

Zavala F, Cochrane AH, Nardin EH, Nussenzweig RS, Nussenzweig V 1983 Circumsporozoite proteins of malaria parasites contain a single immunodominant region with two or more identical epitopes. J Exp Med 157:1947-1957

Zavala F, Tam JF, Hollingdale MR et al 1985a Rationale for development of a synthetic vaccine against *Plasmodium falciparum* malaria. Science (Wash DC) 228:1436-1440

Zavala F, Masuda A, Graves PM, Nussenzweig V, Nussenzweig R 1985b Ubiquity of the repetitive epitope of the CS protein in different isolates of human malaria parasites. J Immunol 135:2790-2793

DISCUSSION

Williams: The CS peptide is interesting for another reason, besides its sequence. We spoke earlier about multiple conformations of peptides, which was one problem with understanding the action of linear peptides as antigens. This peptide is one of peculiar restriction because of its composition. Alanine shows very few conformers because it has such a short side-chain. Again, with a large amino acid, such as asparagine, before proline, there is now a big restriction on the geometry of the peptide. Proline is always special in conformational analysis.

A second point is that such repeating sequences look as if they were almost deliberately designed to *stimulate* antibodies. That might seem odd; it might seem to be an unusual protection for the parasite.

V. Nussenzweig: It is a problem why a parasite should maintain such a strongly immunogenic epitope within a molecule essential for its survival in the host. It has been suggested that the repeats are there to fool the immune response; this doesn't make sense to me, because all antibodies against the repeats neutralize parasite activity very effectively, *in vivo* as well as *in vitro*. Therefore the repeats in this instance cannot be a lure designed to deceive the immune system. I would argue that the immune response to the repeats prevents superinfections by the same species of malaria parasite. It protects the host from death and is therefore also beneficial to the parasite. Also, the immune response to sporozoites does not affect the next stage of development of the parasite, which lives and multiplies inside red blood cells.

Williams: My other point was that if one wants to synthesize peptides and to reduce the mobility within a sequence, one way to do it is to include proline, which would lower the normal entropic factor of random polymers.

V. Nussenzweig: Prolines and asparagines are found in reverse turns, so this domain of the CS protein may be a series of reverse turns.

Rothbard: When I first saw the sporozoite sequence with the multiple repeats and obvious turn possibilities, I felt the system was similar to a polymer; in particular, poly(G-A-T). As Dr Nussenzweig says, monoclonal antibodies elicited by the intact protein only bind peptides greater than eight amino acids in length, or two tetramer units. Dr Sela demonstrated 20 years ago that antibodies raised against poly(G-A-T), a helical polymer, did not cross-react with G-A-T until it reached a length where is adopted a helical conformation (Sela 1966). The monoclonal antibodies raised by my collaborators at Walter Reed Army Institute bind this repeat region. When assayed against a nested set of peptides in this sequence, a marked increase in binding occurred when an asparagine was added to the sequence, and again four residues later (Dame et al 1984, Ballou et al 1985). One explanation of this phenomenon is that this sequence forms a 3^{10} helix and the epitope is one edge of the helix composed of every fourth asparagine. Consequently, the antibody would require the peptide to be a minimum length, providing sufficient interactions to stabilize the conformation. Space-fitting models of this structure demonstrate that it is feasible. However, circular dichroism experiments performed in collaboration with Peter Kim at Stanford have not confirmed this hypothesis.

Crumpton: I take it that we know almost nothing about the conformation of this region in the CS protein?

*V. Nussenzweig:*No, except that the Chou–Fasman analysis predicts that the repeat domain consists of random coils with reverse turns (Chou & Fasman 1978).

Lerner: We have done high-field NMR on this peptide, expecting to see some structure, but we saw nothing.

Crumpton: Is the peptide a monomer in solution?

V. Nussenzweig: That is a problem. The dodecamer peptide doesn't behave like a monomer when subjected to molecular sieving chromatography on HPLC. I am not sure why.

Ada: What about its behaviour on ultracentrifugation?

V. Nussenzweig: We haven't done that.

Rothbard: On Sepharose columns the peptide behaves normally, not as an aggregate.

Corradin: Did you add antibody to the peptide and look for a conformational change by CD?

Rothbard: Yes. I prepared a Fab of a monoclonal antibody directed at this region and attempted to see induction of a helical conformation by incubating the Fab with the eight-, 10- and 12-amino acid peptides. We have not been successful because of the technical difficulty of this experiment.

Ada: Dr Nussenzweig, you quoted results from subjects who had increasing concentrations of antibody to the CS antigen (Zavala et al 1985). Do you reach a stage where those people never get infected with malaria? Why do they become infected, when the antibody concentration is so high?

*V. Nussenzweig:*We don't know. It may be a question of the levels of serum antibody attained. The serum with highest titre was from a volunteer who had been vaccinated with X-irradiated sporozoites. That individual was completely protected against malaria infection. To achieve complete protection, you may need these high levels of antibody. However, it can be argued that even if you don't achieve complete protection, by reducing the parasite load you may diminish the severity of the disease, the levels of parasitaemia, which in turn can have important epidemiological consequences. So even an anti-sporozoite vaccine which does not give complete protection but eliminates 99% of the parasite load would be useful.

Gupta: Another possibility may be that a particular subject is bitten by another species of mosquito, and precirculating antibodies may not be able to combat the new infection.

*V. Nussenzweig:*I don't think so, because all strains of *P. falciparum* sporozoites examined have (NANP)$_3$-like epitopes. I hasten to say that although we didn't find variants, they may exist. Also, perhaps variants will appear, under the selective pressure of antibodies generated by a vaccine. But, at present, variants are not frequent. That tells us that this parasite is fortunately not like trypanosomes, which change their coats very quickly. If there is variation in the CS protein repeats, it may be more complicated to achieve, and it's easy to see why. Mutations in a single repeat will be of little consequence unless the others are equally affected. You would have to substitute the whole block of repeats, which may not be so simple.

Brown: In fact, antigenic variation would have built up in the natural situation anyway, judging by the examples of influenza virus and foot-and-mouth disease virus. So if you are not finding antigenic variation, I don't think vaccination will make much difference.

V. Nussenzweig: I am not so optimistic! I hope that is so, but there are reasons for caution, which derive from studies by Drs Enea and Arnot in Ruth's laboratory with *P. cynomolgi*, a monkey malaria parasite. They studied the CS genes of several strains of this parasite which are morphologically and in every other way similar to each other. To our surprise, the nucleotide sequences were almost identical outside the repeats, but differed considerably inside the repeats. That is, the repeat domain evolves more rapidly than the rest of the molecule (Cochrane et al 1985, Enea et al 1984). In the monkey hosts, the parasites are in equilibrium with the host and there is a lot of serum antibody against the repeats. In this case a variant bearing a different repeat would have a selective advantage. We should remember that *P. falciparum* is not in equilibrium with its human host; it kills the host. High levels of anti-repeat antibodies are found only in adults and there may not be enough selective pressure yet for change.

Anders: Your data on the prevalence of antibodies are interesting. As you said, most adults in endemic areas have occasional parasitaemic episodes. You have found that most adults have detectable antibodies against the CS protein repeat sequence, but nevertheless they are all getting infected occasionally.

V. Nussenzweig: But they are more resistant than children.

Anders: Yes, and the infections in adults are usually asymptomatic. We don't know whether that reflects different degrees of virulence in parasites, or suboptimal levels of immunity to the blood stages.

The other interesting point is that in West Africa, only about 40% of 10–14-year-olds have antibodies to this protein, despite having had many parasitaemic episodes, half of which might have been symptomatic.

R.S. Nussenzweig: You imply that adults have malaria continuously. I don't think that is so throughout the population. In fact, in one study the individuals who had the highest anti-sporozoite antibody titres by the fluorescence technique had had no clinical episodes for some long time. Several of these subjects had no antibodies against blood stages. We concluded that these people had reached a complete level of protection against sporozoites, so that the parasites never matured to blood stages and therefore there was no booster effect; so the antibodies to blood stages disappeared.

Anders: Have you any data from a prospective study that indicate that antibodies to the CS protein protect against symptomatic or asymptomatic infections?

V. Nussenzweig: We shall soon have sufficient amounts of the synthetic peptide (NANP)$_3$ to do a prospective study. This was not possible in the past, because only sporozoites could be used as antigen.

Heusser: It is believed that IgE antibody plays a special role in protection towards certain parasites. What are the natural antibodies to the CS protein coat, and what are the isotypes that you induce with these repeats?

V. Nussenzweig: This is a different situation from the usual IgE-mediated antiparasite immunity to nematode worms. Sporozoites circulate in the bloodstream for a few minutes only. The relevant antibody is therefore circulating antibody, and in the case of sporozoite immunity, it is of the IgG class.

REFERENCES

Ballou WR, Rothbard J, Wirtz RA et al 1985 Immunogenicity of synthetic peptides from circumsporozoite protein of *Plasmodium falciparum*. Science (Wash DC) 228:996-999

Cochrane AH, Gwadz RW, Ojo-Amaize E, Hii J, Nussenzweig V, Nussenzweig R 1985 The *Plasmodium cynomolgi* complex of primate malarias: antigenic diversity of the circumsporozoite proteins. Mol Biochem Parasitol 14:111-124

Chou PY, Fasman GD 1978 Empirical predictions of protein conformation. Annu Rev Biochem 47:251-276

Dame JB, Williams JL, McCutchan TF et al 1984 Structure of the gene encoding the immundominant surface antigen on the sporozoite of the human malaria parasite *Plasmodium falciparum*. Science (Wash DC) 225:593-599

Enea V, Arnot D, Schmidt EC, Cochrane A, Gwadz R, Nussenzweig RS 1984 Circumsporozoite gene of *Plasmodium cynomolgi* (Gombak): cDNA cloning and expression of the repetitive circumsporozoite epitope. Proc Natl Acad Sci USA 81:7520-7524

Sela M 1966 Immunological studies with synthetic polypeptides. Adv Immunol 5:29-129

Zavala F, Tam JF, Hollingdale MR et al 1985 Rationale for development of a synthetic vaccine against *Plasmodium falciparum* malaria. Science (Wash DC) 228:1436-1440

Antigenic repeat structures in proteins of *Plasmodium falciparum*

R. F. ANDERS, P-T. SHI*, D. B. SCANLON⁺, S. J. LEACH⁵, R. L. COPPEL, G. V. BROWN, H-D. STAHL and D. J. KEMP

The Walter and Eliza Hall Institute of Medical Research, and ⁺The Ludwig Institute, Melbourne, Victoria 3050, Australia, ⁵The Russell Grimwade School of Biochemistry, The University of Melbourne, Victoria 3052, Australia, and *The Shanghai Institute of Biochemistry, Shanghai, People's Republic of China

Abstract. The majority of malaria antigens that have been cloned contain short sequence repeats which encode antigenic epitopes that are naturally immunogenic. Synthetic peptides have been used to show that natural antibody responses to a strain-specific *Plasmodium falciparum* S antigen are largely directed against epitopes encoded in an 11-amino acid sequence that is repeated approximately 100 times in the molecule. A 16-amino acid peptide conjugated to bovine serum albumin induced antibodies specific for the S antigen of the homologous isolate.

Synthetic peptides have also been used to confirm the natural immunogenicity of epitopes encoded within two blocks of related repeats in the Ring-infected Erythrocyte Surface Antigen (RESA). A 16-amino acid peptide, comprising four repeats of the tetrameric sequence EENV, induced antibodies reactive with the native molecule. Detailed analyses of these anti-peptide antisera indicate that short sequence repeats express more than one epitope, some of which may cross-react with other repeat structures.

1986 Synthetic peptides as antigens. Wiley, Chichester (Ciba Foundation Symposium 119) p 164-183

There is an urgent need to develop a vaccine against malaria, particularly that due to *Plasmodium falciparum*, the cause of the lethal form of the disease. The symptoms of malaria are caused by the cycle of asexual reproduction in erythrocytes and these life-cycle stages are an important target of naturally acquired specific immune responses. Recently, a number of different asexual blood-stage antigens have been cloned (Ardeshir et al 1985, Coppel et al 1983, 1984, 1985, Hall et al 1984, Kemp et al 1983, Koenen et al 1984, McGarvey et al 1984, Ravetch et al 1985, Stahl et al 1985, Hope et al 1985) and the individual antigens are now becoming available for assessment of their potential as vaccine components. As a consequence of the cloning of these antigens a considerable amount of primary structural information on protein antigens of malaria parasites can now be deduced from DNA sequence studies. Remarkably, all the antigens sequenced so far contain regions of the molecule composed of tandem sequence repeats. In this paper we present some of our results with synthetic peptides which show that these repeats encode naturally immunogenic epitopes that are the immunodominant parts of the molecule.

S antigens

The S antigens are heat-stable antigens found in the plasma of individuals infected with malaria and released into the medium when *P. falciparum* is cultured *in vitro*. They exhibit marked serological diversity (Wilson et al 1969, Wilson 1980). Studies in our laboratories have established that this serological diversity reflects different repeating sequences which make up a large central portion of the S antigen polypeptide (Cowman et al 1985).

The genes for two antigenically distinct S antigens, one from Africa (NF7) and the other from Papua New Guinea (FCQ27/PNG[FC27]), have been sequenced; some of the elements of the gene structures are illustrated in Fig. 1. As anticipated from its release or secretion from the parasitized cell, the antigen has a typical signal peptide which is nearly identical in the two S antigens. Between the signal peptide and the start of the repeats there is a sequence of ~70 amino acids, the C-terminal half of which is highly charged. The homology in this region, at the amino acid level, between the two S antigens is only 70% and may encode strain-specific epitopes, but so far we have found no evidence of a natural antibody response to this region of the S antigen molecule.

The repeat regions of the two molecules differ in the sequence of the repeat unit, the length of the repeat, and the number of repeats in the molecule (Table 1). The FC27 repeat is an undecapeptide sequence and although there is variation of the nucleotide sequence amongst the repeats, this is restricted to the third base in the codons and does not result in amino acid sequence changes. Some degeneracy is seen in the repeats at both the N-terminal and C-terminal ends of the repeat block. The NF7 S antigen has an octapeptide repeat in which variation of amino acid sequence occurs at one position, where

TABLE 1 Repeat sequences in two antigenically distinct S antigens

FC27 repeat	PAKASQGGLED	Repeated ~ 100 times
NF7 repeats	ARKSDEAE ALKSDEAE	Repeated ~ 40 times
	SEAGTEGPKGTGGPG	Repeated once

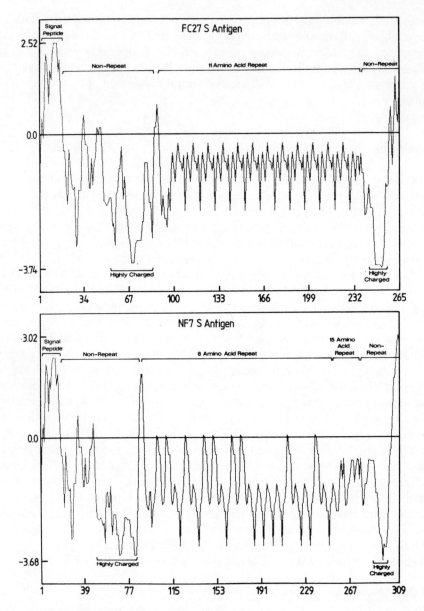

FIG. 1. Computer plots of the FC27 and NF7 S antigens showing the hydropathy profile according to Kyte & Doolittle (1982). The numbers on the vertical axis refer to the hydropathic index; those on the horizontal axis are the sequence numbers.

leucine or arginine may be found. These sequences of eight amino acids are the dominant repeating unit in the NF7 S antigen and, like the repeat of the FC27 S antigen, there is some degeneracy at each end of the block of repeats. However, at the C-terminal end of the block of octapeptide repeats in the NF7 S antigen there is one tandem repeat of a 15-amino acid sequence which contains within it an imperfect nine and six amino acid sub-repeating sequence.

S antigen repeat sequence peptides are antigenic

An 11-amino acid peptide corresponding to one FC27 S antigen repeating unit (Table 2, peptide 1) and two 16-amino acid peptides corresponding to approximately one and a half repeating units (Table 2, peptides 2 and 3)

TABLE 2 Synthetic peptides of the FC27 S antigen repeat

Peptide	Sequence
FC27S-1	QGGLEDPAKAS
FC27S-2	PAKASQGGLEDPAKAS
FC27S-3	LEDPAKASQGGLEDPA

The peptides were synthesized by the Merrifield (1963) solid-phase method. The initial amino acid resin was prepared by esterification of Boc-amino acids to chloromethylated resin (polystyrene–1% divinylbenzene) in dimethylformamide by stirring for 6–8 hours at 80 °C. A two-fold excess of potassium salt over active chloride polymer was found to give almost complete substitution. Substitution was determined to be 0.5–1.0 mmol/g by amino acid analysis.

were synthesized by conventional Merrifield synthesis (Merrifield 1963). Initially, we examined their antigenicity in solid-phase radioimmunoassays (RIA) in which the peptides were used to passively coat the wells of flexible polyvinyl chloride microtitre plates. Each of the peptides bound antibodies in the sera of rabbits that had been immunized with a fused polypeptide (FPAg16), obtained by cloning cDNA corresponding to the FC27 S antigen in the λgt11-Amp3 expression system (Kemp et al 1983, Coppel et al 1983). All peptides also bound antibodies to the FC27 S antigen that are found in the sera of approximately 5% of individuals living in the Madang province of Papua New Guinea, where malaria is endemic. All individuals who reacted in an enzyme-linked immunosorbent assay (ELISA) with S antigen semi-purified from the FC27 culture supernatants also reacted with purified FPAg16 and peptide 2. These results indicated that natural antibody responses to the FC27 S antigen are largely directed against epitopes encoded by the peptide repeat unit. This was confirmed by showing that binding of human antibodies to semi-purified S antigen could be blocked by adding the peptide (peptide

2) to the diluted antibodies before they were added to the S antigen-coated wells (Anders et al, unpublished work 1984). Reactions with peptides 1 and 3 were weaker than with peptide 2 and some of the sera containing anti-FC27 S antigen antibodies did not give signals above background at the dilution of 1:250 at which all these assays were performed (Anders et al, unpublished work 1984).

Mice were immunized with each of the FC27 S antigen peptides conjugated to bovine serum albumin (BSA) using either glutaraldehyde or carbodiimide. In some mice, each of the larger (16-residue) peptides induced antibody responses reactive with S antigen isolated from culture supernatants, but only when conjugated with glutaraldehyde. The resulting antisera when tested by indirect immunofluorescence, or used to probe immunoblots of various culture supernatants, were shown to have the same strain-specificity for the FC27 S antigen as antisera produced by immunizing rabbits with this antigen expressed as a fused polypeptide in *Escherichia coli* (Coppel et al 1983).

The ring-infected erythrocyte surface antigen (RESA)

Antibodies raised against an abundant fused polypeptide, produced by a clone designated Ag13, reacted with an antigen (RESA) that was unusual in that the immunofluorescence pattern indicated an association with the membranes of erythrocytes infected with immature (ring stage) parasites (Coppel et al 1984). Immunoelectron microscopy using the Protein A–gold procedure confirmed the location of RESA at the membrane of the recently invaded erythrocytes and also identifed RESA within merozoites, contained in small vesicles called micronemes (Brown et al 1985). We presume that RESA is released via the apical pore of the merozoite at about the time of merozoite invasion, and may play an important function in the invasion process. No labelling of merozoite surfaces occurred with anti-RESA antibodies, so it appears that RESA is not involved in the initial interaction between the merozoite surface and the erythrocyte membrane.

Immunoblotting of parasite antigens (fractionated by sodium dodecyl sulphate—polyacrylamide gel electrophoresis) with rabbit anti-RESA antibodies identified a dominant antigen of M_r 155 000 (which was sometimes seen as a closely migrating doublet) and a very much less prominent, higher molecular weight antigen which was polymorphic in size (M_r range ~210 000 to 250 000) among different isolates of *P. falciparum* (Coppel et al 1984). Perlmann and collaborators (1984) isolated human antibodies to this antigen by using glutaraldehyde-fixed and air-dried infected erythrocytes as an immunoadsorbent. These antibodies strongly inhibited reinvasion *in vitro* of erythrocytes by merozoites (Wåhlin et al 1984). We have been unable to inhibit parasite reinvasion with antibodies raised against fragments of RESA produced in *E. coli*, but some regions of the molecule have not yet been tested.

RESA contains two separate blocks of repeats

Sequence data derived from a series of clones from two different isolates of *P. falciparum* established that RESA contains two different blocks of repeats that are related in sequence (Cowman et al 1984). Thus, the sequence organization is distinctly different from that of the S antigens (Cowman et et 1985) and of the malaria circumsporozoite proteins (CS proteins) (Godson et al 1983, Dame et al 1984, Enea et al 1984). In RESA there is a series of related 8-, 4- and 3-amino acid repeats at the C-terminus of the polypeptide chain. Towards the N-terminus, and separated by 381 amino acids from the C-terminal repeat, there is a second block of repeats based on an 11-amino acid sequence. Considerable sequence data are now available for isolates FC27 and NF7, and indicate that RESA in two strains of *P. falciparum* from different parts of the world are closely homologous.

Antigenic peptides corresponding to RESA repeats

The three peptides listed in Table 3 were synthesized and their antigenic and immunogenic characteristics examined. When the peptides were coupled

TABLE 3 Sequences and synthetic peptides corresponding to repeats in RESA

Region of RESA	Repeat sequences	Peptides synthesized[a]	
3' repeat	E E N V E H D A (5)[b]	RESA 3'-1	EENVEHDA
	E E N A (1)		
	E E N V (29)	RESA 3'-2	$(EENV)_n$ $(n \sim 4)$
	E E – V (4)		
	E E Y D (3)		
5' repeat	– E E N E E E H T V – (1)		
	D D E H V E E H T – A (1)		
	D D E H V E E P T V A (2)	RESA 5'-1	DDEHVEEPTVAY
	– D E H V E E P T V A (1)		
	– E E H V E E P T V A (1)		
	– E E H V E E P – – A (1)		

[a] Synthesis of peptides was as described in Table 2, except that the RESA 5'-1 peptide was synthesized by the FMOC solid-phase synthesis methodology of Atherton et al (1983) on a Kieselguhr KA resin support.

[b] The numbers in brackets indicate the number of times the respective sequences occur within the blocks of repeats.

to BSA and used as antigens in solid-phase ELISAs, naturally occurring antibodies in the serum of adult Papua New Guineans bound to the dominant tetrameric sequence EENV in the 3' repeat (which had been polymerized in solution to an average of four times) but not to the related 8-amino acid sequence EENVEHDA, which is repeated four times at the start of the 3' repeat (Anders et al, unpublished work 1985).

All the sera that reacted in ELISAs with fused polypeptides corresponding to 3' and 5' repeats reacted with the polymerized tetrameric peptide EENV and also reacted with the 11-amino acid synthetic peptide, DDEHVEEPTVA, corresponding to the canonical sequence in the 5' repeat. No sera judged to be negative in ELISAs on the two fusion polypeptides ($OD_{415} < 0.1$) gave any signal on the RESA synthetic peptide–BSA conjugates over that obtained on BSA alone. It therefore appears that two of the RESA synthetic peptides, one corresponding to 3' repeat sequences and the other corresponding to 5' repeat sequences, express epitopes that are immunogenic in the native molecule. Furthermore, the correspondence in results obtained with peptides and fused polypeptides as target antigens in the ELISAs suggests that no additional, naturally immunogenic epitopes are expressed in these very much larger molecules.

The three RESA synthetic peptides, conjugated to keyhole limpet haemocyanin (KLH), were used to immunize mice. The resulting antisera were assayed against each of the three peptides conjugated to BSA, and against fused polypeptides corresponding to the 3' and 5' repeats of RESA (Fig. 2) and sonicates of infected erythrocytes (Fig. 3). All mice immunized with these peptides produced antibodies that were reactive with the homologous peptide and the fused polypeptide containing that sequence. In addition, peptide RESA 3'-2 (EENV × 4) induced antibodies that also reacted with the other 3' repeat peptide, RESA 3'-1 (EENVEHDA) which has a five-amino acid sequence in common with it. The reverse, however, was not true: anti-RESA 3'-1 antibodies did not react with RESA 3'-2.

When these anti-peptide antisera were assayed on peptide–BSA conjugates there was no apparent cross-reactivity between the 5' and 3' repeats of RESA (Fig. 2). However, assay of the same sera on fused polypeptides revealed that the peptides had induced antibodies that reacted with both repeat structures, although the reaction with the heterologous repeat was very weak in comparison to that with the homologous repeat.

That these reaction patterns reflect multiple epitopes within the repeats is supported by results obtained with monoclonal antibodies raised against FPAg28, the fused polypeptide corresponding to the 3' repeat (Anders et al, unpublished). Two types of monoclonal antibodies have been obtained: one type that reacts with the 3' repeat fused polypeptide but not the 5' repeat fused polypeptide, and a second type that reacts with both fused polypeptides.

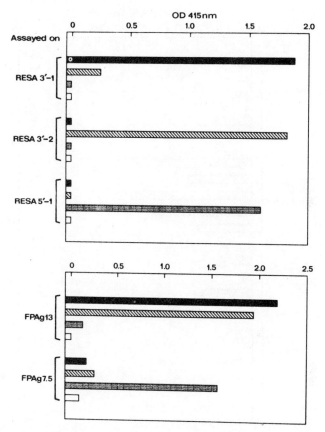

FIG. 2. Antibody responses in mice immunized with RESA synthetic peptides. The peptides, coupled to KLH, were: RESA 3′-1 (solid bars), RESA 3′-2 (hatched bars), RESA 5′-1 (shaded bars), and as a control NF7S-1, a 16-amino acid peptide corresponding to two repeats of the NF7 S antigen (open bars). Mice were immunized with 100 μg of KLH conjugate together with complete Freund's adjuvant and boosted four weeks later with the same amount of conjugate in incomplete adjuvant. The mice were bled two weeks after the boost. Conventional micro-ELISAs were performed in which the bound mouse antibodies were detected with affinity-purified sheep F(ab)₂ conjugated to horseradish peroxidase. The sera were assayed in duplicate at one dilution (1:250) against each of the synthetic peptides conjugated to BSA (upper panel) and fused polypeptides corresponding to the 3′ repeat (FPAg28) and 5′ repeat (FPAg632) of RESA (lower panel). The results are the averages for five mice, except for the group immunized with RESA 5′-1, where only three mice survived.

When two monoclonals, one of each type, were tested for binding to synthetic peptides, we found that the 3′-specific monoclonal (Ag28-5/1 in Table 4) reacted only with one of the two 3′ repeat synthetic peptides, that containing the EENV sequence repeated four times (RESA 3′-2). In contrast, the other

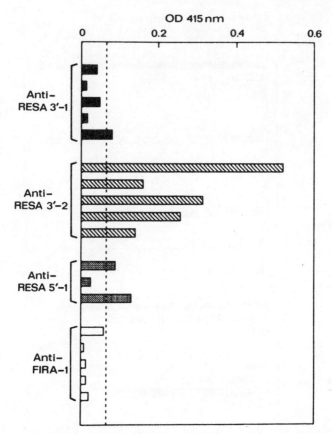

FIG. 3. Reactivity of mouse anti-RESA peptide antisera with a sonicate of erythrocytes infected with *P. falciparum*. Micro-ELISAs were performed as described in Fig. 2. Each bar is the value obtained for an individual mouse.

monoclonal antibody (Ag28-17/1) reacted with both the synthetic peptides containing 3' repeat sequences. Neither monoclonal reacted with the peptide corresponding to a 5' repeat sequence (RESA 5'-1). These results are consistent with the results obtained with the mouse anti-peptide antisera, which

TABLE 4 Specificity of anti-RESA monoclonal antibodies

| Monoclonal antibody | Reactivity on: | | | | |
| | Fused proteins | | Peptides | | |
	3' repeat	5' repeat	RESA 3'-1	RESA 3'-2	RESA 5'-1
Ag28-5/1	+++	−	−	++	−
Ag28-17/1	+++	++	++	++	−

indicate that there is a cross-reacting epitope expressed in both fusion polypeptides and both 3' repeat synthetic peptides, but is not expressed in the 5' repeat synthetic peptide.

Cross-reactions in malaria antigens

The antigenic cross-reactivity between the 3' and 5' repeats of RESA originally observed with antisera to RESA sequences produced in *E. coli*, and now confirmed with antisera to synthetic peptides, is part of a broader network of cross-reactions involving several natural immunogens of *P. falciparum* which contain repeats with related sequences. Included in this network is the Falciparum Interspersed Repeat Antigen (FIRA) (Stahl et al 1985) and possibly also the antigen described by Koenen et al (1984), which contains a nonapeptide repeat sequence EEVVEEVVP. The biological significance of these repeats is not known but we believe that they may in some way modify the host's immune response to the parasite's advantage. The cross-reactions between the repeat structures described here and elsewhere (Hope et al 1985, Coppel et al 1985) may provide a mechanism for such evasion by aborting the normal evolution of a high quality (high affinity) immune response, which clearly depends on selection by antigen of somatic mutations arising during antigen-driven lymphocyte proliferation (reviewed in Manser et al 1985). If this hypothesis is correct, the use of synthetic peptides corresponding to epitopes that are the target of host-protective immune responses, in isolation from multiple cross-reacting epitopes, may provide an avenue leading to the production of an effective vaccine against malaria.

Acknowledgements

We gratefully acknowledge the support of our many colleagues in the Unit of Immunoparasitology at The Walter and Eliza Hall Institute of Medical Research. This work was supported by the National Health and Medical Research Council of Australia, the Rockefeller Foundation Great Neglected Diseases Program, the John D. and Katherine T. MacArthur Foundation and the Australian Biotechnology Grants Scheme.

REFERENCES

Ardeshir F, Flint JE, Reese RT 1985 Expression of *Plasmodium falciparum* surface antigens in *Escherichia coli*. Proc Natl Acad Sci USA 82:2518-2522
Atherton E, Caviezel M, Fox H, Harkiss D, Over H, Sheppard RC 1983 Peptide synthesis. Part 3. Comparative solid-phase syntheses of human β-endorphin on polyamide supports using

t-butoxycarbonyl and fluorenylmethoxycarbonyl protecting groups. J Chem Soc Perkin Trans I 1:65-73

Brown GV, Culvenor JG, Crewther PE, Bianco AE, Coppel RL, Saint RB, Stahl HD, Kemp DJ, Anders RF 1985 Localization of the ring-infected erythrocyte surface antigen (RESA) of *Plasmodium falciparum* in merozoites and ring-infected erythrocytes. J Exp Med 162:774-779

Coppel RL, Cowman AF, Lingelbach KR, Brown GV, Saint RB, Kemp DJ, Anders RF 1983 Isolate-specific S antigen of *Plasmodium falciparum* contains a repeated sequence of 11 amino acids. Nature (Lond) 306:751-756

Coppel RL, Cowman AF, Anders RF, Bianco AE, Saint RB, Lingelbach KR, Kemp DJ, Brown GV 1984 Immune sera recognize on erythrocytes a *Plasmodium falciparum* antigen composed of repeated amino acid sequences. Nature (Lond) 310:789-791

Coppel RL, Favaloro JM, Crewther PE, Burkot TR, Bianco AE, Stahl HD, Kemp DJ, Anders RF, Brown GV 1985 A blood-stage antigen of *Plasmodium falciparum* shares determinants with the sporozoite coat protein. Proc Natl Acad Sci USA 82:5121–5125

Cowman AF, Coppel RL, Saint RB, Favaloro J, Crewther PE Stahl HD, Bianco AE, Brown Gv, Anders RF, Kemp DJ 1984 The ring-infected erythrocyte surface antigen (RESA) polypeptide of *Plasmodium falciparum* contains two separate blocks of tandem repeats encoding antigenic epitopes that are naturally immunogenic in man. Mol Biol Med 2:207-221

Cowman AF, Saint RB, Coppel RL, Brown GV, Anders RF, Kemp DJ 1985 Conserved sequences flank variable tandem repeats in two S-antigen genes of *Plasmodium falciparum*. Cell 40:775-783

Dame JB, Williams JL, McCutchan TF, Weber JL, Wirtz RA, Hockmeyer WT, Maloy WL, Haynes JD, Schneider I, Roberts D, Sanders GS, Reddy EP, Diggs CL, Miller LH 1984 Structure of the gene encoding the immunodominant surface antigen on the sporozoite of the human malaria parasite *Plasmodium falciparum*. Science (Wash DC) 225:593-599

Enea V, Ellis J, Zavala F, Arnot DE, Asavanich A, Masuda A, Quaky I, Nussenzweig RS 1984 DNA cloning of *Plasmodium falciparum* circumsporozoite gene: amino acid sequence of repetitive epitope. Science (Wash DC) 225:628-630

Godson GN, Ellis J, Svec P, Schlesinger DH, Nussenzweig V 1983 Identification and chemical synthesis of a tandemly repeated immunogenic region of *P. knowlesi* circumsporozoite protein. Nature (Lond) 305:29-33

Hall R, Hyde JE, Goman M, Simmons DL, Hope IA, Mackay M, Scaife J 1984 Major surface antigen gene of a human malaria parasite cloned and expressed in bacteria. Nature (Lond) 311:379-382

Hope IA, Mackay M, Hyde JE, Goman M, Scaife J 1985 The gene for an exported antigen of the malaria parasite *Plasmodium falciparum* cloned and expressed in *Escherichia coli*. Nucleic Acids Res 13:369-379

Kemp DJ, Coppel RL, Cowman AF, Saint RB, Brown GV, Anders RF 1983 Expression of *Plasmodium falciparum* blood-stage antigens in *Escherichia coli*: detection with antibodies from immune humans. Proc Natl Acad Sci USA 80:3787-3791

Koenen M, Scherf A, Mercereau O, Langsley G, Sibilli L, Dubois P, Pereira da Silva L, Muller-Hill B 1984 Human antisera detect a *Plasmodium falciparum* genomic clone encoding a nonapeptide repeat. Nature (Lond) 311:382-385

Kyte J, Doolittle RF 1982 A simple method for displaying the hydropathic character of protein. J Mol Biol 157:105-132

Manser T, Wysocki LJ, Gridley T, Near RI, Gefter ML 1985 The molecular evolution of the immune responses. Immunol Today 6:94-101

McGarvey MK, Sheybani E, Loche MP, Perrin LH, Mach B 1984 Identification and expression in *Escherichia coli* of merozoite stage-specific genes of the human malarial parasite *Plasmodium falciparum*. Proc Natl Acad Sci USA 81:3690-3694

Merrifield RB 1963 Solid-phase peptide synthesis. J Am Chem Soc 85:3149-2150

Perlmann H, Berzins K, Wahlgren M, Carlsson J, Björkman A, Patarroyo ME, Perlmann P 1984 Antibodies in malarial sera to antigens in the membrane of erythrocytes infected with early asexual stages of *Plasmodium falciparum*. J Exp Med 159:1686-1704

Ravetch JV, Kochan J, Perkins M 1985 Isolation of the gene for a glycophorin-binding protein implicated in erythrocyte invasion by a malaria parasite. Science (Wash DC) 227:1593-1597

Stahl HD, Crewther PE, Anders RF, Brown GV, Coppel RL, Bianco AE, Mitchell GF, Kemp DJ 1985 Interspersed blocks of repetitive and charged amino acids in a dominant immunogen of *Plasmodium falciparum*. Proc Natl Acad Sci USA 82:543-547

Wilson RJM, McGregor IA, Hall P, Williams K, Bartholomew R 1969 Antigens associated with *Plasmodium falciparum* infections in man. Lancet 2:201-205

Wilson RJM 1980 Serotyping *Plasmodium falciparum* malaria with S-antigens. Nature (Lond) 284:451-452

Wåhlin B, Wahlgren M, Perlmann H, Berzins K, Björkman A, Patarroyo ME, Perlmann P 1984 Human antibodies to a M_r 155,000 *Plasmodium falciparum* antigen efficiently inhibit merozoite invasion. Proc Natl Acad Sci USA 81:7912-7916

DISCUSSION

Lachmann: RESA is an extraordinary hostage for *Plasmodium falciparum* to give to fortune. A good complement-fixing antibody to RESA would stop the infection dead in its tracks.

Anders: The extent to which RESA is exposed on an unperturbed red cell surface is not clear. We initially detected it by indirect immunofluorescence on red cells that were unperturbed in any way, so we think it is somewhat exposed on some cells. But generally you don't see this molecule well unless you perturb the red cell (Perlmann et al 1984). We think that RESA is anchored into the red cell cytoskeleton, because it becomes Triton-insoluble when transferred from the merozoite to the red cell membrane, but it may also span the membrane and be partly exposed on the external surface.

Lerner: When you look at these repeats your eye tends to pick out the exact repeat as the antigen, but it occurs to me that the whole sequence may be relevant. You may need 12 residues rather than four to shift, as it were, the 'frame' of the antigen.

Anders: We have defined two distinct epitopes within the RESA 3′ four-amino acid repeat, and there may be more. But you don't need 12 amino acids (i.e., three repeats) to raise an antibody to the RESA molecule; eight amino acids are enough. However, you might need a 12-amino acid sequence to raise antibodies to the full spectrum of epitopes that such a repeat may encode.

Lerner: It is interesting that whenever you find these repeats, they are strongly antigenic. Another situation where we find repeats is in the Epstein-Barr virus nuclear antigen. That antigen consists of only two amino acids, glycine and alanine, repeated over 200–300 amino acids. That is the strongest antigen in individuals presenting with EBV infection. Only one Gly-Ala combination is the antigenic determinant. In that instance, the exact way in which the antigen is constructed, even though it is made up of only two amino acids, is critical. Perhaps we should try polymerizing the other antigens we have discussed, such as foot-and-mouth disease virus protein, and making repeats of them.

Anders: That would be an interesting exercise. I would predict that antigenicity would be increased.

Brown: This has been done for foot-and-mouth disease virus. The antigenicity is enormously increased and you don't need a carrier to elicit a good response. With FMDV, we added a cysteine residue at each end of the peptide and then air-oxidized it.

Sela: We should distinguish between two situations. On one hand it may be important to have a polymer of a peptide, because then you may get a different conformation produced that is better for cross-reacting with the native immunogen. On the other hand, the fact that you have an epitope which can be repeated means that such a macromolecule may react, for example with a cell receptor, much more strongly, because of the polyvalent interaction.

My other comment is a semantic point. You talk about immunogenic peptides; to me, this means peptides that by themselves, when injected into an animal, lead to an immune response.

Stanworth: When you conjugated the S antigen peptides with carbodiimide the conjugates were not antigenic, whereas those conjugated with glutaraldehyde were. We have had the same experience with other types of synthetic peptides. Is there an immunochemical explanation as to why, if you present the peptide in one way on the carrier, it is more effective than if you present it another way?

Brown: The peptide is linked through different groups. For example, with carbodiimide, the link is through carboxylic acid and amino groups; glutaraldehyde links through two amino groups. That will make a difference to the activity, if an acidic amino acid residue is part of the antigenic site.

Stanworth: On the whole, then, you stand a better chance of producing an immunogenic conjugate by using glutaraldehyde as coupling agent.

Anders: I think so.

Ada: Apart from the fact that you perhaps have a great increase in avidity with these repeat structures, what other advantages do they give to a virus or parasite?

V. Nussenzweig: The malaria parasite has to hit its target in a very short time, and the interaction has to be highly effective, leading to penetration. If its surface molecules contain many copies of the ligand involved in the receptor interaction, the parasite has an important advantage, because its fate will not be altered by random mutations affecting the amino acid sequence of a single copy of the ligand. In other words, the parasite does not have to rely on a single, high affinity interaction to find the appropriate host cell.

Anders: This may be the role of repeats in the CS protein, but it's hard to imagine such a role for the repeats in the S antigen molecule, because the repeats vary so much in different S antigens. All the available evidence indicates that the S antigen system is a complex polymorphism and is not undergoing antigenic variation as is the African trypanosome variable surface glycoprotein (Cowman et al 1985). The most obvious cause of S antigen diversity is selection pressure imposed by the host immune response, but it is not clear that S antigens are targets of protective immune responses. Thus, the probable role of repeats in S antigens and other antigens is somehow to modify the host's immune response, to the parasite's advantage. I have a hypothesis on how this might happen to which I referred briefly (p 173), and could enlarge on here.

All the protein antigens of malaria parasites for which sequence data are available contain elements of a tandem repeat structure which in many cases has been shown to encode dominant, naturally immunogenic epitopes. Recently, we have detected multiple cross-reactions between different epitopes encoded by these repeats. These cross-reactions occur at several different levels. The first level is within one block of repeats—as, for example, in the 3' repeat of RESA (Cowman et al 1984). A second level of cross-reactivities occurs between different blocks of repeats in the one protein as, for example, between the 5' and 3' repeats of RESA and probably between different blocks of repeats in FIRA (Stahl et al 1985). The next level of cross-reactions involves repeats in different proteins. Such cross-reactions are seen between RESA and FIRA (Stahl et al 1985), between the CS protein and an asexual blood-stage antigen (Hope et al 1985), and probably between different histidine-rich proteins. Yet another level of cross-reactions involves antigens such as the S antigen and possibly the 195K protein, which differ in different strains of *P. falciparum*. One epitope may be involved in cross-reactions at several of these levels, giving rise to a network of cross-reactivities.

These characteristics of malaria antigens are so unusual that it seems likely that the cross-reactivities encoded by the repeat structures may be critical to any role they have in modifying the host immune response, and may be responsible for some of the distinctive features of the immune response in malaria, such as marked hypergammaglobulinaemia, slow development of an immunity which is relatively unstable, and autoantibody production.

As we discussed earlier (p 124), high affinity antibody responses probably depend on the selection by antigen of B cells that have accumulated somatic mutations in their surface immunoglobulin receptors (reviewed in Manser et al 1985). Mutations occur at a high rate and, particularly in conditions of limiting amounts of antigen, the minority of mutants with B cell receptors with higher affinities would preferentially proliferate to produce antibody-secreting plasma cells. In normal immune responses, somatic mutants are selected by the epitope that triggered the parental naive B cell to proliferate. However, in immune responses to some malaria antigens there are a large number of structurally related cross-reacting epitopes present in addition to the epitope that triggered the initial response. As a result, a mutated cell that fails to react with the triggering epitope with sufficient affinity to be preserved in the expanding clone may react with one of the cross-reacting epitopes with a much higher affinity and, as a consequence, undergo further proliferation.

These considerations led to the hypothesis that in antimalarial immune responses a higher proportion than normal of B cells accumulating somatic mutations in their surface immunoglobulin will be preserved during clonal expansion. This may be responsible, in part, for the hypergammaglobulinaemia that is a feature of individuals repeatedly infected with malaria parasites. The preservation of a wider range of somatic mutants may also increase the incidence of autoantibodies. More importantly, if the normal evolution of antibody responses is modified in this way, the development of high affinity antibody responses which could be important for effective immunity against malaria may be delayed, because of limits to B cell proliferation (and the number of somatic mutations accumulated in one antibody molecule), imposed by restrictions on the size of the B cell pool or competition among B cells for growth factors.

Humphrey: In the course of hyperimmunization against a defined epitope, as time went on there was a selection for high affinity antibody, but cells were also found that were producing low affinity antibody, at the same time (Werblin et al 1973).

Sela: If you hyperimmunize you generally get a much bigger crop of antibody with time and the average affinity goes up, but so also does the antibody heterogeneity.

Klug: Is it known where these *P. falciparum* antigens are, in the infected cell? Does one of the stages, say the sporozoite, have the repeating structure on its membrane? It is not uncommon to find such structures on cell walls or in coats.

Anders: Antigens with repeats have been located in association with parasite or host cell membranes, or secreted into the plasma.

Klug: So these proteins may also have a structural role; they are not there only to fool the immune system?

Anders: It is hard to imagine a structural purpose for the S antigen. We can't locate this antigen to any parasite structure; it is just released into the plasma when the schizont ruptures.

Klug: These repeating protein sequences remind me of certain bacterial polysaccharides—could they be polysaccharides in disguise? Bacterial polysaccharides show great diversity, yet they are very specific molecules, and have other roles related to the life of the bacterium.

Ada: As Victor Nussenzweig said, although you can make an antibody against CS protein, it may be a mechanism for limiting the infection so that the organism doesn't kill its host. Alternatively, this may be a situation where the organism is diverting the immune system; that is, the resources of the immune mechanism are used up by getting it to do something irrelevant to getting rid of the parasite.

V. Nussenzweig: The various suggested roles for the repeats are not mutually exclusive. CS molecules perhaps interact through the repeats to form the surface coat. At the same time that the repeats participate in the formation of a quaternary structure they can serve as ligands for receptors on the hepatocytes.

In the case of the S antigen, is it possible that before it is secreted, when it surrounds the schizonts, it also forms a coat or a matrix? The S antigen repeats may have a function inside the parasitophorous vacuole, and not be made for export.

Anders: The S antigen is secreted into the parasitophorous vacuole as the schizont matures. I don't know whether it is critical to the maturation of the merozoite coat at that point. Another group have produced a monoclonal antibody to the FC27 S antigen (Saul et al 1985). This monoclonal inhibits merozoite invasion, studied *in vitro*, but whether such antibodies are inhibitory *in vivo* is unknown. However, schizont rupture may be a critical period for the merozoite; a high density of some molecule surrounding it might protect the merozoite surface from antibody attack. If you could lower the 'on-rate' of antibodies, or lower the average affinity or avidity of antibody for that merozoite surface by a small margin, there might be a dramatic increase in the efficiency of reinvasion.

Lerner: If there is still any doubt that an antigen–antibody union can disrupt a structure, it should now be dispersed, because Victor Nussenzweig showed us that after anti-peptide antibody binding, the curved structure of the parasite changes. That is an alteration in protein structure, reflected in a change in the gross anatomy of the organism.

Another reason for this polymorphism, apart from escaping the immune system of the host, could be to match a second polymorphism. For example, suppose the parasite enters a red cell by using a blood group substance. Then the strategy of the parasite could be to match a polymorphic receptor. Is there any particular blood group clustering, or known second polymorphism (perhaps HLA markers), that clusters at the interaction points?

Anders: No. With *P. falciparum* it seems that the species as a whole uses an identical receptor or set of receptors, and therein lies the host-specificity of the different malaria parasites.

Crumpton: The genomic sequence of these antigens will tell us something about the choices available. What is known here?

V. Nussenzweig: The CS protein has one gene, not interrupted.

Anders: There are introns in other malaria antigens, however.

Crumpton: Are there any instances where you find repeats?

Anders: In the S antigen system there seems to be one gene, with multiple alleles in a very complex polymorphism. The gene in different strains may have many different repeats.

V. Nussenzweig: We don't find copies of the repeats elsewhere in the genome. It cannot be excluded, however, that the genome contains a series of precursors of the repeats selected in evolution which are rearranged to make new blocks of repeats.

Anders: We can't rule out the possibility that there are one or two additions of a four-amino acid sequence elsewhere in the genome that become rearranged and amplified.

Klug: These repeating sequences are on a small scale. I don't know how the proteins fold up, but they do not look much like ordinary proteins. As I said before, they look more like some polysaccharides, which have repeats on a small scale. I wonder what the consequences are. If the repeats represent surface features that resemble repeats in polysaccharides, they may generate an immune response more like that evoked by polysaccharides.

Humphrey: The immune response to linear polysaccharides is generally to fairly clearly defined epitopes sticking out from the backbone of the polysaccharide, rather than to the core polysaccharide itself. Soluble polysaccharides are not rigid molecules, so the distance apart of the epitopes can vary quite widely and still permit multipoint binding of them to receptors on the B cell surface. So far as I know, pure polysaccharides have never been shown to elicit T cell help.

Klug: I used the word 'polysaccharide' in a general sense: I didn't mean a simple linear polymer. Many polysaccharides consist of a backbone with branches, sometimes 2–3 sugars long and with a characteristic pattern. It is a small-scale repeating structure. Has anyone looked at short-branched polysaccharides?

Sela: We attached mono- and disaccharides to branched polymers, to see how much they contribute to immunogenicity. The sugars don't contribute anything to immunogenicity but are excellent in terms of antigenic specificity, because they skew the whole specificity of the polymer in the direction of the sugar.

Geysen: We, in conjunction with Robin Anders, have mapped the S antigen for what we define as contact residues for binding to a monoclonal. Interestingly enough, the E and D residues (glutamic acid and aspartic acid) don't form the contact residues; by and large, antibodies are recognizing, in the 11-amino acid repeat, the L and Q (leucine and glutamine) residues.

I would not like to state the minimum number of amino acids for binding. We can show binding to dipeptides, and to single amino acids, as I described earlier. But we can't put an affinity value to it. However, with the sensitivity of modern immunological tests, it is easy to detect these interactions as positive signals. If you are able to see interactions at that kind of level, then, of course, the number of cross-reactions goes up. Normally, where the whole spectrum of amino acids occurs, as in a protein antigen, it is the additional amino acids that preclude the recognition of the more common features. The repeating antigens are not very varied and look uninteresting in terms of the residues present; but those repeat sections and the restricted number of amino acids may allow you to see this multiplicity of cross-reactions, which is purely determined by the amino acid distribution of the proteins.

Crumpton: That cannot be universally true. Many antibodies against carbohydrates are highly specific. With antibodies to the human blood group substances, the distinction between A and B groups is based on single sugar residues (between *N*-acetylgalactosamine for A and galactose for B blood group). These sugars are attached to the same backbone structure. Furthermore, there isn't a great deal of cross-reactivity between an antibody against A blood group substance and a variety of other carbohydrates. So if you reduce interaction to recognition of a single residue, you don't necessarily increase the extent of cross-reactivity.

Geysen: You must do so to some extent, with amino acids, because you have only 20 different possibilities; therefore if you could reduce interactions to a single residue, you would have only 20 possible variants. The further you reduce the number of components making up the antigen, the greater the probability of cross-reaction. I wonder whether the diversity we are seeing is reduced to such an extent that it accounts for the cross-reactivity.

Ada: If Aaron Klug's concept is valid, two questions can be asked. Do we find polysaccharides in these parasites, as well as tandem repeats of amino acids? And do T cells react well with these repeating units?

Lerner: There is an important difference. The whole definition of immunogenicity, as against antigenicity, comes from the carbohydrate field, because of the following situation. If you immunize adult humans with pneumococcal organisms, perfectly good anti-pneumococcal polysaccharide antibodies are produced. So in that context, the polysaccharide is both immunogenic and antigenic. If the free polysaccharide is injected, it is difficult to raise antibody; so it itself is not immunogenic. The fundamental difference is that these peptides are both antigenic and immunogenic.

Anders: We don't know how immunogenic they are. We find abundant antibodies to the repeats of several antigens, in human populations of endemic areas, but these are people who have been infected many times.

Lerner: I am talking about the ability to induce an immune response with a piece of peptide sequence, free from the rest of the organism. You couldn't do that with pneumococcal polysaccharide.

Sela: In the same way in which the pneumococcal polysaccharide is antigenic but not immunogenic, *Bacillus anthracis* has a capsule of poly(γ-D-glutamic acid). When the organism is injected, 100% of the antibodies are against the polymer, but when the polymer is injected, there is no antibody response. However, this is a thymus-independent antigen and if you inject an extremely small amount, you may get immunological paralysis. If you make a polymer of the tetrapeptide or dodecapeptide, not simply attached to a protein, but a large polymer, I would predict from this discussion that it should be thymus-independent.

Anders: Immunization with the CS protein, produced in *E. coli* with different numbers of repeats (16, 32 or 48 tandem copies), resulted in an IgG response (Young et al 1985).

V. Nussenzweig: There are several points to be taken into consideration. The genetically engineered product contains 30 amino acids derived from the plasmid sequences in addition to the repeats, and they may serve as the carrier. Immunization with a polymer of repeats alone has not been tried, to my knowledge. The response to sporozoites—that is, to the intact CS antigen—is thymus-dependent. However, we don't know what part of the molecule is recognized by T cells; it may be the charged areas.

Anders: The other point is that we have been measuring IgG responses in human populations. There is a lot of IgG antibody to many of these repeat structures in the plasma of individuals living in endemic areas.

Corradin: Do you see increased affinity, going from children to adults?

V. Nussenzweig: Affinity has not previously been measured because we did not know the structure of the immunodominant epitope.

Alkan: Coming back to the general rules of immunogenicity, we have shown (Alkan et al 1972), that as a minimum requirement for immunogenicity, in the sense that a molecule induces both T and B cell responses, one needs a minimum of two epitopes. Second, these epitopes can be identical or different. A third rule is that at least one of the epitopes has to be recognized by a T cell. Consider poly(γ-D-glutamic acid) as an example. This is a non-immunogenic molecule; if you inject pure poly(γ-D-glutamic acid) into any given animal with any dose, you never produce an antibody, nor a T cell response (Alkan et al 1971). However, when you put a carrier epitope like azobenzenearsonate-L-tyrosine on this molecule it becomes immunogenic. In this example, the hapten (ABA-T) becomes a carrier and the carrier (polyglutamic acid) becomes a hapten. In other words, one produces high titres of antibody response against polyglutamic acid whereas the T cell response is directed against ABA-T. So I think that a single epitope can induce a T cell response (of course in association with MHC); but for an antibody response a minimum of two epitopes are required. And one of these epitopes has to be recognized by T cells.

Lerner: Should one put arsanyltyrosine on these malaria peptides?

Anders: You don't have to, because the repeats encode more than one epitope. In the full sequence of the CS protein there are four variant repeats which have changed two of the amino acids. In the S antigens there is some degeneracy in every one, and quite a lot in some. And in the RESA molecule there is degeneracy in the 3' and 5' repeats. Thus there is the capacity for multiple epitopes, which was the message I was trying to give. We have shown the multiple epitopes with monoclonals. There is the capacity for T and B recognition of independent epitopes within every repeat looked at.

Lerner: What about a perfect 12-mer?

V. Nussenzweig: To trigger an immune response, two epitopes are needed, but presumably they can be identical. In principle, the epitope recognized by the B cell could be processed and recognized by the T cell.

REFERENCES

Alkan SS, Nitecki DE, Goodman JW 1971 Antigen recognition and the immune response: the capacity of L-tyrosine-azobenzenearsonate to serve as a carrier for a macromolecular hapten. J Immunol 107:353-358

Alkan SS, Williams EB, Nitecki DE, Goodman JW 1972 Antigen recognition and the immune response. Humoral and cellular immune responses to small mono- and bifunctional antigen molecules. J Exp Med 135:1228-1246

Cowman AF, Coppel RL, Saint RB, Favaloro J, Crewther PE, Stahl HD, Bianco AE, Brown GV, Anders RF, Kemp DJ 1984 The ring-infected erythrocyte surface antigen (RESA) polypeptide of *Plasmodium falciparum* contains two separate blocks of tandem repeats encoding antigenic epitopes that are naturally immunogenic in man. Mol Biol Med 2:207-221

Cowman AF, Saint RB, Coppel RL, Brown GV, Anders RF, Kemp DJ 1985 Conserved sequences flank variable tandem repeats in two S-antigen genes of *Plasmodium falciparum*. Cell 40:775-783

Hope IA, Mackay M, Hyde JE, Goman M, Scaife J 1985 The gene for an exported antigen of the malaria parasite *Plasmodium falciparum* cloned and expressed in *Escherichia coli*. Nucleic Acids Res 13:369-379

Manser T, Wysocki LJ, Gridley T, Near RI, Gefter ML 1985 The molecular evolution of the immune response. Immunol Today 6:94-101

Perlmann H, Berzins K, Wahlgren M, Carlsson J, Björkman A, Patarroyo ME, Perlmann P 1984 Antibodies in malarial sera to antigens in the membrane of erythrocytes infected with early asexual stages of *Plasmodium falciparum*. J Exp Med 159:1686-1704

Saul A, Cooper J, Ingram L, Anders RF, Brown GV 1985 Invasion of erythrocytes *in vitro* by *Plasmodium falciparum* can be inhibited by a monoclonal antibody directed against an S antigen. Parasite Immunol, in press

Stahl HD, Crewther PE, Anders RF, Brown GV, Coppel RL, Bianco AE, Mitchell GF, Kemp DJ 1985 Interspersed blocks of repetitive and charged amino acids in a dominant immunogen of *Plasmodium falciparum*. Proc Natl Acad Sci USA 82:543-547

Werblin TP, Young TK, Quagliata F, Siskind GW 1973 Studies on the control of antibody synthesis. III. Changes in the heterogeneity of antibody affinity during the course of the immune response. Immunology 24:477-492

Young JF, Hockmeyer WG, Gross M et al 1985 Expression of *Plasmodium falciparum* circumsporozoite proteins in *Escherichia coli* for potential use in a human malaria vaccine. Science (Wash DC) 228:958-962

Synthetic peptides with antigenic specificity for bacterial toxins

MICHAEL SELA, RUTH ARNON and CHAIM O. JACOB

Department of Chemical Immunology, The Weizmann Institute of Science, Rehovot 76100, Israel

Abstract. The attachment of a diphtheria toxin-specific synthetic antigenic determinant and a synthetic adjuvant to a synthetic polymeric carrier led to production of a totally synthetic macromolecule which provoked protective antibodies against diphtheria when administered in aqueous solution.

When peptides related to the B subunit of cholera toxin were synthesized and attached to tetanus toxoid, antibodies produced against the conjugate reacted in some but not all cases with intact cholera toxin and (especially with peptide CTP 3, residues 50–64) neutralized toxin reactivity, as tested by permeability in rabbit skin, fluid accumulation in ligated small intestinal loops and adenylate cyclase activation. Polymerization of the peptide without any external carrier, or conjugation with the dipalmityl lysine group, had as good an effect in enhancing the immune response as its attachment to tetanus toxoid. Prior exposure to the carrier suppressed the immune response to the epitope attached to it, whereas prior exposure to the synthetic peptide had a good priming effect when the intact toxin was given; when two different peptides were attached to the same carrier, both were expressed. Antisera against peptide CTP 3 were highly cross-reactive with the heat-labile toxin of *Escherichia coli* and neutralized it to the same extent as cholera toxin, which is not surprising in view of the great homology between the two proteins. A synthetic oligonucleotide coding for CTP 3 has been used to express the peptide in a form suitable for immunization. It led to a priming effect against the intact cholera toxin.

1986 Synthetic peptides as antigens. Wiley, Chichester (Ciba Foundation Symposium 119) p 184-199

The availability of synthetic antigens has permitted two independent though related pathways of investigation. In one direction, we attempted to understand certain immunological phenomena better—mainly the molecular basis of antigenicity and immunogenicity, but also such aspects as the genetic control of the immune response, delayed hypersensitivity, and the molecular basis of immunological tolerance (Sela 1966, 1969). Work in the other direction was devoted to more practical applications of the knowledge acquired, and efforts were made towards the development of synthetic vaccines (Arnon

1972, Sela 1974), the specific induction of tolerance, the abolition of autoimmune diseases and the deviation of allergic phenomena.

The spatial folding of proteins plays a decisive role in determining their antigenic specificity, and it has been useful to distinguish between sequential and conformational determinants (Sela et al 1967). In a synthetic model we have shown that the same tripeptide, Tyr-Ala-Glu, may be used to build an immunogen possessing sequential or conformation-dependent antigenic determinants. Attaching it to a branched polymer produced an immunogen triggering the formation of antibodies specific towards the tripeptide. On the other hand, polymerizing the tripeptide led to a high molecular weight polymer possessing the α-helical form in aqueous solution, and the antibodies produced against it reacted well with the polymer but not with the tripeptide Tyr-Ala-Glu or its oligomers (Schechter et al 1971).

We have also shown that a low molecular weight polymer of Tyr-Ala-Glu is not helical, but may be 'transconformed' into a helical shape upon reaction with antibodies to the high molecular weight helical polymer (Schechter et al 1971). This is a clear example of the transconformation occurring when two biologically active macromolecules react via their active sites.

This has also been described for a p-azobenzenearsonate conjugate of the helical polymer (Tyr-Ala-Glu)$_n$ as compared with the conjugate of a random copolymer composed of the same amino acid residues, namely (Tyr,Ala,Glu)$_n$. Only the random conjugate elicited anti-p-azobenzenearsonate antibodies. Moreover, such antibodies would transconform and 'suck-out' the p-azobenzenearsonate moiety from the helical polymer, as readily followed spectroscopically (Conway-Jacobs et al 1970). Another example is the conformational changes induced in anti-polyprolyl antibodies by oligoprolines of different sizes (Forster & Sela 1979).

In globular proteins, most of the antigenic determinants are conformational, as is evident from the loss of reaction with their antibodies after denaturation. It follows that small conformational changes would be expressed as a change in antigenic reactivity that can be detected by antibodies. Antibodies are, therefore, good probes for the conformational state of proteins and there are many reported cases in which antibodies were used to detect different conformations in proteins.

Antibodies to a native protein would be expected to be a mixture of those elicited by rigid, unique conformations (such antibodies would not be expected to cross-react well immunologically with related small synthetic peptides), and those against the more flexible regions within the protein (in which case, the chance of cross-reaction with small peptides would be much higher). Even if a small peptide may potentially be transconformed into an exceedingly large number of possible conformations, it is clear that only a few of these conformations will be thermodynamically the most stable, and thus the number of species of antibodies elicited by such a peptide will be limited. It is, therefore, not surprising that in such cases some of the antibodies cross-react, rather efficiently, via such a flexible region, with the parent native protein. Following this rationale, we chose to study hen egg-white lysozyme, and have shown that an immunopotent region of the molecule (residues 60–83 in the amino acid sequence) is a peptide which we denoted 'loop', as it consists of a polypeptide chain closed through a disulphide bridge. We synthesized this peptide, attached it to a synthetic branched polymer, and after immunization obtained antibodies reacting with native lysozyme through this unique region which is conformation-dependent, as the opening of the disulphide bridge abolished the immune reaction (Arnon & Sela 1969, Arnon et al 1971). Comparable results were obtained with another system, the carcinoembryonic antigen (CEA) of the colon, a glycoprotein of M_r of about 200 000. A synthetic peptide corresponding to the 11 amino acid residues of the N-terminal portion of the molecule, attached to a macromolecular carrier, provoked anti-peptide antibodies that reacted not only with the homologous antigen but also with the intact CEA molecule (Arnon et al 1976), and could serve in an immuno-diagnostic assay for CEA in sera of cancer patients (Arnon et al 1978).

Synthetic vaccines

This work opened up conceptually the road to the synthetic vaccines of the future as it pinpointed the possibility of preparing synthetically relevant determinants of viral coat proteins and bacterial toxins. It also led us to conclude that the antigenic determinants of an immunogenic macromolecule are recognized, and, as it were, the order for the immune response goes out, while this macromolecule is still intact, because otherwise the whole conformation would collapse, and native determinants would not be available.

Vaccination against both bacterial and viral diseases has been one of the major achievements in immunology since the beginning of the last century. However, while existing vaccines have certainly diminished the incidence, morbidity and mortality of many infectious diseases, some of them are still very difficult to prevent and control by prophylactic means. The present mode of vaccination includes the use of killed or live attenuated microbial agents, purified viral proteins or their subunits, and bacterial toxoids. In many cases it has led to successful vaccines, but several major problems still await solution—for example, the lack of sufficient source material, since not all viruses can be cultured and developed into effective vaccines; or safety considerations due to the hazardous effects of some vaccines, caused by insufficient attenuation. Another problem, not yet overcome, is that many existing viruses constantly evolve into new strains, with different serological specificities, thus requiring the continuous development of new vaccines. The synthetic approach offers a potential solution to these problems. According to this approach, vaccines will consist of a synthetic material comprising only the relevant antigenic moiety leading to protective immunity. Such vaccines can be synthesized, either chemically or by genetic engineering, in large amounts, and will not present safety hazards to the individual or the community (Sela 1974, 1983, Sela & Arnon 1981, Arnon et al 1983).

The vaccines of the future should ideally contain within one molecule a specific synthetic antigenic determinant capable of provoking a protective immune response, and a synthetic adjuvant, both covalently attached to a macromolecular synthetic carrier. If possible, several specificities characteristic of different diseases should be linked covalently within the same macromolecule. Ultimately, the choice of the carrier may depend—for optimal results–on the genetic background of the recipient. In order to obtain long-lasting immunity it will be necessary also to take into consideration the correct texture of the synthetic vaccines to be used for immunization.

Appropriate objectives for this type of investigation are the bacterial toxins, immunization against which (e.g. with tetanus, diphtheria or pertussis toxoids) has been used in the past to provide neutralization of toxicity and hence protection.

Diphtheria toxin

This protein consists of a single polypeptide chain of M_r 62 000 with two disulphide bridges. Audibert et al (1981) have shown that active immunization against diphtheria can be achieved by a synthetic peptide attached to a protein carrier. This peptide, a tetradecapeptide consisting of residues 188–201 in the amino acid sequence of the toxin, represents a loop fragment which in the native protein is sustained by a disulphide bridge near the N-terminus of the molecule. Conjugates of this peptide, or the hexadecapeptide 186–201, linked covalently to a protein carrier or to a synthetic polypeptide carrier, elicited in guinea-pigs antibodies which not only bind specifically to the toxin but also neutralize its dermonecrotic activity and lethal effect.

This and several other peptides were also attached to multichain poly-DL-alanine (Audibert et al 1982). When the resulting conjugates were injected into guinea-pigs and mice, either in complete Freund's adjuvant or with N-acetylmuramyl-L-alanyl-D-isoglutamine (muramyl dipeptide, MDP), positive immune responses were obtained. Moreover, a most effective immune response was obtained in mice with a synthetic conjugate comprising both a related octadecapeptide and MDP covalently attached to the synthetic multichain poly-DL-alanine. The completely synthetic immunogen with built-in adjuvanticity induced protective antitoxic immunity when administered in a physiological medium. This was the first report of effective protective immunization against disease-causing bacteria with a totally synthetic vaccine in the absence of Freund's adjuvant.

Cholera toxin

We have used the synthetic approach to provoke antibodies cross-reactive with cholera toxin, that are also capable of partially neutralizing its biological activity. The toxin of *Vibrio cholerae* is composed of two subunits, A and B. Subunit A activates adenylate cyclase, which triggers the biological activity, whereas subunit B is responsible for binding to cell receptors and expresses most of the immunopotent determinants. Antibodies to the B subunits are capable of neutralizing the biological activity of the intact toxin. In view of its immunodominant role, the B subunit was the obvious candidate for this investigation. Moreover, in view of the high level of sequence homology between the B subunits of cholera toxin (CT) and the heat-labile toxin of *Escherichia coli* (LT), we have also investigated whether the same synthetic peptides will also cross-react with the *E. coli* toxin.

Six peptides have been synthesized, corresponding to various segments of the B subunit of cholera toxin (Fig. 1). We selected these particular peptides

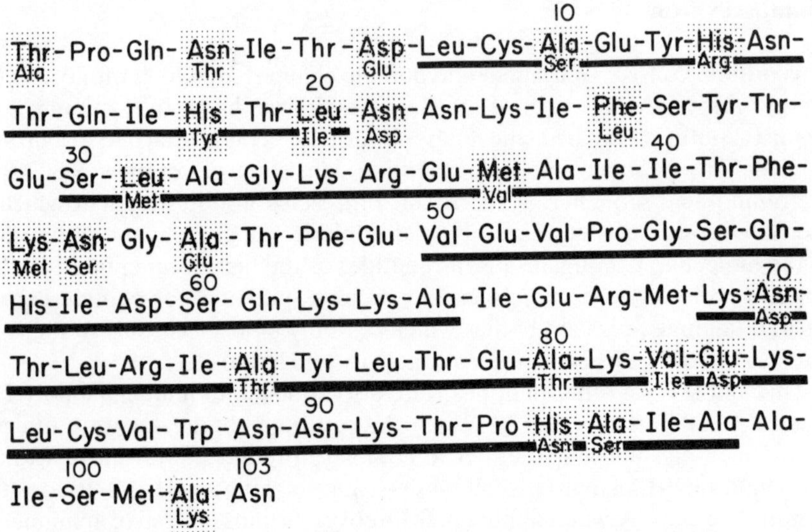

FIG. 1. Primary amino acid sequence of the B subunit of cholera toxin as quoted by Lai (1980). Regions of the protein selected for synthesis are underlined. The residues in the shaded boxes are those which differ in the sequence of the heat-labile toxin of *E. coli*.

on the basis of our preliminary studies with cyanogen bromide fragments of the B subunits, as well as studies from other laboratories on antigenically important regions of this protein. The six peptides, corresponding to sequences 8–20, 30–42, 50–64, 69–85, 75–85 and 83–97, denoted CTP 1 to CTP 6, respectively, were coupled to tetanus toxoid and used to immunize rabbits and mice.

Evaluation of the immunological reactivity of the resultant antisera by radioimmunoassay, immunoprecipitation and immunoblotting indicated that four antisera out of the six that were raised against the appropriate peptides also reacted, to different extents, with the intact B subunit and the native cholera toxin, whereas two peptides, namely CTP 2 and CTP 5, elicited antibodies with specificity limited to the respective peptides (Fig. 2). The antisera against peptides CTP 1 and CTP 6 showed a very high level of reactivity with the respective homologous peptides but reacted only slightly (several orders of magnitude difference) with the intact B subunit or cholera toxin. Incidentally, anti-CTP 1 also reacted with the A subunit of cholera toxin. On the other hand, peptide CTP 3 induced antibodies that, although of lower absolute titre, showed strong cross-reactivity with the intact toxin, very similar in level to the homologous peptide–anti-peptide reaction. This peptide was the only one that also reacted with antiserum against the native cholera toxin.

The CTP 4 and CTP 5 peptides are of interest from another point of view. Antibodies to CTP 5 failed to cross-react with either the B subunit or whole toxin, although they showed appreciable reactivity with the homologous peptide. Elongation of CTP 5 by six amino acid residues resulted in CTP 4,

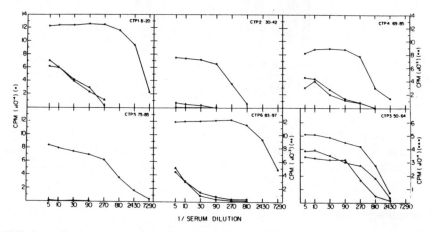

FIG. 2. Antibody response of rabbits to different peptides of the B subunit of cholera toxin. Reactions were carried out with the homologous peptides (●), the B subunit of cholera toxin (▲), and cholera toxin (○). Note the differences in the scales of the reactions with the peptide and the intact proteins for all peptides except CTP 3.

which elicited antibodies cross-reactive with the intact proteins, even though the homologous anti-peptide titre was not significantly higher than with CTP 5.

Of most interest among these peptides were CTP 1 (residues 8–20) and CTP 3 (residues 50–64). Antisera against these two peptides significantly inhibited the biological activity of cholera toxin. The toxic effect of CT can be demonstrated by skin vascular permeation and by fluid accumulation in ligated small intestinal loops, as well as on the biochemical level, by the induction of adenylate cyclase. The anti-peptide sera were inhibitory in all assays of

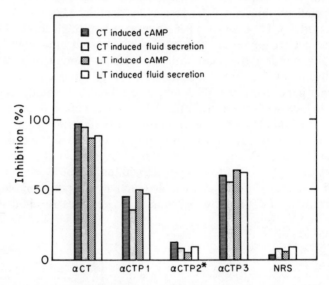

FIG. 3. Inhibition of the biological activity of cholera toxin (CT) and heat-labile toxin of *E. coli* (LT) by rabbit antisera against the synthetic peptides. *Antisera against CTP 4, 5 and 6 had similar effects as anti-CTP 2. NRS, normal rabbit serum.

the biological activity of the toxin, with very good correlation between the biochemical level and the end biological effect of the toxin (Fig. 3). In both cases, inhibition reaches approximately 60% (Jacob et al 1983, 1984a).

Heat-labile toxin of E. coli

The heat-labile toxin (LT) of pathogenic strains of *E. coli* is the causative agent of diarrhoea in many tropical countries and, because of its wide distribution, probably presents a more serious health problem than cholera. As mentioned above, and also demonstrated in Fig. 1, there is a high level of sequence homology between the B subunits of the LT and cholera toxin (CT). Moreover, immunological relationship was demonstrated between the two toxins, with the existence of both shared and specific antigenic determinants (Lindholm et al 1983). We therefore investigated whether the synthetic peptides derived from cholera toxin might cross-react with the LT and/or provide a comparable degree of protection against the heterologous toxin.

In a recent study (Jacob et al 1984b) we have demonstrated that the antiserum elicited by CTP 3 (residues 50–64) is highly cross-reactive with the LT in both radioimmunoassay and immunoblotting. This is not surprising, since in this region the sequence homology between the two toxins is complete (Fig. 1). The antiserum against CTP 1 (residues 8–20) was also cross-reactive with the two toxins, although to a much lower extent. However, antisera to both CTP 1 and CTP 3, which are inhibitory towards cholera toxin, were equally effective in neutralizing the biological activity of the E. coli LT, as shown by significant inhibition of both adenylate cyclase induction and fluid secretion into ligated ileal loops of rabbits (Fig. 3). The inhibition by the anti-CTP 3 was expected, in view of the high level of immunological cross-reactivity.

These results suggest that the two synthetic peptides, corresponding to sequences 8–20 and 50–64 of cholera toxin, may be good candidates for the development of synthetic vaccines since they elicit antibodies that not only cross-react immunologically, but also neutralize the biological activity of the toxin. Any realistic approach to this system must take into consideration the development of adjuvants that are acceptable for use in humans, preferably built-in adjuvanticity, as well as the possibility of inducing effective local immunity. Yet, the clear-cut demonstration that these antisera also cross-react and neutralize the LT of E. coli suggests the potential of these peptides as the basis for a future general vaccine against the coli–cholera family of diarrhoeal diseases.

Effect of carrier on immunogenic capacity

In all the experiments described so far, the carrier for the cholera toxin peptides was tetanus toxoid. In the design of synthetic antigens and synthetic vaccines, primary consideration should be given to the choice of carrier. Since small peptides that are being used as the relevant antigenic determinants are likely to be poor immunogens as such, the augmentation of their immunogenic capacity by the carrier or any other means is crucial for the induction of immunity. On the other hand, the carrier may have a profound effect on the immune response of the host. We have therefore explored several ways of enhancing the immune response to synthetic peptides derived from cholera toxin.

It was interesting to note that for each of the peptides, polymerization without any external carrier, or conjugation to a lipid moiety such as the dipalmityl lysine group, had a comparable effect to that of tetanus toxoid (TT) carrier conjugation in enhancing the specific immune response towards the peptide, as well as in eliciting cross-reactive immunity to the intact toxin (Jacob et al 1985). In most cases the capacity of the antibodies obtained with the different preparations to neutralize the biological activity of the toxin was also similar to the neutralization effected by the antisera against the peptide–TT conjugate (Fig. 4). It is thus apparent that in the foreseeable future the design of an optimal vehicle for synthetic peptide antigens will be feasible.

An extremely important observation is that prior exposure to the carrier alone has a substantial, dose-dependent, epitope-specific suppressive effect on the immune response to the epitopes attached to it (Table 1). In rabbits immunized with TT conjugates, both primary and secondary responses to the peptides were suppressed after pretreatment with tetanus toxoid (Jacob et al 1985). This phenomenon is of special significance and should be borne

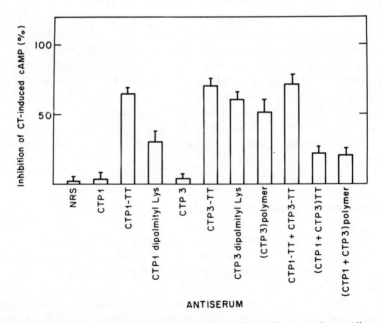

FIG. 4. Inhibition of cholera toxin (CT)-induced cyclic AMP by different antisera. All measurements were made after 3 h incubation of 50 ng CT with 1:10 dilution of the indicated antisera. NRS, normal rabbit serum. Values are means ± SEM.

TABLE 1 CTP 3-specific suppression induced by pretreatment of rabbits with tetanus toxoid (TT) carrier

Group	Pretreatment (Day 0)	Antibody response to immunization with CTP3–TT[a]		Anti-carrier (Day 74)
		Anti-CTP3		
		(Day 44)	(Day 74)	
1	—	1750	59 000	77 000
2	TT (1 μg)	950	61 000	83 000
3	TT (10 μg)	900	53 000	75 000
4	TT (100 μg)	250	21 000	79 000
5	TT (1 mg)	250	2800	81 000

[a]Each rabbit was immunized at Day 30 (primary) and Day 60 (secondary) with 1 mg CTP 3–TT in complete Freund's adjuvant. The values represent the mean c.p.m. in solid-phase radioimmunoassay obtained with a 1:100 dilution of serum.

in mind when one considers TT as a carrier for human use, in view of its worldwide application for anti-tetanus vaccination. The quantities of tetanus toxoid used in human vaccines are usually small and probably below the threshold of suppressive activity. However, caution on this issue, and the continuing exploration of better immunization technologies, are essential for the development of novel effective vaccines towards the bacterial toxins.

Combined use of synthetic peptides and recombinant DNA for priming of anticholera toxin immunity

In parallel to the application of synthetic peptides for the preparation of vaccines as already described, attempts are being made to apply genetic engineering methodology for the insertion of relevant genes into an appropriate vector (e.g. vaccinia virus) that could be used for vaccination (Smith et al 1983). In a recent, unpublished study, we attempted to bridge the synthetic and recombinant DNA approaches by using a product of a synthetic cholera toxin-relevant 'gene' to elicit an anti-cholera immune response. Having identified CTP 3 as a highly relevant epitope, our working hypothesis was that expression of this peptide by bacteria may provide an appropriate agent for the induction of immunity towards cholera and *E. coli* toxins, and that this could be approached by recombinant DNA techniques.

For that purpose we constructed plasmids containing the DNA sequence encoding this peptide, fused in phase to a truncated *lac* Z gene. The CTP 3–β-galactosidase hybrid protein specified by these plasmids was indeed expressed by the transformed *E. coli*. When used to immunize rabbits, a

194   SELA ET AL

single intradermal injection of this protein led to a strong specific priming immunity. Boosted by a minute quantity of cholera toxin, ineffective by itself, it resulted in a substantial level of antibodies reactive with both cholera toxin and heat-labile toxin of *E. coli*. These antibodies efficiently neutralized the biological activities of cholera toxin. We have thus demonstrated that recombinant DNA methodology can be implemented for vaccine development by using synthetic oligonucleotides encoding relatively small peptides, providing that such peptides are endowed with the relevant immunological properties.

In conclusion, we have demonstrated that it is feasible to induce protective immunity against bacterial toxins by the use of synthetic conjugates of immunologically relevant peptides with protein carriers. Such conjugates provoked antibodies that were cross-reactive with cholera toxin and heat-labile toxin of *E. coli*, and also capable of neutralizing their biological activity. Alternatively, polymers of the peptides without any external carrier, or conjugates with a lipid moiety, can lead to efficient protective immunity as well. Moreover, the availability of such relevant synthetic peptides and their utilization as a basis for synthetic vaccines can also be combined with genetic engineering. Although problems still exist, and many improvements have to be introduced, there are several advantages to the application of this approach. Synthetic vaccines can be designed with built in adjuvanticity; they can provide multivalent vaccines with cross-strain specificity for antiviral protection; and, as has been demonstrated here, their high potential as a general vaccine against the coli–cholera family emphasizes their future prospects.

REFERENCES

Arnon R 1972 Synthetic vaccines—dream or reality? In: Kohen A, Klinberg AM (eds) Immunity of viral and rickettsial diseases. Plenum Press, New York, p 209-222
Arnon R, Sela M 1969 Antibodies to a unique region in lysozyme provoked by a synthetic antigen conjugate. Proc Natl Acad Sci USA 62:163-170
Arnon R, Maron E, Sela M, Anfinsen CB 1971 Antibodies reactive with a native lysozyme elicited by a completely synthetic antigen. Proc Natl Acad Sci USA 68:1450-1454
Arnon R, Bustin M, Calef E, Chaitchik S, Haimovich J, Novik N, Sela M 1976 Immunological cross-reactivity of antibodies to a synthetic undecapeptide of carcinoembryonic antigen with the intact protein and human sera. Proc Natl Acad Sci USA 73:2123-2127
Arnon R, Novik N, Haimovich J, Chaitchik S 1978 Viroimmunoassay utilizing a synthetic peptide: a test equivalent to carcinoembryonic antigen radioimmunoassay. Isr J Med Sci 13:1022-1027
Arnon R, Shapira M, Jacob CO 1983 Synthetic vaccines. J Immunol Methods 61:261-273
Audibert F, Jolivet M, Chedid L, Alouf JE, Boquet P, Rivaille P, Siffret O 1981 Active antitoxic immunization by a diphtheria toxin synthetic oligopeptide. Nature (Lond) 289:593-595

Audibert F, Jolivet M, Chedid L, Arnon R, Sela M 1982 Successful immunization with a totally synthetic diphtheria vaccine. Proc Natl Acad Sci USA 79:5042-5045

Conway-Jacobs A, Schechter B, Sela M 1970 Extrinsic Cotton effect and immunological properties of the *p*-azobenzenearsonate hapten attached to a helical amino acid copolymer. Biochemistry 9:4870-4875

Forster HK, Sela M 1979 Conformational changes induced in antipoly(L-prolyl) antibodies by oligoproline haptens of different sizes. Mol Immunol 16:651-656

Jacob CO, Sela M, Arnon R 1983 Antibodies against synthetic peptides of the B subunit of cholera toxin: cross-reaction and neutralization of the toxin. Proc Natl Acad Sci USA 80:7611-7615

Jacob CO, Sela M, Pines M, Hurwitz S, Arnon R 1984a Adenylate cyclase activation by cholera toxin as well as its activity are inhibited with antibody against related synthetic peptides. Proc Natl Acad Sci USA 81:7893-7897

Jacob CO, Pines M, Arnon R 1984b Neutralization of heat labile toxin of E. coli by antibody to synthetic peptides derived from B subunit of cholera toxin. EMBO (Eur Mol Biol Organ) J 3:2889-2893

Jacob CO, Arnon R, Sela M 1985 Effect of carrier on the immunogenic capacity of synthetic cholera vaccine. Mol Immunol, in press

Lai CY 1980 Cholera toxin. CRC Crit Rev Biochem 9:171-207

Lindholm L, Holmgren J, Wikstrom M, Karlsson V, Andersson K, Lycke N 1983 Monoclonal antibodies to cholera toxin with special reference to cross-reactions with *Escherichia coli* heat-labile enterotoxin. Infect Immun 40:570-576

Schechter B, Conway-Jacobs A, Sela M 1971 Conformational changes in a synthetic antigen induced by specific antibodies. Eur J Biochem 20:321-324

Sela M 1966 Immunological studies with synthetic polypeptides. Adv Immunol 5:29-129

Sela M 1969 Antigenicity: some molecular aspects. Science (Wash DC) 166:1365-1375

Sela M 1974 Vaccins synthétiques: Un rêve ou une réalité? Bull Inst Pasteur 72:73-86

Sela M 1983 From synthetic antigens to synthetic vaccines. Biopolymers 22:415-424

Sela M, Arnon R 1981 Immunological approaches to vaccines of the future. In: Bachmann PA (ed) Biological products for viral diseases. Taylor & Francis, London, p 21-37

Sela M, Schechter I, Schechter B, Borek F 1967 Antibodies to sequential and conformational determinants. Cold Spring Harbor Symp Quant Biol 32:537-545

Smith GL, Mackett M, Moss B 1983 Infectious vaccinia virus recombinants that express hepatitis B virus surface antigen. Nature (Lond) 302:490-495

DISCUSSION

Ada: You described the suppressive effect of preimmunization with carrier. Herzenberg & Tokuhisa (1982) also showed this suppression. Have any detailed studies been made, as regards dose of antigen and how long the effect lasts after priming with the carrier? And has Dr Lachmann noticed this with the PPD system?

Lachmann: We have not encountered this problem with PPD, but it is a well-known phenomenon.

V. Nussenzweig: Dr Sela obtained a significant suppressive effect in complete Freund's adjuvant only with 1 mg of tetanus toxoid, a dose that would never be used in a human being, where the dose is normally less than 10 μg (Table 1, p 193).

Secondly, so far as I know, such suppressive effects were not seen when *Haemophilus influenzae* type B polysaccharides were coupled to diphtheria toxoid as a vaccine (M.I. Lepow, personal communication). We also have done competition experiments between determinants on the same molecule (Pincus & Nussenzweig 1969). If you immunize with IgG as antigen and passively transfer antibodies to the Fab part of the molecule, you greatly enhance the response to the Fc portion and suppress the response to Fab. So one can't really predict the outcome of immunization with a peptide–carrier conjugate if the animal is presensitized with the carrier.

Sela: As you correctly say, one normally immunizes against tetanus with microgram quantities. If one injects with milligrams of tetanus toxoid to which various peptide epitopes are attached, the danger may be that paralysis against tetanus is induced in people already immunized to it.

Ada: Is this a theoretical danger, or have you shown it to happen?

Sela: I haven't done this, but Audibert and Chedid mentioned it recently.

V. Nussenzweig: The maximum amount of tetanus toxoid that you can inject into a person without causing ill-effects is about 50 μg (E.H. Relyveld, personal communication). But as a general question: what is the ideal carrier, if it is not tetanus toxoid, diphtheria toxoid, cholera toxin derivatives or PPD?

Lachmann: Work on carrier preimmunization as originally done by Rajewsky et al (1969) and by Mitchison (1971a,b) showed consistent enhancement of antibody response, whereas Roger Taylor obtained suppressor cells (Elson & Taylor 1974). The result seems to depend on what carrier is chosen, how much is given, and by what route. Supra-optimal amounts of priming antigen give rise to suppression (see Claman et al 1980). So, for a successful carrier, one wants an antigen of such a type and given in such a way that it doesn't induce suppression but induces T cell help.

Lerner: Keyhole limpet haemocyanin (KLH) is being used as a carrier in the studies of the synthetic hepatitis vaccine in chimpanzees. You can get enormous antibody responses, of course, to KLH. You also get good antibody responses to the free pre-S peptide, with a switch from 19S to 7S; each time KLH is injected the anti-peptide response is boosted, in the face of overwhelming titres of anti-KLH antibody. So, in this instance, boosting the response does not seem to be a problem.

Lachmann: A trick for enhancing antibody responses was invented in Coons' laboratory (Shek & Coons 1978, Shek et al 1978). The antigen in the first injection is mixed with colchicine, which—since suppressor T cells are the first cells to divide in response to antigen—can prevent their division and thereby give enhanced T cell help. This works well in experimental animals!

Brown: We have done experiments on foot-and-mouth disease virus peptides in which we injected first with carrier and found no effect on the response to the secondary injection. The amount of carrier and the nature of the adjuvant all affect the outcome, as has been said.

Sela: I don't want to generalize from one series of experiments, but I felt I should show it.

Gupta: In answer to Dr Nussenzweig's question of which carrier we should use, Talwar's group have done some interesting experiments. When they inject a particular antigen with a particular carrier, if the antibody response is poor and then later on they give the booster injection using the same antigen on a different carrier, they obtain a good immune response. They have done this using tetanus toxoid as the first carrier and cholera toxoid as the second. They got a very good antibody response to human chorionic gonadotropin (Talwar et al 1985).

Sela: The question really is not what carrier to use, but how to make the peptide express itself efficiently in the immune response. The most obvious way is to find the right carrier, but we know by now that there are other ways, even though each has its disadvantages. I refer to attaching a fatty acid, putting the peptide into a micelle, polymerizing it, and so on. The real problem is to find the best way to immunize to get a good crop of antibodies, and a good specific cellular immune response.

Lerner: One wants a substance that is readily available to use as a carrier. It turns out that a number of plant proteins are useful, especially edestin, which is as good a carrier as KLH. It is cheap, you can get all you want and, as it comes from the seed of *Cannabis sativa*, you can fund your research from the rest of the plant!

McConnell: Presumably we should think of carriers that might lack suppressor determinants. Sercarz and his colleagues (Adorini et al 1979) studied the L_{II} peptide of hen egg-white lysozyme, which is unlike the whole molecule in that it lacks a suppressor determinant. Are there other carriers like this? Is it known whether KLH has suppressor determinants? Perhaps PPD is a bit like the L_{II} region of lysozyme in that it lacks suppressor determinants and therefore makes a good 'universal' carrier.

Sela: I have no simple answer to Dr Nussenzweig's question, but obviously I have a prejudice! Other things being equal I would prefer to use as a carrier a digestible synthetic polymer of amino acids rather than a protein that occurs in Nature and can be cross-reactive with something else. I would be afraid to use non-digestible polymers, because they last too long. Perhaps this is not a real worry, but it's safer to use a digestible one. For many purposes, branched polyalanine is adequate, and it is a very poor immunogen. Generally, in my opinion, the preferred carrier is not KLH or other strong immunogens but a weak immunogen. The plant antigens, like edestin or gliadin, are poor antigens but good carriers. This gives a better chance that the relevant epitope will be able to express itself.

Brown: The information seems to be emerging that you can immunize without a carrier, if you polymerize the peptide in some way. If so, maybe we should be looking towards using no carrier at all in vaccines.

Corradin: You said you can put palmitic acid on the antigen, Dr Sela. What about using liposomes?

Sela: There is a lot of work on liposomes, but would we like to inject them into people? We have to consider where they go, where they stay, and how long they stick around. Liposomes from this point of view are similar to undigestible polystyrene polymers. As research tools they are useful, but I would doubt that liposomes would be the solution as vaccine carriers.

Heusser: We know of the importance of presenting an antigen on a cell surface when we want to amplify the induction of an immune response. Dipalmityl conjugation may well serve as a lipid anchor leading to the attachment of antigen to cells. Thus, the enhanced response observed might well be due to such an optimized antigen-presenting situation.

Alkan: How about using muramyl dipeptide, which serves not only as a carrier but also as an adjuvant, as you showed?

Sela: You mean attaching muramyl dipeptide to the peptide? We have done something on this, but I would still rather polymerize the peptide, attach it to a carrier or cross-link it, and only then attach the muramyl dipeptide.

Lachmann: There are several points to bear in mind when it comes to immunizing people rather than animals. One is that the dose of antigen should be kept low, to avoid Arthus and serum sickness reactions which people tolerate less well than rabbits. This is one reason why I think carrier-free immunization with large doses of weak antigens is likely to be disadvantageous. Furthermore, the occasional subject will have an anaphylactic reaction to almost any antigen, and the dangers of a severe reaction will be reduced by giving small doses of antigen made as highly immunogenic as possible rather than injecting larger amounts. I don't think it is practical, for example, to give repeated injections of KLH; some subjects will develop unpleasant Arthus reactions after the second or later injections.

REFERENCES

Adorini L, Harvey MA, Miller A, Sercarz EE 1979 Fine specificity of regulatory T cells. II. Suppressor and helper T cells are induced by different regions of hen egg-white lysozyme in a genetically nonresponder mouse strain. J Exp Med 150:293-306

Claman HN, Miller SD, Conlon PJ, Moorhead JW 1980 Control of experimental contact sensitivity. Adv Immunol 30:121-157

Elson CJ, Taylor RB 1974 The suppressor effect of carrier priming on the response to a hapten–carrier conjugate. Eur J Immunol 4:682-687

Herzenberg LA, Tokuhisa T 1982 Epitope-specific regulation. I. Carrier-specific induction of suppression for IgG anti-hapten antibody responses. J Exp Med 155:1730-1740

Mitchison NA 1971a The carrier effect in the secondary response to hapten–protein conjugates. I. Measurement of the effect with transferred cells and objections to the local environment hypothesis. Eur J Immunol 1:10-17

Mitchison NA 1971b The carrier effect in the secondary response to hapten–protein conjugates. II. Cellular cooperation. Eur J Immunol 1:18-27

Pincus CS, Nussenzweig V 1969 Passive antibody may simultaneously suppress and stimulate antibody formation against different portions of a protein molecule. Nature (Lond) 222:594-596

Rajewsky K, Schirrmacher V, Nase S, Jerne NK 1969 The requirement of more than one antigenic determinant for immunogenicity. J Exp Med 129:1131-1143

Shek PN, Coons AH 1978 Effect of colchicine on the antibody response. I. Enhancement of antibody formation in mice. J Exp Med 147:1213-1227

Shek PN, Waltenbaugh C, Coons AH 1978 Effect of colchicine on the antibody response. II. Demonstration of the inactivation of suppressor cell activities by colchicine. J Exp Med 147:1228-1235

Talwar GP, Singh O, Sharma NC et al 1985 An improved birth control vaccine inducing antibodies against human chorionic gonadotropin. Proc Natl Acad Sci USA, in press

Use of synthetic peptides as immunogens for developing a vaccine against human chorionic gonadotropin

VERNON C. STEVENS

Department of Obstetrics and Gynecology, Ohio State University, Division of Reproductive Biology, Means Hall, 1654 Upham Drive, Columbus, Ohio 43210-1228, USA

Abstract. Human chorionic gonadotropin (hCG) is a glycoprotein hormone produced by the placental trophoblast soon after conception and is essential for successful gestation in women. A vaccine against this hormone has been developed for the purposes of birth control and the treatment of hormone-related diseases. Synthetic peptides representing the native primary structure of the hCG β subunit have been coupled to protein carriers to produce immunogens. Several peptides, representing varying lengths from the C-terminus of the β subunit, were synthesized and their ability to elicit antibodies reactive to hCG and able to neutralize hCG activity *in vivo* was tested. A peptide representing the 37 amino acids of the C-terminal end of the β subunit was selected as the vaccine antigen and diphtheria toxoid was selected as the carrier for the first prototype vaccine. Procedures for coupling a specified number of peptide molecules to each carrier molecule in a reproducible fashion were developed. The immunogen is mixed with an adjuvant compound and the mixture administered in an oil-in-water emulsion. Significant levels of antibodies to hCG have been elicited in several species and a marked reduction in the fertility of immunized baboons has been observed. Extensive evaluations of vaccine safety have been conducted and Phase I clinical trials have been proposed to test its utility for human birth control. Possible applications of the hCG vaccine to health problems other than birth control are being considered.

1986 Synthetic peptides as antigens. Wiley, Chichester (Ciba Foundation Symposium 119) p 200-225

New methods of birth control are needed to meet the increasing demand for more effective global population regulation. The development of an immunological means of preventing or disrupting human fertility is one of several approaches being used in the search for new antifertility methods. Several strategies are possible for immunological intervention in pregnancy, but the development of a vaccine against the placental hormone human chorionic gonadotropin (hCG) is perhaps the most promising approach for an effective method in the immediate future. As hCG is known to be essential for successful pregnancy in women, a safe and effective vaccine against it would offer many advantages over existing methods of birth control.

The chemical similarities between hCG and several hormones secreted by the pituitary have required the use of hormone fragments as immunogens to elicit specific immune responses to hCG. Extensive studies have been conducted during the past several years to define peptide antigens of the hCG molecule suitable for vaccine development. Methods of coupling peptides to carrier molecules, the selection of the most effective carriers and adjuvants, and the formulation of vaccine delivery systems have also been addressed. A prototype vaccine has been obtained for preliminary clinical evaluation.

Antigen selection

hCG is a glycoprotein with a relative molecular mass (M_r) of 38 000. The hormone contains two non-covalently linked dissimilar subunits (α and β). The α subunit is about 14 500 in M_r and contains 28% carbohydrate, while the β subunit has an M_r of 22 000 with 32% carbohydrate. The α subunit is identical in structure to the α subunits of pituitary glycoprotein hormones (luteinizing hormone, LH; follicle-stimulating hormone, FSH; and thyrotropin, TSH). The β subunit is receptor-specific for target tissues, whereas the α subunit has no hormone-specific properties.

Antisera raised to the intact hCG molecule cross-react highly with other hormones, particularly hLH, whereas antisera to the hCG β subunit react poorly with hLH. Reports of this selective reactivity with hCG by antisera to β-hCG, with low reactivity of these antisera against hLH (Vaitukaitis et al 1972), suggested that the β subunit of hCG could be used to develop an antifertility vaccine. However, subsequent studies showed that immunization with β-hCG consistently elicited antisera with some reactivity to hLH. Reports later appeared describing the amino acid sequences of hCG and hLH (Morgan et al 1973) and revealing extensive homology in the primary structures of the β subunits of hCG and hLH. However, the hCG subunit contains 30 more amino acids on its C-terminus than β-hLH. Also, few residues were identical in both hormone subunits beyond the last common cysteine residue at position 110 of the 145 residues in β-hCG (Fig. 1). The availability of these sequences provided an opportunity to evaluate peptides at the C-terminus of β-hCG for development of a vaccine specific for hCG.

Epitopes on β-hCG

To date, only continuous determinant sites on the C-terminus of the β-hCG molecule, not related to β-hLH sequences, have been assessed as immunogens.

202   STEVENS

AMINO ACID SEQUENCE OF β hCG & β hLH

```
        I                          10                          20              25
                                  (CHO)
β-hCG   H₂N-Ser-Lys-Glu-Pro-Leu-Arg-Pro-Arg-Cys-Arg-Pro-Ile-Asn-Ala-Thr-Leu-Ala-Val-Glu-Lys-Glu-Gly-Cys-Pro-Val-
β-hLH   H₂N-   -Arg-  -  -  -  -   -Trp-  -His-  -  -  -   -Ile-  -  -  -Gln-  -  -  -  -  -  -

        26                 30                                40                          50
                          (CHO)
β-hCG   Cys-Ile-Thr-Val-Asn-Thr-Thr-Ile-Cys-Ala-Gly-Tyr-Cys-Pro-Thr-Met-Thr-Arg-Val-Leu-Gln-Gly-Val-Leu-Pro-
β-hLH   -  -  -  -  -  -  -  -  -  -  -  -  -  -  -  -  -Arg-Met-Leu-  -  -Ala-  -  -  -

        51                          60                          70              75
β-hCG   Ala-Leu-Pro-Gln-Val-Val-Cys-Asn-Tyr-Arg-Asp-Val-Arg-Phe-Glu-Ser-Ile-Arg-Leu-Pro-Gly-Cys-Pro-Arg-Gly-
β-hLH   Pro-  -  -  -Pro-  -  -Thr-  -  -  -  -  -  -  -  -  -  -  -  -  -  -  -  -  -

        76              80                          90                          100
β-hCG   Val-Asn-Pro-Val-Val-Ser-Tyr-Ala-Val-Ala-Leu-Ser-Cys-Gln-Cys-Ala-Leu-Cys-Arg-Arg-Ser-Thr-Thr-Asp-Cys-
β-hLH   -Asp-  -  -  -  -Phe-Pro-  -  -  -  -  -Arg-  -Gly-Pro-  -  -  -  -  -Ser-  -  -

        101             110                         120             125
                                                                  (CHO)
β-hCG   Gly-Gly-Pro-Lys-Asp-His-Pro-Leu-Thr-Cys-Asp-Asp-Pro-Arg-Phe-Gln-Asp-Ser-Ser-Ser-Ser-Lys-Ala-Pro-Pro-
β-hLH   -  -  -  -  -  -  -  -  -  -  -Pro-Gln-His-Ser-Gly-COOH

        126             130                         140             145
              (CHO)                 (CHO)                    (CHO)
β-hCG   Pro-Ser-Leu-Pro-Ser-Pro-Ser-Arg-Leu-Pro-Gly-Pro-Ser-Asp-Thr-Pro-Ile-Leu-Pro-Gln-COOH
```

FIG. 1. Amino acid sequences of the β subunit of hCG (upper letters) and hLH (lower letters), aligned by the positions of cysteine residues. Where no residue is indicated on the hLH sequence, it is identical to that of hCG. Carbohydrate groups are indicated by CHO.

Discontinuous sites, believed to exist, may require the successful crystallization of the molecule for definition. Crystallization of hCG has proved difficult, because of its high carbohydrate content, and the clear definition of discontinuous antigenic sites on the hCG molecule awaits further investigation.

The epitopes on the C-terminal end of β-hCG (C-terminal peptide, CTP) have been studied by various techniques. Antisera have been raised to natural and synthetic peptides of increasing lengths from the C-terminus; their reactivity to hCG, and their ability to neutralize hCG *in vivo*, have been assessed. Antisera to short peptides (20 residues or less) bind hCG but fail to neutralize it *in vivo* while antisera to 35-residue peptides both bind and neutralize hCG. Studies using competition radioimmunoassay (RIA) have suggested that antisera to short CTPs are reactive to a single epitope on the native molecule, whereas antisera to longer ones bind to at least two determinants on intact hCG. The regions on the peptide representing β-hCG 111–145 which may contain antibody-binding sites are 111–118 and 131–145. More than one epitope may be represented in each region; recent studies by others using monoclonal antibodies have suggested that four epitopes exist in this 111–145 segment of the β-hCG molecule (Bidart et al 1985).

We have investigated whether simultaneous immunization with peptide fragments, suspected of containing two separate immunological determinants on peptide 111–145, elicits antibodies reactive to the full-length peptide with levels equal in magnitude to those evoked by intact 111–145. We injected rabbits intramuscularly three times at three-week intervals with peptides 111–118, 138–145, 111–118 mixed with 138–145, and a hybrid peptide, 111–118-Pro-Pro-Lys-Pro-Pro-138–145. All peptides were conjugated to tetanus toxoid and administered in complete Freund's adjuvant. The hybrid peptide was conjugated to a carrier via the lysine residue connecting the two small peptide fragments. All immunizations resulted in high levels of antibody reactive to the immunizing antigen. None produced levels of antibody reactive to peptide 111–145 or hCG as high as those produced by immunization with the 111–145 peptide (Table 1). These results imply, but do not prove, that

TABLE 1 Binding of ^{125}I-labelled peptides and hCG to antisera raised to the β-hCG peptide 111–145, fragments of this peptide, and a hybrid peptide containing both fragment sequences (values are means of four sera)

Antisera to hCG-β peptide sequence:	Antigen bound (mol/l × 10^{-10})			
	β-hCG 111–118	β-hCG 138–145	β-hCG 111–145	hCG
111–118	1725.4	0.1	127.5	15.2
138–145	5.7	2234.9	231.0	19.7
111–118 + 138–145[a]	1511.3	1822.3	194.2	23.4
110–118-Pro-Pro-Lys-Pro-Pro-138–145	4546.0	7742.0	171.5	25.4
111–145	264.7	436.1	865.4	727.6

[a] Individual conjugates mixed (w/w) before immunization.

the full-length C-terminal peptide is required to produce a structural configuration of the antigen necessary for the antibodies raised to be highly reactive to it or to the analogous peptide within the intact hCG molecule.

As the evidence from these immunological studies suggests a tertiary structure to CTPs, and as there are numerous proline and serine residues in the β-hCG CTP, we studied peptide structure by obtaining circular dichroic spectra of 35- and 37-residue peptides. In aqueous solutions or in trifluorethanol the spectra were consistent with the occurrence of Type II β-turns, but no evidence was found for α-helicity or β-structure (Puett et al 1982). The single phenylalanine residue at position 115 contributed to the circular dichroic spectra and may be involved in an immunological determinant in the 111–118 region. Using structural predictive rules and a computer program (Chou & Fasman 1978), β-turns have the greatest probability of occurring between residues 110–115, 117–122, 125–128, 130–133, and 134–140 (Fig. 2). Should these Type II β-turns actually exist on the 111–145 peptide, our data would

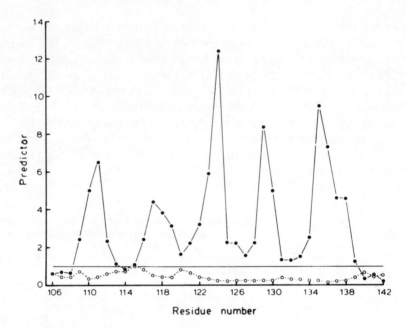

FIG. 2. Probability of occurrence of β-turns (●) and α-helices (○) for the β-hCG sequence 106–145. Each ith point shown for β-turns refers to the tetrapeptide of residues i, i + 1, i + 2 and i + 3. The solid horizontal line at predictor = 1 is an arbitrary cut-off, with points below this value indicating a low probability of occurrence. Predictions were also made for β-structure and this, like the α-helix, had a very low probability of occurrence.

suggest that the N- and C-terminal turns contain the most immunogenic sites of the peptide molecule.

These findings have been compared with predictive plots of the antigenic sites on the β-hCG CTP using the hydrophilicity values assigned by Hoop & Woods (1981). Using a moving average of the values for successive pentapeptides we obtained the pattern of predicted antigenic sites shown in Fig. 3. An amazing similarity between these predictions and the empirical results obtained experimentally is seen. The highest peak on the plot surrounds the 112 residue, with a secondary peak including residues 118–124 and two smaller peaks in the 131–142 residue region. There are however some discrepancies with other findings. For example, other results suggested that the 131–145 region contained the dominant determinant on CTP, whereas the hydrophilicity plot suggests that this is subordinate to those in the 110–116 and 118–124 regions. Another difference between this plot and the one reflecting Type II β-turns according to the Chou & Fasman rules is the lack of an antigenic site in the 125–130 residue region on the plot of hydrophilicity values. The

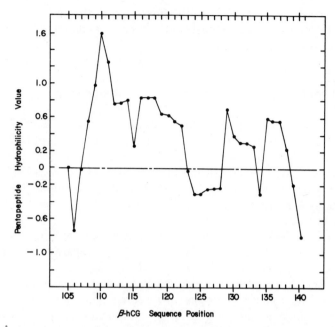

FIG. 3. The hydrophilicity profile of β-hCG peptide 105–145. Hydrophilicity values plotted at each ith point represent the mean of the ith residue, $i^{th} - 1$, $i^{th} - 2$, $i^{th} + 1$ and $i^{th} + 2$ residues. Arbitrary hydrophilicity values for amino acids assigned by Hoop & Woods (1981) were used for this plot.

reason for these differences in the suggested location of the antigenic sites of β-hCG CTP is still unresolved.

The influence of the four carbohydrate moieties, all associated with serine residues, on this segment of the β subunit is not known. There is evidence that intact sugar moieties with a sialic acid residue as their terminal component are not antigenic, but that they help to determine the immunological properties of CTPs (Birken et al 1982). As these rather bulky moieties are attached at serine residues 121, 127, 132 and 138, this could account for the apparent absence of a dominant antigenic site in the 125–130 sequence region and the apparent dominance of the 110–116 region. The moiety located at residue 138, by this reasoning, should not have permitted the 133–145 region to express a dominant antigenic determinant, as revealed by the earlier experiments. However, one should keep in mind that the peptides used to generate antibodies in those studies were either desialylated natural fragments of β-hCG or synthetic peptides. Thus the lack of carbohydrate or the denaturing of its native structure could have destroyed its usual regulation of the immunological properties of the CTP sequence. The lack of data suggesting the role of these carbohydrate moieties in the formation of the antigenic sites on the β-hCG CTP is perhaps the greatest void in our understanding of the immunological properties of these peptides.

Evaluation of C-terminal peptides of β-hCG as immunogens

Peptides representing regions of the C-terminal portion of β-hCG were prepared by digesting the purified subunit with trypsin, chymotrypsin or thermolysin. The purified peptides were used to immunize rabbits. The resulting antisera reacted with hCG, but not at all with hLH (Stevens 1977). The C-terminal region of the subunit thus represented an immunologically specific area of the hCG molecule and peptides of this sequence seemed to be suitable antigens for vaccine development.

Yields of purified peptides from the enzymic cleavage of native β-hCG were very low and the time and cost required to prepare large supplies for development work were prohibitive. In order to acquire a supply of peptides for evaluating this approach to vaccine development, we prepared several peptides by solid-phase synthesis procedures and then compared them with native peptides as immunogens. Using conjugates of peptides with foreign protein molecules, we showed that native and synthetic peptides elicited antisera with similar titres, affinity and specificity (Powell et al 1980). Small differences in the reactivity of antisera to synthetic peptides and to native peptides with hCG were found, since the latter contained four serine-linked carbohydrate moieties not present on the synthetic molecules. However, these differences were slight and, subsequently, we have used synthetic peptides in all our vaccine development studies.

Numerous peptides of various lengths representing residues within positions 105–145 of the subunit were synthesized and tested; our findings on the immunogenicity, specificity, affinity and hCG biological activity-neutralizing capacity of antisera to these peptides will be briefly summarized here. Peptides with fewer than 20 amino acids or more than 40 amino acids (from the C-terminal end of β-hCG) elicited low quantities of antibodies reactive with intact hCG. Although high levels of antibodies could be generated to the peptides after conjugation to carriers, the population of antibodies reactive to the native hormone was smaller ($P < 0.05$) than for peptides of 35–37 residues (position 109–145 or 111–145 of β-hCG). Also, synthetic peptides representing residues 109–145 contain a cysteine at position 110 which was convenient for coupling to carrier molecules (see later). Another criterion important for antigen selection was the ability of antisera to peptides to neutralize the biological activity of hCG in vivo. When antisera to various peptides were assessed for neutralizing capacity, we found that sera raised to 35 or

37 residues blocked hCG action very effectively. On the basis of these and other results, to be presented later in this paper, the synthetic peptide representing β-hCG 109–145 was selected for further vaccine development.

Antigen presentation

In the initial immunization of animals with C-terminal peptides we conjugated the peptides to various proteins (bovine gamma globulin, keyhole limpet haemocyanin, tetanus toxoid, and others) using conventional cross-linking agents (such as carbodiimide, glutaraldehyde and isocyanates) and administering them in complete Freund's adjuvant. These procedures yielded antisera adequate for the assessment of immunogenicity, antibody specificity and affinity, and hCG biological activity-neutralizing capacity, but few of them were acceptable for preparing a vaccine immunogen for clinical application. Conventional coupling procedures yielded a variety of products consisting of polymers of peptides, carriers and conjugates which could not be controlled for quality. Some proteins used were not suitable for injection into women and, clearly, Freund's adjuvant could not be used. As all these features are important for the safe and effective presentation of the peptide antigen, we had to do extensive studies to arrive at a clinically acceptable vaccine.

Chemical coupling of peptides to carriers

A method of coupling peptides to macromolecular carriers that permits covalent conjugation in a predictable fashion was developed. Peptides representing hCG β subunit residues were coupled to a variety of protein carriers. Carrier compounds, containing amino groups but devoid of SH groups, were reacted with 6-maleimidocaproic acyl N-hydroxysuccinimide ester (MCS) under conditions that result in this bifunctional reagent being attached to carrier amino groups via the active ester, with the stable maleimido group remaining free. Subsequently, peptides containing SH groups (exposed after dithiothreitol reduction) were reacted with the reagent-modified carrier. The peptides became coupled to the carrier via the reaction between SH groups on the peptide and the maleimido group on the carrier, as shown in Fig. 4. Peptides devoid of SH groups were thiolated using homocysteine thiolactone or other thiol compounds. The efficiency of coupling was confirmed by amino acid analysis and sodium dodecylsulphate (SDS)–polyacrylamide gel electrophoresis. The results indicated that the coupling of peptides to protein carriers could be regulated by the number of moles of MCS reacted with the carrier to yield free maleimido groups. The SH group reaction with maleimido groups

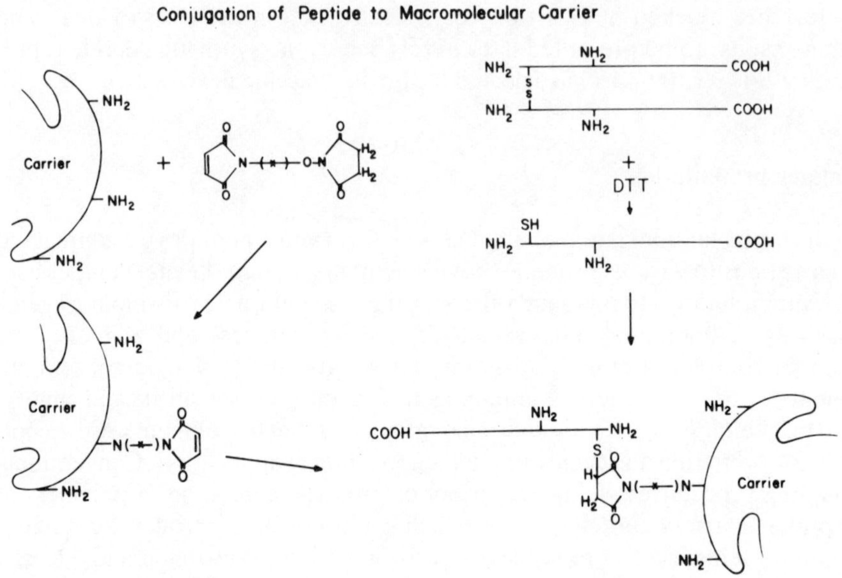

Conjugation of Peptide to Macromolecular Carrier

FIG. 4. Scheme of steps in the chemical conjugation of peptides to proteins carriers. Amino groups of the carrier are reacted with the N-hydroxysuccinimide ester of the bifunctional coupling reagent. After purification, the maleimido groups of the reagent are reacted with the free SH groups exposed when the peptide dimer is reduced by dithiothreitol (DTT).

was stoichiometric. Details of this procedure are reported elsewhere (Lee et al 1980). Conjugates prepared by this method were used to immunize rabbits with the C-terminal peptide 109–145 for further vaccine development.

Selection of a carrier

The criteria used to select a carrier for a vaccine against hCG were: (1) effectiveness in enhancing immune responses to peptides, (2) acceptability of injections into humans, (3) the smallest number of side-effects, and (4) low cost of materials. A series of conjugates were prepared using β-hCG C-terminal peptides with different macromolecules as carriers. The same conjugation method was used for all preparations and rabbits were immunized to each conjugate under identical conditions. Antibody levels attained in animals receiving the various conjugates were used as the indicator of carrier efficacy.

The results of some of these experiments are shown in Table 2. The highest antibody levels were observed in rabbits injected with conjugates of bovine

TABLE 2 Effects of different carrier molecules on the immunogenicity of conjugates of the β-hCG subunit peptide in rabbits

| | Maximum antigen-binding levels $(mol/l \times 10^{-10})$ | | | |
| | $^{125}I\text{-}hCG$ | | $^{125}I\text{-}109\text{-}145\ peptide$ | |
Carrier molecule	Mean[a]	SD	Mean[a]	SD
Bovine gamma globulin	497.2	402.5	552.3	410.8
Diphtheria toxoid	365.3	176.8	423.3	189.3
Tetanus toxoid	339.3	95.5	417.6	106.2
Corynebacterium parvum	215.9	121.5	255.4	131.6
Flagellin	210.4	157.5	244.6	198.1
Pneumococcal polysaccharide	135.7	102.8	153.7	113.0
Meningococcal protein	97.9	107.6	118.4	122.6
Poly(Tyr,Glu), poly(Ala,Lys)	29.9	22.6	37.3	35.5
Ficoll	10.6	8.3	13.0	9.0
Poly(D,L-Ala,Lys)	8.6	4.7	12.2	7.5

Conjugates were injected intramuscularly in complete Freund's adjuvant, three times at three-week intervals.
[a] Four rabbits per group.

gamma globulin, tetanus toxoid or diphtheria toxoid. Moderate amounts of antibody were raised to conjugates with bacteria or bacterial proteins as carriers but very low levels were found when synthetic polypeptides or carbohydrates were used.

As it was believed that bovine gamma globulin would probably not be found safe for human use, the most efficacious conjugates acceptable for human vaccines were tetanus and diphtheria toxoids. We investigated which of these provided the fewest side-effects from repeated injection. Diphtheria toxoid elicited many fewer delayed-type hypersensitivity reactions than tetanus toxoid and was selected for further vaccine development.

Site of conjugation and antigen density

The region of β-hCG CTP selected for vaccine development was essentially the portion of the molecule beyond the last cysteine residue at position 110. Minor variations in peptide length (110 ± 2 residues) did not yield differences in the immunological similarity to intact hCG. Sequences modified to provide a thiol group at different sites for coupling to carriers have been prepared. In addition, spacer molecules (six proline residues) have been introduced at the N- or C-terminus of the peptide for theoretically better antigen presentation. All these modified peptides, as well as the native sequence 109–145, were coupled to the same carrier (tetanus toxoid) and antibody levels in rabbits after immunization with each were compared. Immunization conditions were the same as those used for carrier selection. The immunogenicity of all the peptides was similar, except that coupling at the Lys-122 position of peptide 111–145 elicited lower antibody levels than the native 109–145 peptide or other modified sequences. As the cost of preparing extended peptides or peptides with blocking groups is greater than that of synthesizing the native 109–145 sequence, the latter process was chosen for further vaccine development.

After selection of the synthetic peptide, the number of peptide molecules per molecule of carrier which elicits the highest antibody response to the peptide was determined. Conjugates containing 5–33 peptides per 10^5 daltons of carrier were prepared and rabbits were immunized with each. The antibody levels attained by each group are shown in Fig. 5. Evidently, fewer than 16 peptides/10^5 daltons of carrier were not as effective as higher ratios. Increasing the ratio to 40 : 1 (data not shown) caused a decrease in antibody levels to the peptide. Thus a range of 20–30 peptides/10^5 daltons of carrier was optimum for this antigen (Stevens et al 1981a).

Selection of adjuvant and vaccine vehicle

Many of the results discussed here were obtained by injecting peptide immunogens into rabbits in complete Freund's adjuvant (CFA). This adjuvant produces severe lesions at the site of injection and under no circumstances could be used in a vaccine administered to humans. In order to develop a vaccine that could be safely tested in women, we have done extensive studies in rabbits of other commercially available adjuvants.

Very weak responses were obtained when immunogens and adjuvants were administered in saline or in emulsions of water and vegetable oils (peanut oil or soybean oil). However, when the vaccine components and adjuvants were contained in an emulsion of water and mineral oil (incomplete Freund's adjuvant, IFA), many experimental compounds promoted high antibody levels to peptides. We assessed antibody responses in rabbits to a conjugate injected in a CFA–water emulsion and to the same conjugate given in other adjuvants contained in mineral oil (IFA)–water emulsions (Stevens et al 1981b). Some of the adjuvant compounds (muramyl dipeptide analogues) were clearly equivalent or superior to CFA in eliciting antibodies to the conjugate in rabbits, and one of these, CGP-11637, was selected for further vaccine work.

Although these data encouraged us to think that effective adjuvants suitable for human use might become available for development of an hCG vaccine,

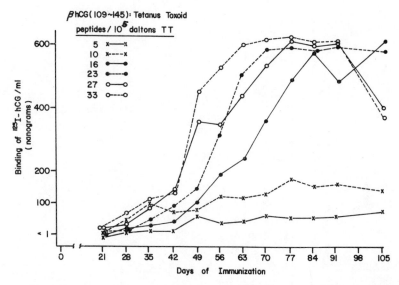

FIG. 5. Mean antibody levels measured by binding to ^{125}I-hCG in six groups of four rabbits each, immunized with varying densities of synthetic β-hCG peptide 109–145 coupled to tetanus toxoid. Three injections were given at three-week intervals using complete Freund's adjuvant. No significant differences in antibody levels were found at 42 days of immunization between the six groups ($P > 0.05$), but at Day 63 there were significant differences between groups receiving conjugates with 23 or more peptides per 10^5 daltons of carrier and those conjugates with lower peptide densities ($P = 0.028$). At Day 84 of immunization there was no difference in the levels of antibodies in groups of animals receiving conjugates with densities of peptide of more than 16 per 10^5 daltons of tetanus toxoid ($P = 0.05$), while significant differences were observed between these groups and those injected with conjugates of lower peptide density ($P = 0.028$). These studies were conducted before the selection of diphtheria toxoid as the preferred carrier, but subsequent experiments using a conjugate containing 25 peptides per 10^5 daltons of tetanus toxoid and a conjugate containing 25 peptides per 10^5 daltons of diphtheria toxoid elicited equivalent antibody levels (data not shown).

the injection of mineral oil into humans was unacceptable. Obviously, a suitable substitute had to be identified for delivering the vaccine components to the immune system. As the mechanism underlying the efficacy of mineral oil as a vehicle for immunogens is not known, the identification of a substitute has required considerable study. A variety of oil–water emulsions and other vehicles, potentially acceptable for human use, were investigated. The vehicle providing the most consistently high antibody response was an emulsion of squalene and water, with mannide monooleate as the emulsifier (Table 3). Since these studies, all further vaccine development has been done with this vehicle.

TABLE 3 Comparison of antibody levels in sera from rabbits immunized with β-hCG (Cys-Pro$_6$-111–145): tetanus toxoid conjugate and synthetic adjuvant DT-1 incorporated into four different vehicles. Peak antibody levels, together with those from one week earlier and one week later, were pooled for evaluation

Vehicle	n	Antibody level (mol/l × 10^{-10})				95% confidence interval	SD	P*
		Minimum	Median	Maximum	Mean			
CFA (reference vehicle)	12	52.4	150.8	320.2	161.3	101.7–220.9	93.7	
Squalene–Arlacel emulsion	11	189.0	312.6	833.7	400.1	225.7–574.4	226.7	0.01
Squalane–Arlacel emulsion	11	44.2	150.6	290.0	168.5	114.5–222.5	80.4	NS
Peanut oil emulsion	9	12.5	22.5	27.1	21.3	17.5–25.1	4.9	0.001
Alum precipitate	12	5.8	8.4	16.1	9.9	7.9–11.9	3.2	0.001

* Probability, compared with CFA. NS, not significant ($P < 0.05$).

Antifertility testing in baboons

Adult baboons have been immunized with several different conjugates made up of a variety of carriers and peptides. In our early studies, these immunogens were administered in complete Freund's adjuvant. The antibody levels to peptide and to hCG varied widely, and very low levels of antibodies were reactive with baboon CG. (Binding of ^{125}I-labelled baboon CG by antisera was only 2–10% of binding by ^{125}I-hCG.) Females were mated with males of proven fertility. A significant reduction in their fertility rate was observed after immunization, compared with that of untreated or carrier-immunized controls. However, the number of animals in each group receiving a particular conjugate formulation was small (usually four) and it was therefore not possible to demonstrate a statistically valid antifertility effect of the immunization.

When we had made the final selection of the peptide, carrier, adjuvant and delivery system to be used in the first prototype vaccine, we conducted antifertility studies of this vaccine in baboons. The vaccine consisted of a conjugate of diphtheria toxoid and synthetic β-hCG peptide 109–145 mixed with a muramyl dipeptide adjuvant. These were dissolved in saline and the solution was emulsified with squalene with the aid of mannide monooleate. The vaccine was injected intramuscularly at 28-day intervals, five times or until pregnancy occurred. The experimental design was 15 females in the control group, injected with carrier, and 15 females receiving the vaccine. All animals were mated three times each. Levels of antibodies reactive with hCG, baboon CG and β-hCG peptide are shown in Table 4. Antibodies against the peptide immunogen were only about 4.0% as reactive with baboon CG as with hCG. After the matings, a reduction in the fertility rate of the immunized baboons was obvious: 70.0% of the matings in the control group resulted in pregnancy whereas only 4.6% of the matings in the vaccinated group yielded pregnancies (Table 5).

It is recognized that an antifertility method yielding a pregnancy rate of 5% is not likely to be attractive in human populations, but it should be remembered that these were heterologous immunizations of baboons with the human antigen and that the reactivity of the antibodies with baboon CG was very low. Should the vaccine elicit similar antibody levels reactive to hCG in women, a much lower pregnancy rate is likely to be observed.

Acknowledgement

The costs for the development of the hCG vaccine described here were provided by The Special Programme on Research and Research Training in Human Reproduction of the World Health Organization.

TABLE 4 Antibody levels produced by female baboons against β-hCG (109–145) peptide, hCG and baboon chorionic gonadotropin after immunization with β-hCG (109–145): diphtheria toxoid conjugate. Values determined from serum collected during the early luteal phase of each menstrual cycle after immunizations during Days 1–5 of each cycle. Animals mated during cycles 3–5

Antibody reactive to:	Antigen binding $(mol/1 \times 10^{-10})$ in menstrual cycles:				
	1	2	3	4	5
β-hCG (109–145) peptide					
Mean	41.4	186.0	205.6	252.0	284.1
95% confidence interval	25.6–57.3	139.4–232.5	168.3–243.0	186.1–317.7	226.5–341.7
Human chorionic gonadotropin					
Mean	31.9	160.0	172.1	205.5	224.8
95% confidence interval	18.7–45.2	117.0–203.1	141.6–202.5	145.5–265.4	172.0–276.6
Baboon chorionic gonadotropin					
Mean	0.7	3.7	5.5	7.7	9.0
95% confidence interval	0.3–1.0	1.9–5.6	3.6–7.3	5.0–10.4	6.3–11.8
Number of animals	15	15	15	15	14

TABLE 5 Comparison of fertility rates of female baboons immunized with diphtheria toxoid with those immunized with diphtheria toxoid conjugated to β-hCG (109–145) synthetic peptide[a]

	Fertility observed in mating cycle:			
Baboons immunized with:	1	2	3	Total
Diphtheria toxoid				
Number mated	15	4	1	20
Number pregnant	11	3	0	14
Fertility rate (%)	73.3	75.0	0	70.0
Diphtheria toxoid: β-hCG (109–145)				
Number mated	15	15	14	44
Number pregnant	0	1	1	2
Fertility rate (%)	0	6.7	7.1	4.6

[a] Matings commenced during the third menstrual cycle after immunization had been started.

REFERENCES

Bidart JM, Ozturk M, Bellet DH et al 1985 Identification of epitopes associated with hCG and the β-hCG carboxyl terminus by monoclonal antibodies produced against a synthetic peptide. J Immunol 134:457-464

Birken S, Canfield R, Agosto G, Lewis J 1982 Preparation and characterization of an improved β-COOH terminal immunogen for generation of specific and sensitive antisera to human chorionic gonadotropin. Endocrinology 110:1555-1563

Chou PY, Fasman GD 1978 Empirical predictions of protein conformation. Annu Rev Biochem 47:251-276

Hoop TP, Woods KR 1981 Prediction of protein antigenic determinants from amino acid sequences. Proc Natl Acad Sci USA 78:3824-3828

Lee AC, Powell JE, Tregear GW, Niall HD, Stevens VC 1980 A method for preparing β-hCG COOH peptide–carrier conjugates of predictable composition. Mol Immunol 17:749-755

Morgan FJ, Birken S, Canfield RE 1973 Human chorionic gonadotropin: a proposal for the amino acid sequence. Mol Cell Biochem 2:97-99

Powell JE, Lee AC, Tregear GW, Niall HD, Stevens VC 1980 Characteristics of antibodies raised to carboxy-terminal peptides of hCG beta subunit. J Reprod Immunol 2:1-13

Puett D, Ryan RJ, Stevens VC 1982 Circular dichroic and immunological properties of human choriogonadotropin-β carboxyl terminal peptides. Int J Pept Protein Res 19:506-513

Stevens VC 1977 Actions of antisera to hCG-β: in vitro and in vivo assessment. In: James VHT (ed) Proc Fifth Int Congr Endocrinol. Excerpta Medica, Amsterdam (International Congress Series no. 402) vol 1:379

Stevens VC, Cinader B, Powell JE, Lee AC, Koh SW 1981a Preparation and formulation of a human chorionic gonadotropin antifertility vaccine. Selection of a peptide immunogen. Am J Reprod Immunol 1:307-314

Stevens VC, Cinader B, Powell JE, Lee AC, Koh SW 1981b Preparation and formulation of a human chorionic gonadotropin antifertility vaccine. Selection of adjuvant and vehicle. Am J Reprod Immunol 1:315-321

Vaitukaitis JL, Braunstein GD, Ross GT 1972 A radioimmunoassay which specifically measures human chorionic gonadotropin in the presence of human luteinizing hormone. Am J Obstet Gynecol 113:751-758

DISCUSSION

Skehel: Is it clear that the difference in the baboon antibody response (Table 4, p 214) is due to a sequence difference between baboon and human CG, or is it just a species response difference?

Stevens: It is most likely to be due to a sequence difference in baboon and human CG. We haven't been successful yet in sequencing baboon CG by conventional biochemical methods. A collaborator in Melbourne has sequenced one gene from baboon placenta but it was not the gene expressing the secreted CG of pregnancy. There were about 10 amino acid differences in the last 40 residues of the β subunit but, as this sequence was not from a gene expressing baboon CG, we do not know for sure the differences between the human and baboon hormone structure. Eventually, we expect to define these differences.

V. Nussenzweig: You presented a ranked series of vehicles (Table 3, p 212), the last one being alum precipitate. Did you boost the same rabbits with the antigen in alum?

Stevens: Yes; we gave the same number of injections of each vehicle, at the same interval, using the same dose of antigen and adjuvant compound.

V. Nussenzweig: I am surprised by the result, because with several antigens given in aluminium hydroxide, after the first dose the antibody titres may be low, but when you boost, the response can go quite high.

Stevens: I agree that other workers have used alum successfully. I have seen examples in the literature where alum was a good adjuvant/vehicle with certain antigens, but not with others.

Gupta: I would like your comments on some observations made by others. Louvet et al (1974) and Matsuura et al (1978, 1979) studied the C-terminal peptide antisera and showed that they have very low biological neutralization properties. In fact, antibodies against the 23- amino acid C-terminal peptide do not neutralize the biological activity of hCG *in vivo*. Moreover, antibodies generated against the C-terminal peptides by-and-large have very low affinity for the native hormone (Chen et al 1980). A third observation, from Talwar's group, is that the C-terminal peptides do not recognize the hCG receptor (Ramakrishnan et al 1978a). In view of these observations, do you think that your vaccine, based on the C-terminal peptide, will be effective in clinical trials?

Stevens: We have raised antibodies to a 20-residue C-terminal peptide as well as to shorter peptides. I agree that antibodies to the C-terminal 23-residue peptide do not neutralize hCG, but we are not using 22- or 23-residue peptides; we are using 37-residue ones. It is necessary to go beyond about 35 residues; any shorter, and the antibodies raised do not neutralize. Of course, we don't know whether neutralizing capacity of the antibodies is necessary to produce an antifertility effect after immunization. We know that there is CG on the preimplantation blastocyst, and that immunization allows many antibodies to be present in the uterine fluid surrounding the blastocyst. John Hearn has shown that antisera to chorionic gonadotropin arrest implantation and embryonic development in the marmoset monkey, both *in vivo* and *in vitro* (Hearn et al 1984). It may not be necessary, therefore, to generate a neutralizing antibody. However, we want to assure efficacy of the immunizations, so we plan to use a peptide that will elicit neutralizing antibodies.

We have also found that affinity is not correlated with biological neutralization. If we are using an immunological method that doesn't depend on neutralization as a mechanism of action, affinity may be more important. Some of our lowest affinity antibodies are some of the best neutralizers. We think the mechanism of neutralization involves having at least two epitopes on an hCG peptide, so that an antibody population is produced of at least two qualitatively different specificities that react with the hCG molecule at different points and cause more rapid clearance of the hormone. Thus high affinity, which we normally think of as desirable, may not be critical when we are talking about neutralization.

On your third point, we are glad that the C-terminal peptide antibodies don't react with the hCG receptor-binding site. Certainly, if you administered a monoclonal antibody to a single epitope that reacts with the hormone at the point of its receptor binding, you would have an efficient way of blocking hormone function. The hazard from this is that you may induce antibody damage to the receptor as well as to the hormone. If the hormone is bound to the receptor at the time of antigen–antibody reaction, autoimmune damage could result. So we are pleased that we are not using a peptide that induces antibodies reacting with the receptor-binding site. We shall have to wait either until clinical trials in women reach the point that we can establish antifertility efficacy, or until we can perform a trial of a homologous CG vaccine in baboons where it will be possible to titrate the minimum level of antibodies necessary to be effective in blocking fertility.

Gupta: You have chosen the 37 amino acid-long C-terminal peptide in order to make a specific vaccine against this polypeptide hormone. There is apprehension in some quarters as to whether one should have a specific vaccine, or not; to resolve this, a study was undertaken by scientists at the Indian Population Council. Rhesus monkeys were immunized with the β subunit of ovine luteinizing hormone (oLH), which elicits an antibody response that reacts with monkey LH and also with monkey chorionic gonadotropin (CG). The purpose was twofold: (i) to see whether antibodies reactive with the species' own gonadotropin can indeed prevent fertility, and (ii) to evaluate the side-effects of antibodies cross-reactive with pituitary LH. No obvious cytotoxic effects were seen (Thau et al 1979, 1983, Thau & Sundaram 1980). Effective anti-β-oLH titres did not interfere with ovulation and regular menstrual cycles. Cross-reaction of antibodies with the monkey pituitary LH resulted in shortening of the luteal phase, which could even be beneficial and certainly is not a harmful effect. So specificity is perhaps not a major criterion. The important point is to induce enough immune response to neutralize the bioactivity of hCG, so as to terminate pregnancy. If you induce an immune response which cannot neutralize the biological activity of the hormone completely, you may have more problems than if you induce a good antibody response with a minor cross-reaction with LH.

Stevens: I agree with you that fears of autoimmune damage by LH antibodies may have been unwarranted. When we started these studies we had no way to know whether it would be safe to raise an antibody reactive to pituitary hormones. In the studies you cited, there appeared to be no consequences, at least over four years, of having antibodies circulating to LH. I don't agree, however, that reducing ovarian function, even slightly, is necessarily a positive effect. It certainly is useful in terms of keeping a woman from becoming pregnant, but the long-term consequences of reduced ovarian function are less certain. A supply of ovarian steroids is needed for various metabolic functions and where progesterone levels are diminished, allowing unopposed oestrogen stimulation to the breast or vagina, this is thought by some to lead to neoplastic states resulting in carcinoma.

There is no question that immunization with the whole β subunit will have a better chance of being effective, because this procedure elicits attacks on many different targets, not only of the conceptus but of the maternal organism. The question is whether it will be as safe as the use of hCG-specific peptides. Conversely, the peptide approach, which is no doubt a safer method, may not induce high enough hCG antibody levels and will not attack enough targets to be effective.

Lerner: In medicine, specificity is always good, whether you think you need it or not. You don't ever know what are the consequences of non-specificity.

We should be cautious about using the word 'neutralization'. The term derives from studies of viruses, and it means a hit by an antibody that destroys biological activity by altering the structure or function of the protein to which it binds. As you implied, hCG might be more rapidly cleared when bound to antibody. If you injected a second antibody into the individual, clearance might be better still, but one cannot do that.

Stevens: We have shown that after the injection of ^{125}I-labelled hCG into rabbits immunized with an hCG antigen, the labelled hormone is cleared from the circulation much faster than from a non-immunized rabbit (unpublished results).

Lerner: To come back to a point raised earlier, many people wonder whether they should choose peptide synthesis *per se* as a way of making peptides, or should they make the gene and express the peptide on the end of a fusion protein. The problem there is that since *E. coli* organisms or yeast don't know how to make branched-chain amino acids, you end up with one molecule of synthetic immunogen for one molecule of carrier, as it were (the fusion protein). But you showed in Fig. 5 (p 211) that even five molecules of peptide per molecule of carrier is not very effective. One is therefore left with the chemical synthesis, if one wants to control the number of molecules of immunogen per molecule of carrier. If you wanted to, you could engineer repeats, as Fred Brown said (p 176, 198).

Stevens: Yes. That is under way!

Lerner: A general question that is bound to be asked is whether one will make a vaccine that eventually induces autoimmunity. This is an ethical hurdle which may be higher than the scientific hurdle.

Ada: One point relevant to this approach is that the antigenic determinant here is a transient one that is seen only at certain times.

Lerner: Like a virus! There is certainly a fine line separating the parasitic invader and the occasional invasion of self by self. People might baulk at the distinction between those two.

Ada: A recent meeting at the World Health Organization laid down criteria for the selection of an antigen with which to make a vaccine for controlling human fertility. One criterion was that the chosen antigens should appear transiently and be confined to gametes. (See Ada et al 1985.)

Sela: We have been concentrating on the use of synthetic peptides as ingredients of potential vaccines, but synthetic peptides could also be used as suppressors against autoimmune diseases, or against the production of antibodies of certain classes. Thus, the peptides may be designed to provoke an immune response or to eliminate another such response.

Ada: Tissues from baboons exposed to the 37-residue C-peptide have been examined for pathological reactions, and John Humphrey reported on the findings.

Humphrey: The sera of the baboons, immunized with repeated doses of the peptide conjugate much larger than would be used in human beings, were examined for autoantibodies. Control animals were immunized with the vehicle oil, the adjuvant and the carrier diphtheria toxoid. These sera were tested by immunofluorescence for binding of Ig to conventional sections of thyroid, pancreas, skin and other rat and monkey tissues. Several weak reactivities were observed, but the only significant autoantibodies that appeared to be induced by the complete immunogen, as opposed to being already present or induced by immunization with diphtheria toxoid rather than the conjugate, were antibodies against smooth muscle. These antibodies appeared to be absorbable with the C-terminal peptide conjugated to diphtheria toxoid. In other words, if they were induced at all, as opposed to being due to polyclonal stimulation, they were induced by some configurational change that occurred when the C-peptide was attached to the diphtheria toxoid. Low titres of smooth muscle antibodies are not regarded as a cause for serious concern. There was no real evidence that the antibodies persisted for long after the immunization course was completed, and that they were associated with pathological changes. The conclusion was that apart from at the sites of injection, where you would expect a certain amount of granuloma formation even from the squalene and Arlacel, there was nothing which a histologist would regard as abnormal. It was interesting that some other apparent autoantibodies at quite low titres appeared to result from diphtheria toxoid. Millions of people have received diphtheria toxoid with no ill-effects—but of course no one has ever thought to examine whether autoantibodies were stimulated thereby!

Lachmann: How long do the granulomas at the site of injection last when you inject squalene and Arlacel, Dr Stevens?

Stevens: They persist for 2—3 months. The detailed histological studies were done in rabbits, using a standard irritancy test. These studies used a much larger injection volume than is used in a typical immunization, and therefore induced a much greater reaction than you would find in practice. There was some residual scar left at the deep muscle site where the emulsion was deposited. In the planned clinical trials we will start at one-fortieth of that dose and work up to perhaps one-tenth. There is no way to know in advance whether these injections are painful. Also, we are not considering using this vehicle in a vaccine designed for widespread use. Its use will be limited to Phase I trials. That is why it is necessary to develop better delivery systems soon, so that if we have promising results from a limited clinical trial, we can have available a more suitable delivery system for expanded trials.

Lerner: There is from time to time a search for a non-irritating adjuvant (as opposed to carrier). A senior immunologist said to me, and I think it's true: 'you show me something that is not an irritant and I'll show you something that is not an adjuvant'. You probably cannot have such a thing as a non-irritating adjuvant, because adjuvants call forth the cells that respond to irritation, among other things.

McConnell: It depends on how you think an adjuvant works. One view of an adjuvant could be as something that promotes clonal expansion; a desired property of an adjuvant is therefore that it causes the release of interleukin 2, which can produce further clonal expansion. Another type of adjuvant would be recombinant interleukin 2 on its own. The latter, of course, would have to be delivered to the correct site at the right time, but it would presumably be a non-irritant adjuvant which will induce clonal expansion.

Lerner: One has also to discriminate between the 'depot' effect and the adjuvant effect.

Stevens: We define the adjuvant as the muramyl dipeptide analogue. The oil-in-water emulsion is the delivery system, or vehicle, and the carrier is the toxoid. We showed from studies using an osmotic pump system that persistent antigen release is required to obtain a good antibody response. If you use these pump systems without any oil-in-water emulsion (i.e., using saline) but include MDP, you obtain good titres. We are hoping that biodegradable polymer delivery systems, not known themselves to cause any inflammation, will also be satisfactory. I agree that you can probably never obtain as high a response from non-inflammatory delivery systems as you can from inflammatory ones.

Geysen: If you vaccinate with a peptide, do you expect the hormone itself to boost the response? If so, are you ever going to be able to turn the response off, if you want to do so?

Stevens: That is a very important question, particularly in contradistinction with what most people here are trying to do. We want an immunization that will not be irreversible so that when pregnancy occurs after a fall in titre there won't be a boost of the antibody level from CG secretion and hence a complete sterilization of the subject. We don't know yet what happens in people, but our animal studies suggest that a foreign molecule must be coupled to the antigen in order to break T cell tolerance and obtain antibodies in an homologous immunization. The return of natural hormone secretion does not boost the response. You must administer the altered antigen again to boost the response.

We are beginning to study reversibility. We think one might be able to override the effect of hCG immunization by supplying the reproductive hormone, progesterone, at the time conception is expected to occur. This depends on the yet-undefined mechanism of action of the vaccine. If the conceptus is destroyed before it implants, this procedure will not be effective and we shall have to find another way of turning off the immune blockage of fertility. The immunization will probably be reversible when antibody titres decline to low levels, which we expect to occur after one to three years in immunized women. If this happens, the method would not allow for precise family planning! In this situation, one couldn't predict precisely when fertility would return.

Geysen: And you really don't think that the hormone will boost at all, to keep antibody levels up?

Stevens: No. I think Dr Gupta has some direct evidence on this point.

Gupta: Talwar's group confirmed that the native hormone does not lead to a booster effect in rhesus monkeys immunized with β-hCG linked to tetanus toxoid as carrier (Ramakrishnan et al 1978b). In baboons immunized with β-hCG linked to tetanus toxoid, when the antibody response went down, the females became pregnant on mating and delivered normal babies, thereby demonstrating that the phenomenon is reversible.

Geysen: That's not a homologous system; the test will be the human trial.

Gupta: I agree. Talwar's group observed that hCG alone did not boost the immune response, in limited Phase I clinical trials. Moreover, women with very low antibody titres became pregnant (Talwar 1984).

Ada: May we turn to the broader question of antigen persistence and whether it is undesirable, or whether it is necessary for generating long-lived memory cells, in order to prepare a successful vaccine. Another related question is the extent to which antibodies to peptides react with the parent molecule, and what factors determine this.

Sela: I have always said that persistence of antigen is desirable until the moment when the message goes out. In other words, a conformational determinant on a protein must be recognized while it is still in the protein, so at that moment it still persists. Once the message to initiate the immune response starts, it is desirable to remove the antigen, because if it persists at that level it may cause immunological paralysis.

Ada: Is there any evidence for paralysis? That would surely require a large amount of antigen. We are thinking of using small amounts of antigen, as far as possible, in vaccines.

Sela: I am thinking more about the immune response, rather than long-term persistence, but if you want to see when antigens produce the best immune response, this is when they can still display the epitope in its native state. If you are asking whether it is advantageous that the antigen should be present 20 years later, the question is: where? John Humphrey could tell us whether it's necessary that the antigen should remain in the lymphocyte. I think the answer is probably 'no', but does one need an active virus somewhere around to trigger an immune response?

Humphrey: It depends on the sort of immune response required. If you want continuous antibody production, to keep the levels up, that is different from having memory cells that are able to respond again at short notice.

Ada: Let's look at the second question, then, because for many vaccines against infectious disease organisms we are aiming to prime a person to respond to the disease when it comes along, which might be tomorrow or several years hence.

Humphrey: John Skehel would say that if you want to immunize against polio or influenza, you test the level of circulating antibody. You regard people as being protected who have more than a certain level. That's not to say that a reinfection does not evoke a rapid increase in antibody, or that immunization by, say, attenuated virus does not boost the response. But for the forms of protection for which existing immunizing agents are designed, not only are they evaluated by a level of antibody which is considered to be protective, because this level is found to be so in epidemiological surveys, but this is what is aimed for.

There is also no doubt that even if the antibody can prevent the virus or toxin attaching to its target (provided it is there in sufficient quantity, at the right time and in the right place), once the agent has penetrated into cells, antibodies do not cure the infected cells—even if, as in the case of measles, they can destroy them. To get rid of infected cells you often need the second line of defence, either cytotoxic T lymphocytes capable of recognizing the affected cell at a reasonably early stage of infection and killing it, or natural killer (NK) cells and other killer cells which act on antibody-coated targets. Elicitation of cell-mediated immunity is distinct from antibody production. I know of one study (Miller 1964) showing that for six months after tritiated thymidine had been given to immunized rats, occasional plasma cells still contained the label, and some appeared to secrete antibody for three months. It must be rare for a cell at the height of antibody secretion to go on living for a long time, unless it's a myeloma or lymphoma cell.

I certainly accept that continuing antibody production is antigen-driven. Whether it is due to persisting exogenous antigen or whether, after a while, the stimulus is anti-idiotype (which can resemble the original immunizing epitope) is unclear. It is certainly possible to elicit antibodies against a given antigen by immunizing with antibodies specifically reactive with the binding site of anti-bodies against the original antigen. A good recent example is the use of an anti-idiotype vaccine to protect rats against experimental schistosomiasis (Grzych et al 1985). However, we must also remember that antigens can persist as complexes for a very long time at the surface of follicular dendritic cells in germinal centres.

Skehel: It is true that the mechanism of the persistence of immunity after a virus infection is unclear. There certainly is persistence, but whether it is antigen-driven or anti-idiotype-driven is not known. In some infections the virus itself may persist, for instance after measles infection, and in these cases persistence of immunity may result from the presence of antigen. In others, for example influenza, where there is no evidence that virus persists, it has been thought that immunity is short-lived. However, when the H_1 variant of influenza arrived in 1977, nobody above the age of 25 years was infected; so immunity even in these cases lasts for over 20 years, since the H_1 viruses were prevalent only before 1957. The basis for this persistent immunity is unknown.

Ada: I thought antibody was found, in some people?

Skehel: Yes, but rarely and at a low level. As John Humphrey says, normally you would correlate protection with the level of serum antibodies.

Brown: We are in a different situation with synthetic antigens. I was interested in Michael Sela's evidence on priming with a peptide. I know of only one other report of priming with a peptide so that a secondary injection of the complete virus raised a lot of neutralizing antibody. That was with poliovirus in rabbits. That experiment has not been repeated, with polio or with the structurally similar foot-and-mouth disease virus, and I wondered what other evidence there is that after priming with a peptide, one obtains a boost with the complete protein or the complete organism. With hCG, Dr Stevens doesn't get any boost either, after peptide sensitization.

Sela: The priming was not with the peptide, in fact, but with the protein from *E. coli* which includes the peptide (p 193–194).

Brown: Then is there any evidence that peptides prime for the complete organism?

Ada: Dr Eckard Wimmer gave several injections of large amounts of the poliovirus peptide in complete Freund's adjuvant—not a realistic situation.

Brown: That is the case I was referring to. Wimmer obtained either no antibody or very little neutralizing antibody with the peptide. Then he gave a subimmunizing dose of poliovirus particles and obtained an enormous boost; but this hasn't been repeated by others.

Lerner: There is evidence the other way, in fact; immunologically, the intact molecule and the peptide are handled differently. Workers at Scripps have a strain of mice that cannot respond to the intact surface antigen of hepatitis B (HBsAg). If a synthetic piece of the antigen is given, a perfectly good antibody is made that reacts with the native particle. I suggest that you may be tolerant to your own folded proteins but not tolerant at all to a synthetic piece of such a protein. This has numerous implications, and the inverse is what we are discussing here. You may not be able to prime a response to the whole protein with a synthetic piece. Suppose you have a piece of the influenza virus to which under no circumstances do you make an antibody—say, the C-terminus of the HA1 antigen. What good would it do to prime against that?

Ada: You might prime a T helper cell population. If Wimmer's work has an explanation, it would presumably be that he had done this.

Sela: In the case I mentioned (p 193–194), of a large protein isolated from *E. coli*, which may be hooked on β-galactosidase or something like this, both the labile toxin of *E. coli* and cholera toxin can boost the response, so there is priming by a protein which includes the synthetic peptide.

Brown: Both Ruth Arnon and Fritz Melchers claim to prime with influenza peptides and to boost with the complete virus. This is important in terms of what has been said about not having a peptide or synthetic antigen that persists for a long time in the body. If it is not going to prime for the complete protein, I don't see what the problem is. We know that peptides will prime for peptides.

Stevens: Dr Humphrey, it is important for immunological memory to have complement present at the site of antigen injection. Some chemical groups have been shown to be effective in inducing complement. What are the implications for vaccines?

Humphrey: The best way to elicit B memory cells is to have complement-attached antigen–antibody complexes on follicular dendritic cells in the spleen and lymph nodes. This is not necessarily the only way, but it is so much more efficient than any other method in the animals in which it has been tried, that it must be biologically significant. If the complexes don't fix complement, they don't elicit memory (summarized in Klaus et al 1980).

REFERENCES

Ada GL, Basten A, Jones WR 1985 Prospects for developing vaccines to control fertility. Nature (Lond) 317:288-289

Chen HC, Matsuura S, Ohashi M 1980 Limitation and problems of hCG specific antisera. In: Segal SJ (ed) Chorionic gonadotropin. Plenum Press, New York, p 231

Grzych JM, Capron M, Lambert PH, Dissous C, Torres S, Capron A 1985 An anti-idiotype vaccine against experimental schistosomiasis. Nature (Lond) 316:74-76

Hearn JP, Gems S, Hodges JK, Wennink C 1984 The role of chorionic gonadotropin during embryonic attachment and implantation *in vivo* and *in vitro*. Proc Soc Study Fertil 72A:48 (abstr)

Klaus GGB, Humphrey JH, Kunkl A, Dongworth DW 1980 The follicular dendritic cell: its role in antigen presentation in the generation of immunological memory. Immunol Rev 53:3-28

Louvet JP, Ross GT, Birken S, Canfield RE 1974 Absence of neutralization effect of antiserum to the unique structural region of human chorionic gonadotropin. J Clin Endocrinol Metab 39:1155-1158

Matsuura S, Chen HC, Hodgen GD 1978 Antibodies to carboxyl-terminal fragment of human chorionic gonadotropin β-subunit: characterization of the antibody recognition sites using synthetic peptide analogs. Biochemistry 17:575-580

Matsuura S, Ohashi M, Chen HC, Hodgen GD 1979 A human chorionic gonadotropin-specific antiserum against synthetic peptide analogs to the carboxyl-terminal peptide of its β- subunit. Endocrinology 104:396-401

Miller JJ III 1964 An autoradiographic study of plasma cell and lymphocytic survival in rat popliteal lymph node. J Immunol 92:673-681

Ramakrishnan S, Das C, Talwar GP 1978a Recognition of the β-subunit of human chorionic gonadotropin and sub-determinants by target tissue receptors. Biochem J 176:599-602

Ramakrishnan S, Das C, Talwar GP 1978b Progesterone levels in monkeys immunized with Pr-β-hCG-TT after injection of hLH and hCG during luteal phase. Contraception 18:51-58

Talwar GP 1984 Structural vaccines for control of fertility and communicable diseases. Crit Rev Trop Med 2:245-269

Thau RB, Sundaram K 1980 The mechanism of action of an antifertility vaccine in the rhesus monkey: reversal of the effects of antisera to the β-subunit of ovine luteinizing hormone by medroxyprogesterone acetate. Fertil Steril 33:317-320

Thau RB, Sundaram K, Thornton YS, Seidman LS 1979 Effects of immunization with the β-subunit of ovine luteinizing hormone on corpus luteum function in the rhesus monkey. Fertil Steril 31:200-204

Thau RB, Yamamoto Y, Sundaram K, Spinola PG 1983 Human chorionic gonadotropin stimulates luteal function in rhesus monkeys immunized against the β-subunit of ovine luteinizing hormone. Endocrinology 112:277-283

The use of synthetic peptides in the delineation of immunoglobulin antigenic epitopes and Fc effector functions

D. R. STANWORTH, D. S. BURT and G. Z. HASTINGS

Rheumatology and Allergy Research Unit, Department of Immunology, The University of Birmingham, The Medical School, Birmingham, B15 2TJ, UK

Abstract. As an alternative strategy to the use of proteolytic and chemical cleavage in the production of fragments of immunoglobulins retaining Fc effector functions, peptides representative of amino acid sequences constituting the putative active sites have been synthesized and assessed for biological activity in various *in vitro* systems. This approach has been adopted in attempts to define more precisely the autoantigenic epitope on human IgG against which anti-γ-globulin antibodies (the so-called general 'rheumatoid factors'), found in the sera and joint fluids of patients with rheumatoid arthritis, are directed. Synthetic peptides representative of ε-chain sequences are being used in the production of antibodies (polyclonal and monoclonal) directed against specific epitopes within the Fc regions of human and rat IgE. The ability of these antisera to influence the *in vitro* functional properties of IgE anaphylactic antibodies is now under investigation, with particular attention being focused on cytophilicity and mast cell triggering. Preliminary findings suggest that certain of the antisera might be capable of inhibiting mast cell sensitization by IgE antibodies, and therefore might form the basis of a new type of anti-allergy compound.

1986 Synthetic peptides as antigens. Wiley, Chichester (Ciba Foundation Symposium 119) p 226-244

Although synthetic peptides are being used increasingly in the production of antibodies against specific epitopes (antigenic determinants) on a wide range of globular proteins, this approach has so far found only limited application in the study of the antigenic determinants of immunoglobulin (Ig) molecules. This is somewhat surprising, in view of the potential immunopathological importance of anti-γ-globulin antibodies encountered in rheumatoid arthritis and other conditions; quite apart from the generally held assumption that such anti-antibodies play important physiological roles in the feedback control of immunoglobulin synthesis.

As part of a long-term research programme aimed at delineating various Fc effector sites of human IgG (see Stanworth 1982, 1984a), peptides comprising $C_\gamma2$ and $C_\gamma3$ domain sequences of the IgG heavy chain have been synthesized in attempts to locate the position of the autoantigenic site against which so-called general rheumatoid factor is directed. As will be indicated, comparative studies on monoclonal rheumatoid factors isolated from the sera of patients with lymphoproliferative disorders have revealed a quite different antigen-specificity profile. The possible immunological significance of these findings will be discussed.

Another major aspect of our peptide work has been concerned with the synthesis of ε-chain peptides representative of putative Fc effector sites involved in the sensitization and triggering of mast cells by anaphylactic antibodies of the IgE class (Stanworth 1984b). Polyclonal and monoclonal antibodies are now being raised against such peptides, to provide another dimension to these studies. We hope that such an approach will lead ultimately to the development of more effective anti-allergy agents.

Synthesis of immunoglobulin heavy chain peptides

The selection of human immunoglobulin heavy chain sequences for synthesis has been based on preliminary evidence, obtained from studies of IgG fragments, of the location of putative Fc effector sites; and, in the case of mast cell-triggering ε-chain peptide, on the results of initial structure–activity studies on model basic polypeptides. More recently, potentially immunogenic rat ε-chain peptides were selected on the basis of the primary sequence of the parent immunoglobulin heavy chain, and its predicted tertiary and quaternary structure, according to the criteria proposed by Lerner (1982).

Peptides have been synthesized by the solid-phase method of Merrifield (1963), involving the sequential coupling of t-butoxycarbonyl (Boc)-amino acid derivatives to benzhydrylamine resin using appropriate coupling and deprotecting procedures. On completion, peptides were cleaved from the resin with hydrogen fluoride and purified by gel filtration (on Bio-Gel P2), eluting with either 0.1 M-ammonium bicarbonate (pH 8.0) or 0.05 M-acetic acid and monitoring at 280 nm and/or 260 nm. Eluates containing the absorbance peaks were pooled, lyophilized, and stored over P_2O_5 in a vacuum desiccator at 4 °C. Peptides thus synthesized were characterized by HPLC, TLC and quantitative amino acid analysis (after hydrolysis in 6 M-HCl for 24 h at 110 °C). Preparations were usually found to possess amino acid compositions consistent with their expected structures; if not, they were not used in the types of study to be described.

Identification of the autoantigenic site on human IgG

Of the various types of antigenic determinant expressed by human IgG molecules, that responsible for autoantigenicity as reflected by the formation of general rheumatoid factor (RF) is probably the most interesting from both the immunochemical and immunopathological standpoints. For instance, how does 'self' IgG apparently thus become autoimmunogenic in conditions such as rheumatoid arthritis, and are the consequences of this beneficial or detrimental to the patient?

Our early IgG fragmentation work (see Stanworth & Stewart 1976) had shown that the autoantigenic determinant was located within the Fc region of human IgG; but later Fc sub-fragmentation studies failed to show evidence of a clear-cut association of RF reactivity with either the $C_\gamma2$ or $C_\gamma3$ domains. Indeed, in this connection, it is interesting that RF reactivity appeared to be lost on cleavage between these two domains (Stewart et al 1978). But other, chemical substitution studies in our laboratory (Hunneyball & Stan-

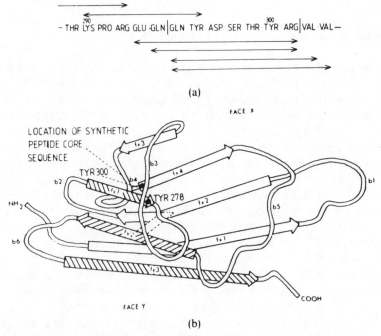

(a)

(b)

FIG. 1. (a) 'Core' human γ-chain sequence (295–301) and related structures synthesized by the solid-phase procedure. (b) Location of the 'core' sequence within the three-dimensional structure of the $C_\gamma2$ domain (adapted from Edmundson et al 1975). (Reproduced from Stanworth 1982, with permission.)

worth 1976), involving the selective citraconylation or carbamylation of lysyl side-chains or the nitration of tyrosyl residues, suggested that the autoantigenic determinant was located towards the C-terminal end of the $C_\gamma 2$ domain of human IgG (and the cross-reactive rabbit IgG).

The use of synthetic peptides representative of sequences constituting this part of the human γ-chain (see Fig. 1) obviously appeared to offer an alternative strategy which might be expected to pin-point more precisely the location of the autoantigenic sequence. Consequently, 7–12-residue linear chain peptides were synthesized spanning this region of the $C_\gamma 2$ domain, notably between amino acid residues 274 and 303, and focusing particularly around the aspartic acid residue of position 297 to which an oligosaccharide unit is conjugated in native human IgG molecules.

An inhibition-haemagglutination method, based on the use of sheep red cells coated with baboon IgG, which had been developed in our laboratory to determine the RF reactivity of cleavage fragments of human IgG, proved not to be sensitive enough for assaying the autoantigenicity of such peptides. Consequently, this was established by means of a radioimmunoassay procedure involving measurement of the capacity of the peptides to inhibit the binding of ^{125}I-labelled purified RF to IgG–Sepharose in mini-columns. As will be noted from Fig. 2, the autoantigenic site appeared to be located within

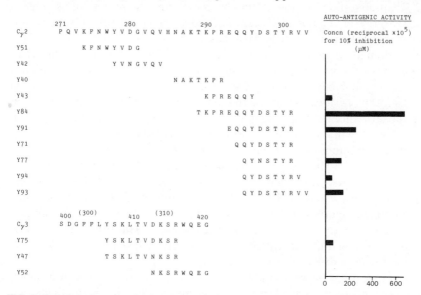

FIG. 2. Relative autoantigenicities of synthetic human γ-chain peptides, determined by the capacity to inhibit binding of radiolabelled general RF to IgG–Sepharose. The one-letter notation for amino acid sequences is used. Numbers in parentheses indicate the equivalent positions in $C_\gamma 2$.

the region incorporating amino acid residues 291–303 of the human γl heavy chain: a peptide (Y84) consisting of the sequence Thr-Lys-Pro-Arg-Glu-Gln-Tyr-Asp-Ser-Thr-Thr-Arg proved to be most reactive with general RF.

The observed inactivity of one of the synthetic peptides consisting of a sequence within this region, namely peptide Y71, comprising residues 294–301, is difficult to explain, particularly as a peptide composed of the equivalent sequence within the rabbit γ-chain (i.e. Glu-Phe-Asn-Ser-Thr-Ile-Arg) showed some reactivity with the same purified RF preparations.

Control peptides consisting of other γ-chain sequences (i.e. 497–506 and 505–515) proved to be non-reactive with isolated RF; as did a human $C_\gamma 3$ domain peptide (Y52) comprising residues 412–420 of the human γl heavy chain sequence, a derivative (Y47) of the sequence 406–416, a nonsense peptide (Tyr-Tyr-Ser-Glu-Thr-Asp-Arg) and a peptide comprising the partial gastrin sequence Gly-Trp-Met-Asp-Phe-Gly. Yet, surprisingly, another peptide, made up of the $C_\gamma 3$ domain sequence Tyr-Ser-Lys-Leu-Thr-Val-Asp-Lys-Ser-Arg, also showed some reactivity with isolated RF (see Fig. 2). Possibly this reflects the presence of anti-γ-globulins with specificities other than that of general RF within the preparations (isolated by immunoadsorption) used in our peptide inhibition radioimmunoassay procedure.

Interestingly, parallel peptide inhibition studies with ^{125}I-labelled monoclonal RF preparations, rather than the polyclonal RF preparations referred to above, revealed a quite different antigen-specificity profile. Of the various synthetic γ-chain peptides tested (of those listed in Fig. 2), only that containing the $C_\gamma 3$ domain sequence spanning residues 413–420 (Y52) proved to be active. This points to a different mechanism being responsible for the formation of such monoclonal RFs, found in the sera of some patients with lymphoproliferative disorders; besides suggesting that an antibody raised in experimental animals against this peptide might offer a satisfactory alternative reagent to monoclonal RF in the routine measurement of circulating immune complexes in various conditions of clinical interest.

Obviously, it will be desirable to look further into the question of the reactivity of human IgG with general RF using peptides composed of other γ-chain sequences: both C-terminal to the region within the $C_\gamma 2$ domain on which attention has been particularly focused, and other regions of the $C_\gamma 3$ domain. Nevertheless, on the basis of the evidence obtained so far from this approach, we conclude that the autoantigenic site on human IgG is located within or includes the region 289–303 of the γ-chain.

The implications of this tentative conclusion are far-reaching. For instance, at the immunochemical level, it could be significant that the site on the human γl-chain identified as the likely location of the autoantigenic determinant includes the asparagine residue at position 297 to which a complex-type biantenary oligosaccharide, composed of $\alpha(1 \rightarrow 3)$ and $\alpha(1 \rightarrow 6)$ arms, is N-linked through a glycosylamine bond. Recent collaborative studies with Dwek and his associates in Oxford (Parekh et al 1985) have provided evidence of changes in the extent of galactosylation of this oligosaccharide in IgG preparations isolated from patients with rheumatoid arthritis. It is possible that glycosylation of the human IgG molecule renders it structurally asymmetric, thus accounting for the puzzling finding that rheumatoid factor–IgG interactions are invariably monovalent, despite the apparent polypeptide structural symmetry of the IgG molecule.

Moreover, one could then envisage that an abnormality in glycosylation of one of the two oligosaccharide sub-units on rheumatoid IgG would lead to exposure of a single underlying peptide 'self' determinant, responsible for stimulating autoantibody formation. The resultant rheumatoid factor directed against this altered form of human IgG might induce the native immunoglobulin to adopt the conformation of the altered form (a possibility consistent with the views of Crumpton, this volume, on the importance of conformation in antigenicity). This might explain why general rheumatoid factor reacts readily with normal as well as rheumatoid human IgG (Normansell & Stanworth 1966).

From the immunopathological standpoint, the findings from our γ-chain peptide studies appear to have potentially important ramifications. For instance, it seems significant that synthetic peptides composed of sequences within the same part of the human γ1 heavy chain have been found by us to inhibit the binding of human IgG to homologous monocytes (Ratcliffe & Stanworth 1982) and to inhibit antibody-dependent cell-mediated cytotoxicity (Sármay et al 1984) (Fig. 3). Furthermore, the region of the human chain

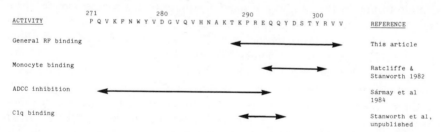

FIG. 3. Comparison of location of various effector functions within the human $C_\gamma 2$ domain, as revealed by synthetic peptide studies. ADCC, antibody-dependent cell-mediated cytotoxicity.

in question includes the tetrapeptide sequence (Thr-Lys-Pro-Arg) of the synthetic peptide, tuftsin, shown to possess phagocytosis-stimulating activity (Nishioka et al 1972). It is not inconceivable that the production of general rheumatoid factor, directed against an autoantigenic epitope located within a similar region of the $C_\gamma 2$ domain, could interfere with the ability of a patient's IgG antibody to mediate essential phagocytic and killer cell functions.

Immunogenic ε-chain peptides

Until recently, the main emphasis of our laboratory's work on ε-chain peptides has been on elucidating the signal for mediator release which is transmitted to target mast cells when IgE antibodies, bound to Fc receptors on their surface, are cross-linked by specific antigen (allergen). Following our structure–activity studies on model histamine-releasing polypeptides (ACTH and melittin) and their derivatives (Jasani et al 1973, 1979), we synthesized peptides consisting of sequences within the $C_\varepsilon 4$ domain of human IgE and showed them to be capable of eliciting the non-cytolytic releases of histamine from normal mast cells in a manner essentially similar to that mediated by anaphylactic anti-body–antigen interaction (Stanworth et al 1979). Subsequent more detailed studies, involving the synthesis of analogues of a decapeptide based on the human ε-chain sequence 497–506, and an octapeptide based on the sequence 497–504, have revealed the precise structural requirements for this direct triggering of rat peritoneal mast cells (Stanworth et al 1984).

We had hoped that the inactive analogues of the human ε-chain peptide, demonstrated in this study, might be capable of antagonizing histamine release effected by the active ε-chain decapeptide, and even by IgE antibody–antigen interaction, thereby forming the basis of a new type of anti-allergy compound. But, so far, such peptide derivatives have shown only very limited evidence of such a potential. A likely explanation for this has been provided by the results of recent collaborative investigations undertaken with Richard Cherry and his associates at Essex University (Dufton et al 1984), based on measurement of the capacity of the various synthetic analogues of the human ε-chain peptide to inhibit the rotation of band 3 protein within a model erythrocyte membrane system. These results have suggested (see Stanworth 1984) that the effective mast cell-triggering ligand, Lys-Thr-Lys-Gly-Ser-Gly-Phe-Phe-Val-Phe-NH$_2$, constituting residues 497–506 of the human ε-chain (like substance P, Arg-Pro-Lys-Pro-Gln-Gln-Phe-Phe-Gly-Leu-Met-NH$_2$, a histamine-releasing neuropeptide) consists of a cationic N-terminal region separated by three spacer residues from a hydrophobic C-terminal region. In other words, it possesses what can be regarded as 'second grade' specificity, rather than being composed of a particular primary sequence.

Consequently, we have recently been placing more emphasis on an alternative strategy aimed at producing antibodies directed against specific epitopes within the Fc region of IgE (Burt et al 1985) which might constitute that part of the antibody molecule involved in binding to mast cell Fc(ε) receptors.

Rabbits have been immunized with keyhole limpet haemocyanin (KLH)-conjugated peptides made up of linear sequences within the $C_\varepsilon 4$ domain of rat IgE, predicted to be located within accessible regions of the immunoglobulin molecule, on the assumption of a three-dimensional structural homology between the rat $C_\varepsilon 4$ domain and the human $C_\gamma 3$ domain (defined by the X-ray studies of Deisenhofer 1981). For instance, polyclonal antibodies have been produced in rabbits against the ε-chain sequences spanning His 542–Lys 557 (P123) and Tyr 459–Arg 472 (P124), which are located in accessible regions of the $C_\varepsilon 4$ domain of rat IgE (see Fig. 4). The antisera were tested for reactivity with free ε-chain peptides and whole rat IgE by inhibition ELISA (enzyme-linked immunosorbent assay) and shown to be entirely specific for the immunizing peptide (giving dilution titres of $1/64\,000$ to $1/312\,000$), while proving unreactive with other synthetic peptides (γ and ε) of similar chain length and composition. Moreover, the antisera against ε-chain peptides P123 and P124 were shown to bind specifically to purified rat myeloma IgE (IR162) and IgE in whole serum (giving titres of greater than $1/6400$), while showing no reactivity with normal rat serum and only very weak cross-reactivity with purified human myeloma IgE. In addition, the binding of anti-peptide sera to rat IgE could be completely inhibited with either homologous peptide or purified rat IgE, but not by other peptides or by purified human IgG.

Rabbit antibodies have also been produced against peptides representative

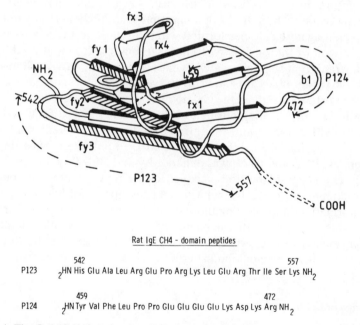

Rat IgE CH4 - domain peptides

542   557
P123 $_2$HN His Glu Ala Leu Arg Glu Pro Arg Lys Leu Glu Arg Thr Ile Ser Lys NH$_2$

459   472
P124 $_2$HN Tyr Val Phe Leu Pro Pro Glu Glu Glu Glu Lys Asp Lys Arg NH$_2$

FIG. 4. The $C_H 4$ ($C_\varepsilon 4$) domain of rat IgE represented schematically by the $C_H 3$ domain model for human IgG (adapted from Edmundson et al 1975). The presumed locations of the synthetic peptides P123 and P124 are shown together with their amino acid sequences. The broken segment at the C-terminus represents the additional decapeptide sequence present in rat IgE.

of other parts of the rat $C_\varepsilon 4$ domain as well as to sites within the $C_\varepsilon 3$ domain. Fig. 5 shows the ability of such anti-peptide antisera to bind ^{125}I-labelled affinity-purified rat (IR162) and human (WT) IgE using a totally solution-phase radioimmunoassay. The anti-peptide sera bound rat IgE to various extents compared with its inactivity with normal rabbit serum. Interestingly, only antibodies against P129 (Ser 414–Gly 428), a $C_\varepsilon 3$ domain sequence, bound both rat and human IgE. A comparison of the primary structure of rat and human IgE in this region shows 60% sequence homology, which accounts for this cross-reactivity. These results demonstrate the ability of anti-peptide antibodies to interact specifically with IgE at sites on the native molecule of which the synthetic peptides are representative.

Obviously, as already implied, we hope that this approach will lead to the production of specific anti-ε-chain peptide antibodies capable of modulating IgE-mediated hypersensitivity reactions. So far, we have been unsuccessful in raising antibodies directed against the human ε-chain decapeptide which our earlier studies have shown possesses potent mast cell-stimulating activity. Some of the antisera raised against other regions of the rat IgE molecule would seem to be potentially capable of inhibiting the binding of rat IgE to Fc receptors on mast cells. For instance, we have indirect evidence to suggest that certain of the anti-$C_\varepsilon 4$ domain peptide antibodies already referred to are directed against epitopes located within or close to the heat-sensitive cytophilic region of the rat IgE molecule (see Fig. 6). It is well established that heating rat IgE at 56 °C abrogates its mast cell-binding activity (Stanworth & Kuhns 1965), an effect attributed to irreversible conformational changes occurring almost exclusively in the $C_\varepsilon 4$ domain (Dorrington & Bennich 1973). As shown in Fig. 6B, heating purified rat IgE for one hour at 56 °C reduced its reactivity with a rabbit anti-rat IgE (Fc) antiserum; whereas binding of the same preparation of rat IgE heated at 56 °C to antisera against the $C_\varepsilon 4$ chain peptides, P123 and P124, was enhanced 4-fold and 60-fold respectively (Fig. 6A). This suggests that these sequences are representative of epitopes in the $C_\varepsilon 4$ domain of native IgE which as a consequence of heating at 56 °C adopt conformations approaching those of the peptide immunogens. Furthermore, the ability of these anti-$C_\varepsilon 4$ chain antisera to detect subtle alterations in the conformation of IgE on heating suggests that they may be directed to a region of the immunoglobulin molecule involved in its heat-sensitive cytophilicity.

Concluding comments

The use of synthetic heavy chain peptides in two very different approaches to the study of the antigenic epitopes of the Fc region of the Ig molecule has been outlined.

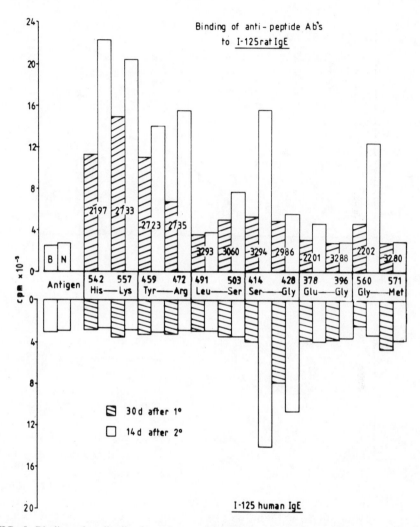

FIG. 5. Binding of antibodies in various anti-peptide sera to affinity-purified rat and human ^{125}I-labelled IgE. Rabbits were immunized by two subcutaneous injections of KLH–peptide conjugate (500 μg). The first was given in complete Freund's adjuvant and the second in incomplete adjuvant, 44 days later. Antisera (final dilution, 1 in 6) were incubated with 300 000 c.p.m. of ^{125}I-IgE in a total volume of 30 μl for 2 h at 20 °C. IgE bound to rabbit antibodies was precipitated with 50 μl 10% *Staphylococcus aureus* Protein A. Sera were isolated and tested from bleeds taken 30 days after the primary (hatched columns) and 14 days after the secondary (open columns) injection. Binding of ^{125}I-IgE to normal rabbit serum (N) and in the absence of serum (B) is also shown. In the same assay, similar dilutions of rabbit antisera specific for the Fc regions of rat and human IgE bound 60 000 c.p.m. and 160 000 c.p.m. respectively of their radiolabelled immunizing IgE preparations. Results are expressed as the mean of triplicate determinations.

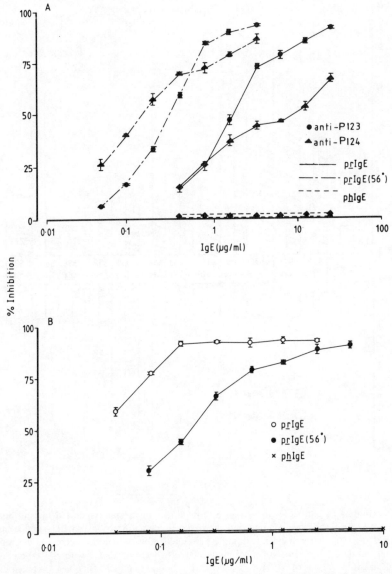

FIG. 6. Binding of antisera to rat IgE heated at 56 °C for 1 h using inhibition ELISA. A. Antisera (1/500 dilution) raised against synthetic peptides P123 (●) and P124 (▲) representative of sequences 542–557 and 459–472 respectively in the rat $C_\varepsilon 4$ domain were preincubated with various concentrations of three purified IgE preparations: rat, ———; rat, heated at 56 °C for 1 h, —·—·—; and human, ---. Aliquots were transferred to microtitre plates coated with 1 μg/ml purified rat IgE and binding was measured by ELISA. B. Rabbit anti-rat IgE (Fc) (1/12 500 dilution) was preincubated with either purified rat IgE, heated (●) or not heated (○), or purified human IgE (×). Other conditions as for A.

We have used synthetic γ-chain peptides to try to locate more precisely than was possible from our earlier strategies the autoantigenic determinant against which spontaneously occurring general rheumatoid factor is directed. An even more comprehensive coverage of sequences including the putative autoantigenic site than that represented by the γ-chain peptides synthesized by us would be needed to obtain more definitive evidence. It will also be necessary to exclude the possibility that the antigenic site in question is a conformational one. Nevertheless, our proposal that this site is contained within, or includes, residues 289–303 in the $C_\gamma 2$ domain is attractive from a conformational stand-point, particularly since this sequence includes an asparagine residue at position 297, to which is linked an oligosaccharide unit thought to have a crucial influence on inter-$C_\gamma 2$ domain spacing. If we are correct in our fixing of the position of the IgG autoantigenic site, an antibody produced experimentally against a peptide incorporating this sequence of the human γ1 chain might be expected to possess rheumatoid factor-like activity.

The approach adopted in our work on ε-chain peptides has been different, in that we have synthesized peptides which, from primary and tertiary structural considerations, would be expected to include antigenic epitopes within the $C_\varepsilon 3$ and $C_\varepsilon 4$ domains of the IgE antibody molecule. Moreover, the polyclonal antisera so far produced against such peptides would seem to offer a potentially new way of modulating IgE-mediated hypersensitivity reactions. The observation that subjecting rat IgE to a form of heat treatment known to abrogate mast cell-sensitizing activity (i.e. 56 °C for one hour) led to a marked increase in its reactivity with anti-$C_\varepsilon 4$ domain peptide antibodies might be interpreted as evidence that the peptides in question are located within or close to the Fc(ε) receptor-binding site(s) on the rat IgE molecule. We are now ascertaining whether such anti-peptide antisera are capable of blocking the *in vivo* sensitization of rat mast cells by IgE antibody, by passive cutaneous anaphylaxis (PCA) testing, as well as the binding of radiolabelled rat IgE to isolated rat peritoneal mast cells *in vitro*. Recently produced polyclonal rabbit antisera against other ε-chain peptides, representative of rat $C_\varepsilon 3$ domain sequences, are being likewise assessed; in view of the claim that sites within both the $C_\varepsilon 3$ and $C_\varepsilon 4$ domains of IgE antibodies are involved in their binding to mast cells. Obviously, we are planning to screen all the polyclonal anti-rat ε-chain peptide antibodies that we are producing (as well as parallel mouse monoclonal ones now under production) for their capacity also to influence mast cell triggering; either positively, by cross-linking cell-bound IgE molecules, or negatively by blocking the signal thought to be provided to a 'second receptor' by a region of the $C_\varepsilon 4$ domain other than that involved in Fc(ε) receptor binding (Stanworth 1984b).

The lines of investigation discussed here indicate that there is scope for anti-peptide antibody production in other important areas besides the development of new forms of vaccine; notably, as far as immunoglobulin chain peptides are concerned, in the elucidation and perhaps eventual modulation of Fc effector functions to the benefit of the host.

Acknowledgements

Our present work on the production and characterization of anti-peptide antibodies is receiving generous financial support from The Wellcome Trust. Financial support for our previous peptide work referred to here was kindly provided by the National Development Corporation and the Medical Research Council. The supervision of the solid-phase synthesis of the peptides by Dr John Fox of the Macromolecular Service Laboratory, University of Birmingham, is gratefully acknowledged.

REFERENCES

Burt DS, Hastings GZ, Stanworth DR 1985 Use of synthetic peptides in the production and characterisation of antibodies directed against predetermined specificities in rat immunoglobulin E. Mol Immunol, in press
Crumpton MJ 1986 The importance of conformation and of equilibria in the interaction of globular proteins and their fragments with antibodies. This volume, p 93-101
Deisenhofer J 1981 Crystallographic refinement and atomic models of a human Fc fragment and its complex with fragment B of protein A from *Staphylococcus aureus* at 2.9- and 2.8-Å resolution. Biochemistry 20:2361-2370
Dorrington KJ, Bennich H 1973 Thermally induced structural changes in immunoglobulin E. J Biol Chem 248:8378-8384
Dufton MJ, Cherry JW, Coleman JW, Stanworth DR 1984 The capacity of basic peptides to trigger exocytosis from mast cells correlates with their capacity to immobilize band 3 proteins in erythrocyte membranes. Biochem J 223:67-71
Edmundson AB, Ely KR, Abola EE, Schiffer M, Panagiotopoulos N 1975 Rotational allomerism and divergent evolution of domains in immunoglobulin light chains. Biochemistry 14:3953-3961
Hunneyball IM, Stanworth DR 1976 The effects of chemical modification on the antigenicity of human and rabbit immunoglobulin G. Immunology 30:881-894
Jasani B, Stanworth DR, Mackler B, Kreil G 1973 Studies on the mast cell triggering action of certain artificial histamine liberators. Int Arch Allergy Appl Immunol 45:74-81
Jasani B, Kreil G, Mackler BF, Stanworth DR 1979 Further studies on the structural requirements for polypeptide-mediated histamine release from rat mast cells. Biochem J 181:623-632
Lerner RA 1982 Tapping the immunological repertoire to produce antibodies of predetermined specificity. Nature (Lond) 299:592-596
Merrifield RB 1963 Solid phase peptide synthesis. I. The synthesis of a tetrapeptide. J Am Chem Soc 85:2149-2154
Nishioka K, Constatopoulos A, Saton PS, Najjar VA 1972 The characteristics, isolation and synthesis of the phagocytosis stimulating peptide tuftsin. Biochem Biophys Res Commun 47:172-179
Normansell DE, Stanworth DR 1966 Ultracentrifugal studies of the reactions of rheumatoid factors with native human γ-G-globulin. Immunology 10:527-533

Parekh RB, Dwek RA, Sutton BJ, Fernandes DL, Leung A, Stanworth D, Rademacher TW, Mizuochi T, Taniguchi T, Matsuta K, Takeuchi F, Nagano Y, Miyamoto T, Kobata A 1985 Association of rheumatoid arthritis and primary osteoarthritis with changes in the glycosylation pattern of total serum IgG. Nature (Lond) 316:452-457

Ratcliffe A, Stanworth DR 1982 The use of synthetic gamma chain peptides in the localisation of the binding site(s) on human IgG1 for the Fc receptors of homologous monocytes and heterologous mouse macrophages. Immunol Lett 4:215-221

Sármay G, Benczur M, Petranyi GY, Klein E, Kahn M, Stanworth DR, Gergely J 1984 Ligand inhibition studies on the role of Fc receptors in antibody-dependent cell-mediated cytotoxicity. Mol Immunol 21:43-51

Stanworth DR 1982 Application of synthetic peptides representative of immunoglobulin sequences to the delineation of receptor binding and signalling processes. Mol Immunol 19:1245-1254

Stanworth DR 1984a Use of synthetic peptides with immunoglobulin-heavy chain sequences in the delineation of Fc effector function. Biochem Soc Trans 12:747-754

Stanworth DR 1984b The role of non-antigen receptors in mast cell signalling processes. Mol Immunol 21:1183-1190

Stanworth DR, Kuhns WJ 1965 Quantitative studies on the assay of human skin sensitising antibodies (reagins). I. An examination of factors affecting the accuracy of the Prausnitz-Küstner (P-K) test. Immunology 9:139-150

Stanworth DR, Stewart GA 1976 Biological activities located within the Fc region of immunoglobulins. In: Hemmings WA (ed) Maternofoetal transmission of immunoglobulins. Cambridge University Press, London, p 7-24

Stanworth DR, Kings M, Roy PD, Moran JM, Moran DM 1979 Synthetic peptides comprising sequences of human immunoglobulin E heavy chain capable of releasing histamine. Biochem J 180:665-668

Stanworth DR, Coleman JW, Khan Z 1984 Essential structural requirements for triggering of mast cells by a synthetic peptide comprising a sequence in the $C_e 4$ domain of human IgE. Mol Immunol 21:243-247

Stewart GA, Várro R, Stanworth DR 1978 The influence of enzymatic cleavage of human and rabbit IgG on their reactivity with staphylococcal protein A. Immunology 35:785-791

DISCUSSION

Skehel: The hydrophobic sequence which follows the basic residue in the neuropeptide substance P is analogous to the N-terminal hydrophobic sequence in the Sendai virus fusion glycoprotein; in IgE the hydrophobic sequence is analogous to the sequence in the influenza virus fusion glycoprotein, the haemagglutinin. Is it conceivable that one or all of those basic residues are sites for proteolytic processing in IgE?

Stanworth: That is very interesting. I have wondered if such a proteolytic cleavage process would be restricted to the sites of arginyl residues. It would be very exciting if mast cell-bound IgE is cleaved in this manner. There is a precedent for this type of process, as indicated by the work of Weigle's group on macrophage–T cell interaction, where part of the C_H3 domain of IgG appears to be cleaved to provide a fragment which induces T cell-dependent B cell activation (Hobbs et al 1985). One could postulate that something similar happens here, namely that a protease is activated in the mast cell plasma membrane as a result of immunological triggering. I showed the Lys-Thr-Lys-Gly-Ser-Gly-Phe-Phe-Val-Phe histamine-releasing ε-chain peptide sequence; the next N-terminal residue is an arginine, and then at the C-terminal end there is a valine and then another arginine residue. If one examines the whole of the Fc region sequence of the human IgE molecule, this is the only stretch between two arginyl residues which fulfils the criteria that we have defined as being essential for mast cell triggering, namely a cluster of basic amino acids, the absence of acidic ones, and nearby hydrophobic residues (Stanworth 1979). Cleavage of the IgE Fc region by a tryptic protease (i.e. at both lysyl and arginyl residues) would be expected to lead to sacrifice of the most important of these structural features. But is it possible that a mast cell membrane protease is activated during immunological triggering which cleaves only at arginyl residues?

Skehel: The two viral glycoproteins involved in fusion are synthesized as inactive precursors and are activated by proteolytic cleavage at basic residues which immediately precede these hydrophobic sequence analogues.

Crumpton: I have two questions in relation to the proposed mechanism for mast cell triggering by IgE. Firstly, there are many instances where monoclonal antibodies against receptors act as ligands. Are there any instances where monoclonal antibodies against IgE receptors cause triggering? If there are, then this would argue for a single signal from the cell surface.

Stanworth: There are antisera which do this, and this is the basis of the claims by the Ishizaka group (Ishizaka & Ishizaka 1978) that all that is needed to initiate mast cell triggering is to cross-link Fc(ε) receptors. We produced an antiserum against rat mast cell Fc(ε) receptor that will initiate histamine release from pleural but not peritoneal mast cells (Batchelor & Stanworth 1980). The antibodies produced by the Ishizakas were directed against receptors on certain basophil leukaemic cell lines. But their findings do not necessarily denigrate the mechanism of mast cell triggering which I am proposing, because there are many other ways in which one can 'fire' mast cells artificially. One can use an ionophore to get calcium ions into the cell, for example, and thereby induce histamine release.

Crumpton: That is my next question, and it relates to your use of melittin. This is a sodium ionophore, at least in some cells (Rozengurt et al 1981). Furthermore, in these cells there is evidence that an increase in intracellular sodium concentration precedes the increase in calcium concentration. I understand that a rise in intracellular calcium concentration is believed to act as the primary trigger for histamine release. So are you suggesting that there is a portion of the Fc domain of IgE that somehow, on binding to receptor, inserts itself in the mast cell membrane and acts like a sodium ionophore?

Stanworth: Yes, and perhaps mobilizes cytosolic calcium in the process. One has to remember that we tend to use these cations under rather artificial experimental conditions, and the important part of the contribution of calcium ions to mast cell triggering might be the mobilization of intracellular calcium. I would suggest that there would be scope for the type of peptide ligand which I am proposing to have such an effect, particularly if it is selectively cleaved from mast cell-bound IgE antibody.

Crumpton: Has anybody looked for changes in the intracellular sodium ion or proton concentrations in these cells?

Stanworth: Evidence has been obtained (Cochrane & Douglas 1976) that calcium influx occurs during mast cell triggering as the result of a Ca^{2+}/Na^{+} ion exchange process, which is sensitive to extracellular sodium ions. Consequently, when the extracellular medium is depleted of sodium ions, mast cells will release histamine spontaneously.

Geysen: With reference to your rheumatoid factor studies, 18 months ago we synthesized all the hexapeptides corresponding to the published sequence of an IgG; that is, more than 500 peptides. We were then unable to continue our studies because, whereas in any other system, preimmune or unrelated sera do not react with the synthesized set of peptides, all sera reacted with this set. Reactions were generally with those peptides corresponding to the Fc region of the molecule, and no reaction was observed with peptides corresponding to the hypervariable regions. This indicates that sera from each of the animals tested contain the equivalent of autoantibodies, and reactions from sera containing rheumatoid factor did not stand out sufficiently to allow identification of peptides corresponding to the epitopes being recognized.

Stanworth: One must define what one means by rheumatoid factor. There are many anti-γ-globulins that are referred to as 'rheumatoid factors'; for example, the anti-allotypes found in the sera of patients who have received many blood transfusions. I am talking about what is usually called 'general rheumatoid factor', identified by Allen & Kunkel (1966), directed against an antigenic determinant called 'Ga' present on three of the four isotypes of human IgG. In this case, do your sera react with the IgG3 subclass?

Geysen: The rheumatoid arthritis sera were supplied from a Melbourne hospital. Before we tested these on the synthesized hexapeptides we collected sera from people in the laboratory, and found reactions in every case. As I said, reactions obtained from some of the rheumatoid arthritis sera didn't seem to differ from the normal type of non-specific reaction. This is the only case where we have found this. When we made the set of peptides for the hepatitis antigen, we found any number of human sera that were uniformly negative.

Lachmann: You made the valid point that there is only a single antigenic site in an intact IgG molecule able to react with IgM rheumatoid factor to form a 22S complex. Then you said that peptides produced from a single Fc chain react with rheumatoid factor. Those statements at first sight seem incompatible.

Stanworth: Not peptides synthesized from a single Fc chain, but representative of a specific part of the $C_{\gamma}2$ domain. There is potentially an autoantigenic site on both heavy chains; the idea I am invoking (and this has been neglected in the symposium so far) is that if some of the proteins we have been discussing are in fact glycoproteins, we have to recognize the contribution of the oligosaccharide to the availability of peptide antigenic determinants. The amino acid sequence in question will be present in both γ-chains; but it might be accessible in only one, because of their asymmetric glycosylation.

Lachmann: I thought the asymmetric glycosylation was found only in rabbit IgG?

Stanworth: The Oxford group have evidence that the same applies to human IgG.

Williams: The sequencing of the sugars of glycoproteins can be done now, for example by Dwek and his colleagues in Oxford; theirs is the only laboratory in the UK which has the skills necessary (see Parekh et al 1985).

Humphrey: Is the oligosaccharide longer on one chain than on the other?

Stanworth: Yes, slightly. There is some chemical difference. The rigid $\alpha(1\rightarrow3)$ arm of at least one of the paired oligosaccharides is always devoid of galactose, thereby exposing its outer-arm $\beta(1\rightarrow2)$-linked N-acetylglucosamine residue, which then interacts directly with the $Man\beta(1\rightarrow4)$ GlcNac segment of the opposing carbohydrate chain.

Humphrey: So you would have an 'umbrella' over one chain but not over the other?

Stanworth: Yes! This is very much speculation, but it offers a plausible explanation for the puzzling fact that monomeric IgG seems to be univalent with regard to its autoantigenic determinant.

Humphrey: Does this apply to all the IgG in the rheumatoid sera?

Stanworth: So far, as near as possible, total IgG has been isolated, and used in the Oxford study to which I have referred. We now want to break that down into subclasses. We have independent evidence (Leung 1983) that there is no substantial change in overall subclass composition between rheumatoid and normal IgG.

Skehel: In relation to the suggested shielding of antigenic sites by carbohydrate side-chains, it is known for the influenza virus haemagglutinin that a monoclonal antibody selects for a variant which is additionally glycosylated. In this case antibody–antigen interaction is prevented by glycosylation of the variant antigen.

Edmundson: In most of the IgG molecules that have been examined crystallographically, there is an axis of two-fold symmetry down the middle of the molecule. This implies that in a myeloma protein, at least, there has to be symmetry in the carbohydrate moieties. Are you saying that only in rheumatoid factors is there asymmetry in the carbohydrates?

Stanworth: No, the asymmetry is found in normal human IgG as well. But one has to be careful in extrapolating from myeloma proteins, because each myeloma protein of the same IgG subclass appears to have a distinctive oligosaccharide pattern, and it would therefore be dangerous to generalize. We are saying that there is a quantitative difference between normal, osteoarthritic and rheumatoid IgG, in the extent of galactosylation of their asparagine-linked oligosaccharides. There is no overlap in the oligosaccharide pattern shown by the IgG from these three groups of subjects.

Edmundson: In rabbit immunoglobulins the normal state seems to be heterogeneity in the carbohydrate moieties.

Stanworth: The Oxford group have confirmed this. I don't know whether the fact that rheumatoid factor cross-reacts with rabbit IgG is influenced by the oligosaccharide composition of this immunoglobulin.

Williams: There is a further problem about the sugars in Ig molecules, that the sequences previously used and fitted on some of the crystallographic maps are wrong; so there might be sufficient disorder in the sugar part of the molecule for it not to make much difference to the crystallographic fitting of sequence and electron density. We have to wait for the full story on the sugars in these antibodies from Dwek and his co-workers.

Edmundson: I agree with that, but the crystallographic studies done on Ig in the rabbit system have been on the Fc region, which is inherently non-symmetric when crystallized.

Stanworth: Smyth & Utsumi (1967) showed that there is a single N-acetylglucosamine residue attached to threonine within the hinge region of just one of the two chains in a proportion of rabbit IgG molecules. The Oxford workers have now confirmed this, so there is certainly that amount of heterogeneity of one of the oligosaccharide units of rabbit IgG.

Rothbard: Are there sequence variations between different subclasses of immunoglobulins in the region which you believe interacts with the receptor involved in antibody-dependent cellular cytotoxicity? Can you rationalize from the different sequences why IgG2a is more effective than the other subclasses?

Stanworth: There is no substantial primary structural difference between the subclasses in that region of the human γ-chain.

Rothbard: Do you find that disturbing?

Stanworth: Yes; but one could incriminate the oligosaccharide here again and suggest that it can also influence the binding of IgG molecules to Fc receptors. There is evidence, for instance, that oligosaccharide prosthetic groups can influence the catabolism of IgG molecules in this manner.

Rothbard: It would be interesting to see whether any of the peptides corresponding to these regions can compete with the immunoglobulin in your assays.

Stanworth: Yes; we have data on the homology in that region of the γ-chain.

Lerner: Incidentally, it might be interesting to check the lytic peptides which you have cast aside for possible antibiotic activity, or anti-yeast activity. We have seen some peptides which seem to be bacteriocidal.

REFERENCES

Allen JC, Kunkel HG 1966 Hidden rheumatoid factors with specificity for native gamma globulins. Arth Rheum 9:758-768

Batchelor KW, Stanworth DR 1980 A comparison of the histamine-releasing properties of rat pleural and peritoneal mast cells. Immunology 41:271-278

Cochrane DE, Douglas WW 1976 Histamine release by exocytosis from rat mast cells on reduction of extracellular sodium: a secretory response inhibited by calcium, strontium, barium or magnesium. J Physiol (Lond) 257:433-448

Hobbs MV, Morgan EL, Weigle WI 1985 Bifunctional lymphocyte regulation by human Fcγ fragments and a synthetic peptide, p23, derived from the Fc region. Immunol Lett 9:201-206

Ishizaka T, Ishizaka K 1978 Triggering of histamine release from rat mast cells by divalent antibodies against IgE-receptors. J Immunol 120:800-805

Leung A Y-T 1983 PhD Thesis, Birmingham University

Parekh RB, Dwek RA, Sutton BJ, Fernandes DL, Leung A, Stanworth D, Rademacher TW, Mizuochi T, Taniguchi T, Matsuta K, Takeuchi F, Nagano Y, Miyamoto T, Kobata A 1985 Association of rheumatoid arthritis and primary osteoarthritis with changes in the glycosylation pattern of total serum immunoglobulin G. Nature (Lond) 316:452-457

Rozengurt E, Gelehrter TD, Legg A, Pettican P 1981 Melittin stimulates Na entry, Na–K pump activity and DNA synthesis in quiescent cultures of mouse cells. Cell 23:781-788

Smyth DS, Utsumi S 1967 Structure at the hinge region in rabbit immunoglobulin-G. Nature (Lond) 216:332-335

Stanworth DR 1979 Molecular basis of mast cell triggering processes. Monogr Allergy 14:271-280

Characterization of the human c-*myc* protein using antibodies prepared against synthetic peptides

GERARD I. EVAN, DAVID C. HANCOCK, TREVOR LITTLEWOOD and C. DAVID PAUZA*†

*Ludwig Institute for Cancer Research and *MRC Laboratory of Molecular Biology, MRC Centre, Hills Rd, Cambridge CB2 2QH, UK*

Abstract. Synthetic peptides with amino acid sequences based on inferred sequences encoded by the human c-*myc* proto-oncogene have been used as immunogens to produce polyclonal and monoclonal antibodies. These peptide-specific antibodies have then been used to identify the intact human c-*myc* protein. By immunoprecipitation and immunoblotting analysis we have defined the human c-*myc* protein as a phosphoprotein with an apparent molecular mass of 62 kDa on a sodium dodecyl sulphate–polyacrylamide gel. The protein is present in both normal and transformed cells but the steady-state levels of p62$^{c\text{-}myc}$ are elevated in the transformed cells by comparison with normal ones.

We have used our anti-c-*myc* peptide antibodies to study the subcellular localization of p62$^{c\text{-}myc}$. We find the protein to be loosely associated with cell nuclei by an interaction which is highly sensitive to variations in ionic strength within the physiological range. In response to *in vitro* or *in vivo* heat-shock the protein becomes sequestered in an insoluble complex associated with the nucleus. This complex contains a discrete subset of nuclear proteins, of which p62$^{c\text{-}myc}$ is a member. Immunofluorescence microscopy of p62$^{c\text{-}myc}$ shows it to be localized in a defined and previously unobserved subnuclear structure. A role for p62$^{c\text{-}myc}$ as an intracellular messenger is suggested.

1986 Synthetic peptides as antigens. Wiley, Chichester (Ciba Foundation Symposium 119) p 245-263

Modern recombinant DNA technology has made the isolation, characterization and sequencing of interesting genes relatively straightforward. However, identifying the proteins encoded by these genes has for long been a difficult task.

Two main methods exist for raising antibodies specific for undefined proteins

---

† *Present address:* The Salk Institute for Biological Sciences, PO Box 85800, San Diego, California 92138, USA.

whose genes are well characterized. One strategy is to clone part or all of the gene into a bacterial expression vector. The vector is used to transform bacteria and the expressed heterologous polypeptide ('xenoprotein') is purified and used as an immunogen. Antibodies raised against such xenoproteins have proved useful in identifying oncogene proteins. The other strategy is to synthesize peptides whose amino acid sequences are determined by the DNA sequence of the gene of interest. These synthetic peptides are then used as immunogens to raise antibodies which cross-react with the intact gene product.

We have used the second strategy (the synthetic peptide approach) to identify and study the protein product of the human proto-oncogene c-*myc*.

The myc oncogene

The oncogene *myc* was first identified as the transforming sequences of the avian myelocytomatosis viruses, which mainly cause acute myelocystic leukaemia in chickens, as well as a number of other neoplasms. Four independent isolates of avian myelocytomatosis virus have been described—MC29, OK10, MH2 and CM II. All contain *myc* oncogene sequences in various forms. More recently, *myc* sequences have been identified in naturally occurring acutely transforming feline retroviruses. Viral *myc* (v-*myc*) genes are not required for the life cycle of retroviruses and appear to have been acquired at the expense of part of the retrovirus's normal genetic complement. Since retroviruses contain only three genes, each necessary for viral replication, retroviruses containing v-*myc* sequences are therefore invariably replication-defective. It is now thought that v-*myc* sequences are derived from host cell genes by viral transduction. Retroviruses are particularly prone to acquiring host genes by transduction, perhaps because integration into the host genome is an obligatory part of their life cycle. A number of other genetic sequences, unrelated to *myc*, are also actively oncogenic in retroviruses and these sequences constitute the known viral oncogenes (v-*oncs*). The v-*oncs* all appear to have been derived from host genes (Bishop 1983).

Normal host cell genes, homologous with the v-*myc* sequences of avian myelocytomatosis virus, have been identified in many eukaryotic genomes. Indeed, like all the 'cellular oncogenes', *myc* sequences are probably present in all eukaryotic organisms, from yeast to man. The degree of evolutionary conservation shown by the cellular oncogenes suggests that each encodes a protein which is a vital component of *normal* eukaryotic cellular machinery. It is probably only when the expression of a cellular oncogene is altered in some way that it is capable of inducing neoplastic transformation. Cellular oncogenes therefore have the potential to transform cells, but this is not their normal function. For this reason, many prefer the term 'proto-oncogene' to describe these sequences. Alteration in oncogene expression is an inevitable consequence of transduction into a retrovirus, because the transduced gene is placed under the control of a viral promoter instead of normal cellular control elements. In addition to viral transduction, however, other mechanisms have now been identified by which normal cellular *myc* (c-*myc*) gene expression may be altered in a cell. (For a review of viral and cellular oncogenes, see Bishop 1983 and Müller & Verma 1984.)

The c-myc proto-oncogene and cancer

Several observations suggest that the c-*myc* proto-oncogene has a role in the aetiology of human neoplasia.

(1) Integration of a retrovirus next to, or in the vicinity of, the host cell's c-*myc* gene can occur during the natural course of infection by some retroviruses. The strong promoter and enhancer elements of the integrated retrovirus may lead to over-expression of the c-*myc* gene, with cell transformation as a consequence. This is the process of 'promoter insertion' (Hayward et al 1981, Payne et al 1982).

(2) The c-*myc* gene lies at the site of chromosomal breakage and translocation observed in various haemopoietic tumours, in particular Burkitt's lymphoma in man (Adams et al 1983). Such translocations may alter the control or structure of the c-*myc* gene, giving rise to a transformed phenotype. The precise relationship betweeen chromosomal translocation, c-*myc* expression and malignancy is, however, still obscure.

(3) A number of human tumour cell lines lines have an amplified c-*myc* gene (reviewed in Stark & Wahl 1984, Alitalo 1985). This amplification has, in many of these cell lines, been localized to an homogeneously staining region of one chromosome, or to double minute chromosomes. C-*myc* gene amplification considerably increases the expression of c-*myc* mRNA. A related gene, N-*myc*, is also amplified in several tumours of probable neuroectodermal origin (Schwab et al 1983).

(4) Induction of c-*myc* expression is a common feature when cells progress from a resting state to a dividing state (Kelly et al 1983). Expression of c-*myc* is therefore associated with cell growth and division. The de-regulation of c-*myc* expression may thus be a cause or component of cellular transformation. In fact, most naturally occurring human tumours show significant c-*myc* expression.

(5) A variety of polar organic compounds, such as retinoic acid, dimethyl sulphoxide and butyric acid, induce some tumour cell lines to differentiate terminally (e.g. Filmus & Buick 1985). C-*myc* expression is abruptly repressed

when differentiation is induced. A consequence of uncontrolled c-*myc* expression might therefore be that cells are prevented from progressing along their normal differentiation pathway. A cell in which differentiation is arrested would be a constantly self-renewing clone with many of the characteristics of a transformed phenotype.

All these observations suggest possible roles for the c-*myc* gene in human tumours. The next step is to identify the c-*myc* gene product and to discern its function in the normal and transformed cell.

Structure of the human c-myc gene

The detailed structure and nucleotide sequence of the human c-*myc* gene have been elucidated (e.g. Colby et al 1983). The gene contains three exons, of which the second and third encode the c-*myc* protein. The function of the first, non-coding, exon is unknown, though a role in post-transcriptional regulation of the gene has been proposed. Exons 2 and 3 encode a 439-amino acid protein with an inferred molecular mass of about 48 kDa. This expressed protein is presumably responsible for all the activities associated with the c-*myc* gene.

To study the c-*myc* protein in detail, we prepared antibody probes which specifically recognize the protein and can be used to identify and characterize it and to investigate its function.

Production of antibodies specific for the human c-myc protein

We used the synthetic peptide approach to prepare antibodies specific for the human c-*myc* oncoprotein. Initially, seven peptides were synthesized, each containing sequences of the human c-*myc* protein inferred from the open reading frame present in exons 2 and 3 of the gene. Each peptide was from a different and non-overlapping region of the sequence (Ramsay et al 1984). The peptides were conjugated to keyhole limpet haemocyanin (KLH) using *N*-maleimidobenzoyl hydroxysuccinimide ester. When these conjugates were injected into rabbits, either separately or in various combinations, a number of antisera were obtained with anti-peptide activities. Most of these sera also immunoprecipitated a phosphoprotein of 62 kDa apparent molecular mass from human cells expressing c-*myc*. This protein was shown to be the human c-*myc* product, p62$^{c\text{-}myc}$ (Ramsay et al 1984).

To obtain a continuous supply of good anti-p62$^{c\text{-}myc}$ antibodies, we also immunized mice with each of the seven synthetic peptide–KLH conjugates. In the mouse strain used, BALB/c, only two peptides (D and G) induced respectable antibody titres. The sequences of peptides D and G, together with those of the homologous regions of the mouse c-*myc* and chicken c- and v-*myc* proteins, are shown in Table 1. Splenocytes from mice immunized with peptides D and G were fused with SP2 myeloma cells to produce hybridomas. Culture supernatants were screened by a solid-phase enzyme-linked immunosorbent assay (ELISA) and positive hybridomas were cloned and recloned. Three monoclonal antibodies (MAbs) specific for peptide D and three specific for peptide G were finally isolated (Table 2).

These six MAbs were tested for their abilities to immunoprecipitate p62^{c-myc} from radiolabelled lysates prepared from the cell line Colo 320 HSR, a human colonic apudoma containing an amplified c-*myc* gene located in an homogeneously staining region of the X chromosome. As a positive control for anti-p62^{c-myc} antibody we used a rabbit polyclonal anti-peptide G antibody, shown

TABLE 1 Sequences of synthetic peptide immunogens and homologous sequences in mouse and chicken myc proteins

Peptide D	(amino acid residues 171–188)
Human c-*myc* (immunogen)	C S T S S L Y L Q D L S A A A S E C
Mouse c-*myc*	C S T S S L Y L Q D L T A A A S E C
Chicken c-*myc*	A A S A G L Y L H D L G A A A A D C
Chicken v-*myc*	A A S A G L Y L H D L G A A A A D C

Peptide G	(amino acid residues 408-439)
Human c-*myc* (immunogen)	A E E Q K L I S E E D L L R K R R E Q L K H K L E Q L R N S C A
Mouse c-*myc*	A D E H K L T S E E D L L R K R R E Q L K H K L E Q L R N S G A
Chicken c-*myc*	S D E H R L I A E K E Q L R R R R E Q L K H K L E Q L R N S R A
Chicken v-*myc*	S D E H K L I A E K E Q L R R R R E Q L K H N L E Q L R N S R A

TABLE 2 Characteristics of anti-myc peptide monoclonal antibodies

Monoclonal antibody	Peptide specificity	Ig subclass	Binding to:		
			Human p62^{c-myc}	Mouse p64/66^{c-myc}	Chicken p110^{c-myc}
Myc1-8F9	D	IgG$_1$.k	+	+	−
Myc1-3C7	D	IgG$_1$.k	+	+	−
Myc1-6E10	D	IgG$_1$.k	+	+	−
CT14-G4	G	IgG$_1$.k	+	−	−
CT9-B7	G	IgG$_1$.k	+	−	−
Myc1-9E10	G	IgG$_1$.k	+(IB)[a]	−	−

[a]IB = binds only immunoblotted p62^{c-myc}.

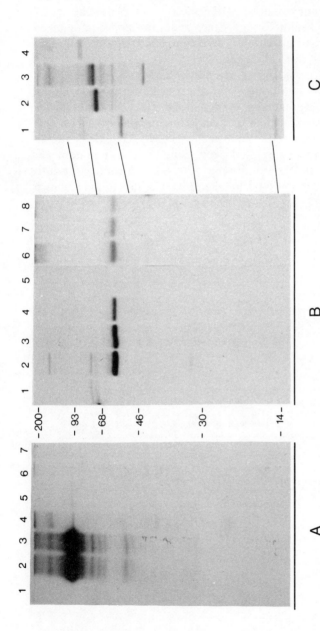

FIG. 1. Immunoprecipitation of *myc* proteins from human, mouse and quail cells. MC29 virus-transformed quail fibroblasts (panel A), human Colo 320 HSR cells (panel B and panel C, tracks 1 and 2) and mouse Rec2A fibroblasts (panel C, tracks 3 and 4) were all labelled with ^{3}[H]lysine for one hour. Cells were lysed in RIPA buffer and aliquots of each cell lysate were immunoprecipitated with antibodies. Purified antigens were fractionated on a 12.5% sodium dodecylsulphate–polyacrylamide gel and detected by autoradiography. The antibodies used were as follows:

Panel A. Track 1, preimmune rabbit serum; track 2, rabbit anti-peptide G antibody; track 3, rabbit antibody to chicken *myc* proteins; track 4, MAb CT9-B7; track 5, MAb CT14-G4; track 6, MAb Mycl-8F9; track 7, MAb Mycl-6E10.

Panel B. Track 1, preimmune rabbit serum; track 2, rabbit anti-peptide G antibody; track 3, MAb CT9-B7; track 4, MAb CT14-G4; track 5, MAb Mycl-9E10; track 6, MAb Mycl 8F9; track 7, MAb Mycl-3C7; track 8, MAb Mycl-6E10.

Panel C. Track 1, W6/32 monoclonal anti-HLA antibody; track 2, MAb Mycl-8F9; track 3, MAb Mycl-8F9; track 4, MAb W6/32 anti-HLA. Tracks 1 and 2 are immunoprecipitates from human cells, tracks 3 and 4 from mouse cells. Molecular weight markers were myosin (200 kDa), phosphorylase *b* (93 kDa), bovine serum albumin (68 kDa), ovalbumin to recognize the human c-*myc* protein. Five of the six MAbs immunoprecipitated a 62 kDa antigen (Fig. 1B). Three of these (Myc1-8F9, Myc1-6E10 and Myc1-3C7) are specific for peptide D and two (CT14-G4 and CT9-B7) are specific for peptide G. By means of *Staphylococcus aureus* V8 protease mapping of each 62 kDa antigen recognized by both polyclonal and monoclonal antibodies, we showed that all the 62 kDa antigens were indeed the same protein, p62^{c-myc}. Only one MAb, peptide G-specific Myc1-9E10, failed to immunoprecipitate p62^{c-myc}. The three peptide D-specific MAbs also recognize a 64 kDa protein in mouse cells which we believe to be the murine c-*myc* protein (Table 2 and Fig. 1C). The mouse c-*myc* was not recognized by any of the antibodies specific for peptide G. None of the MAbs recognized the 110 kDa *gag-myc* fusion protein expressed by MC29 virus-transformed quail fibroblasts (Fig. 1A).

We then assayed the ability of each of the six monoclonals to recognize human p62^{c-myc} in cell lysates which had been electrophoretically fractionated on sodium dodecyl sulphate–polyacrylamide gels and electroblotted onto nitrocellulose paper. All six MAbs bound electroblotted p62^{c-myc}, including Myc1-9E10, which does not recognize native p62^{c-myc}. Indeed, in our experience, Myc1-9E10 is the best probe of all the six MAbs for detection of p62^{c-myc} by immunoblotting.

Immunoblotting analysis was then used to estimate the relative amounts of p62^{c-myc} in different human cell lines with MAb Myc1-9E10 as probe. As expected, cell lines with amplified c-*myc* genes had the highest steady-state levels of p62^{c-myc}. The lowest p62^{c-myc} levels were in non-transformed cell lines possessing finite lifespans *in vitro* (Fig. 2). Surprisingly, transformed cell lines such as HeLa and CCRF-CEM also demonstrated high levels of p62^{c-myc}, even though these cells do not possess amplified c-*myc* genes. High levels of p62^{c-myc} can therefore accumulate without c-*myc* gene amplification; this seems to be a common feature in transformed cells.

Subcellular localization of p62^{c-myc}

Extensive analyses of the subcellular localization of the avian v-*myc* proteins have been documented. All show a primarily nuclear location for v-*myc* proteins. Immunofluorescence microscopy suggests a fairly even distribution throughout the nucleus with exclusion of v-*myc* proteins from nucleoli (Alitalo et al 1983). During metaphase, v-*myc* proteins become dispersed throughout the cell and show no obvious association with condensed chromosomes (Winqvist et al 1984).

The subcellular distribution of c-*myc* proteins might be expected to be similar to that of v-*myc* proteins. However, cells expressing v-*myc* do so at a

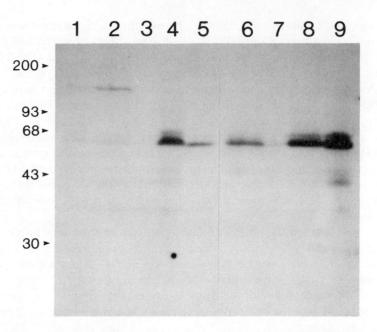

FIG. 2. Comparison of p62$^{c\text{-}myc}$ levels in various human cell lines by immunoblotting. 10^6 cell equivalents of each cell type were fractionated on a 10% SDS–polyacrylamide gel and electroblotted onto nitrocellulose paper. The blot was probed with MAb Mycl-9E10 for p62$^{c\text{-}myc}$. The cells analysed were: track 1, MRC-5 (human fibroblast); track 2, Detroit 532 (human foreskin fibroblast); track 3, Flow 4000 (human embryonic kidney); track 4, HeLa (human cervical carcinoma); track 5, CCRF-CEM (human T cell leukaemia); track 6, HL60 (human promyelocytic leukaemia) (before addition of dimethyl sulphoxide to growth medium); track 7, HL60 (3 h after adding 1.2% dimethyl sulphoxide to growth medium); track 8, Colo 320 HSR (human colonic apudoma); track 9, SCCL-N417 (human small cell lung carcinoma). Molecular weights were estimated by reference to the positions of prestained protein markers (see legend to Fig. 1).

level many times higher than the level at which c-*myc* is expressed, even in cells with c-*myc* gene amplification. Perhaps, therefore, the vast excess of v-*myc* protein in virus-transformed cells leads to the abnormal accumulation of v-*myc* proteins in certain regions of the cell. We decided to analyse the subcellular location of p62$^{c\text{-}myc}$, using our p62$^{c\text{-}myc}$-specific monoclonal antibodies.

Initially we analysed p62$^{c\text{-}myc}$ localization in human cells by immunofluorescence microscopy. Even in cells expressing high levels of p62$^{c\text{-}myc}$ we were unable to see bright nuclear fluorescence, using either our monoclonal or polyclonal antibodies specific for p62$^{c\text{-}myc}$ peptides. This is in stark contrast to the bright nuclear staining observed upon immunofluorescence microscopic analysis of v-*myc* proteins, as outlined above. However, on closer inspection of the cells we saw small, ring-shaped structures within the nuclei of cells which stained brightly with anti-p62^{c-myc} antibodies (Fig. 3A). This staining is specifically blocked by preincubating the antibodies with the appropriate synthetic peptide immunogen. In different cell lines, the brightness and size of the ring structures correlates perfectly with the steady-state levels of p62^{c-myc} in each cell, as judged by immunoblotting. The ring structures appear to lie on the surface of the nucleus, and are visible only within a very tight focal plane. Treatment of fixed, permeabilized cells with the enzyme Pronase reveals that the ring structures may be part of a larger reticular nuclear structure. Possibly, this more diffuse structure also contains p62^{c-myc} in a form which is not normally accessible to antibodies but is exposed by the mild proteolytic digestion (Fig. 3B). In mitotic cells, the ring structures vanish and anti-p62^{c-myc} antibodies stain the entire interior of the cell except for the region containing condensed chromosomes (Fig. 3C). This diffuse pattern of immunofluorescence in mitotic cells is characteristic of a number of proteins associated with the interphase nucleus and is also shown by v-*myc* proteins (Winqvist et al 1984).

The conclusion from our immunofluorescence microscopic data is that p62^{c-myc} is localized in a discrete subnuclear compartment located at, or near the surface of the nucleus. To our knowledge, the ring-shaped structures containing p62^{c-myc} are unlike anything previously observed, and we can only guess at their significance. Because of the possibility that the rings might be artifacts, perhaps caused by fixation conditions or by cross-reacting antibody specificities, we sought some biochemical evidence to corroborate our idea that p62^{c-myc} exists in a discrete subnuclear compartment.

Subcellular fractionation of p62^{c-myc}

In order to establish the nuclear location of p62^{c-myc} unequivocally we fractionated cells in hypotonic buffers, generating cytoplasmic and nuclear fractions. The fractions were assayed by immunoprecipitation and immunoblotting for the presence of p62^{c-myc}. Under all conditions of hypotonic cell lysis, whether with or without non-ionic detergents, virtually all the p62^{c-myc} was associated with the nuclear fraction (Persson & Leder 1984, Eisenman et al 1985, Evan & Hancock 1985).

Subnuclear fractionation

The ultrastructure of the interphase nucleus is largely unknown. In non-ionic detergents and high salt buffers, nuclease-treated nuclei can be depleted of

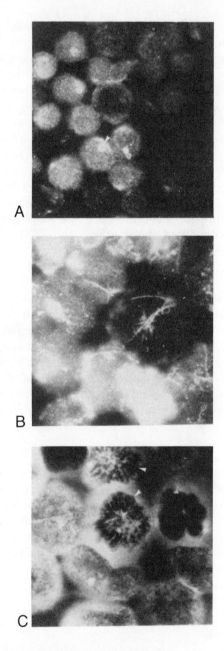

FIG. 3. Immunofluorescence microscopic analysis of p62$^{c\text{-}myc}$.

A. Mid log-phase human colonic apudoma cells (Colo 320 HSR) were centrifuged onto an untreated glass microscope slide for 5 min at 400 r.p.m. in a cytocentrifuge (Shandon Southern

the majority of their chromatin components, leaving a residual 'nuclear matrix' that retains some of the gross morphological features of intact nuclei. The matrix consists of the nuclear lamina (three related proteins forming a proteinaceous shell around the nucleus), plus a number of other poorly defined proteins, probably attached to the lamina by metalloprotein interactions (Lewis et al 1984). A number of nuclear functions, including transcription, DNA replication and control of RNA processing, have been associated with the nuclear matrix. We therefore wanted to determine in which of the two nuclear fractions, chromatin or matrix, $p62^{c\text{-}myc}$ is located. Such information might suggest a function for this protein.

Unfortunately, the composition of the nuclear matrix is difficult to define and appears to vary according to the precise method of preparation and the cell type used as its source. We prepared nuclear matrices by several established methods, all following the basic pattern of nuclease treatment followed by extraction in high salt (2 M NaCl) buffers. We then assayed matrix and chromatin fractions for $p62^{c\text{-}myc}$ by immunoblotting, using MAb Myc1-9E10 as probe. Curiously, $p62^{c\text{-}myc}$ cofractionated with the matrix (i.e. was insoluble in high salt buffer) by some methods but cofractionated with the chromatin (i.e. was soluble in high salt buffer) in others. The key variable affecting the behaviour of $p62^{c\text{-}myc}$ was found to be the temperature at which the nuclei were digested with nuclease; $p62^{c\text{-}myc}$ becomes insoluble in high salt buffers whenever isolated nuclei are exposed to temperatures of 37 °C (Fig. 4).

Further analysis showed that the digestion of DNA was irrelevant and that $p62^{c\text{-}myc}$ becomes insoluble in 2 M NaCl buffers at 37 °C even in isolated nuclei not treated with nuclease. The critical temperature for this insolubilization was found to be 35 °C. Insolubilization of $p62^{c\text{-}myc}$ did not occur below 35 °C, even after long incubations, but above 35 °C $p62^{c\text{-}myc}$ rapidly became resistant to high salt extraction. The insolubilization process is thus critically dependent on a small variation in temperature.

Cytospin). The cells were immediately fixed in fresh 3.5% paraformaldehyde in phosphate-buffered saline (PBS). Cells were permeabilized with PBS containing 0.1% NP40 detergent and incubated in rabbit anti-peptide G serum (Ramsay et al 1984), followed by affinity-purified donkey anti-rabbit antibody conjugated with Texas Red (Amersham UK). Immunofluorescence was observed under incident UV light using a Zeiss Universal microscope with a III RS rhodamine filter set. The arrowhead indicates a $p62^{c\text{-}myc}$-containing ring structure.

B. Mid log-phase Colo 320 HSR cells were centrifuged onto glass microscope slides, fixed in paraformaldehyde, permeabilized, and treated for 2.5 minutes with a solution containing 10 mg/ml Pronase. Cells were then washed and stained with rabbit anti-peptide G antibody, followed by Texas Red-conjugated anti-rabbit antibody. Arrowheads indicate intact ring structures surviving the proteolytic digestion.

C. A G_2/M population of Colo 320 HSR cells was isolated on the basis of cell size in a FACS II cell sorter. Cells were fixed, permeabilized, and stained with anti-$p62^{c\text{-}myc}$ antibody as described for A and B. Arrowheads indicate the positions of condensed chromosomes.

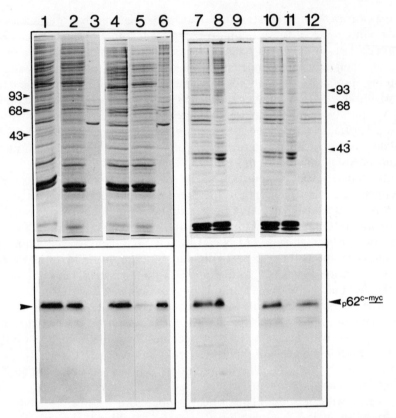

FIG. 4. Analysis of Colo 320 HSR and HeLa nuclear fractions. Purified Colo 320 HSR and HeLa cell nuclei were incubated in RSB (10 mM Tris HCl pH 7.4, 5 mM MgCl$_2$, 0.1% digitonin, 1% thiodiglycol, 0.1 mM phenyl methyl sulphonyl fluoride) containing 50 μg/ml DNase I at either 4 °C for one hour (tracks 1–3 and 7–9) or 37 °C for 10 minutes (tracks 4–6 and 10–12). Half the nuclei from each incubation were used directly and half were extracted with high salt buffer containing 0.1% digitonin (Lewis et al 1984). High salt extracts, residual pellets and total nuclear fractions were each then dissolved in SDS gel sample buffer and fractionated on a 12.5% (Colo 320 HSR) or a 10% (HeLa) SDS–polyacrylamide gel. Total protein in each extract, stained with Coomassie brilliant blue, is shown in the upper panels, and immunoblots of each fraction probed for p62^{c-myc} with MAb Mycl-9E10 are shown in the lower panels. Tracks 1–6 are from Colo 320 HSR cells; tracks 7–12 are from HeLa cells.

Fig. 4 (Tracks 6 and 12) shows that other nuclear proteins also become insoluble in high salt buffers when isolated nuclei are exposed to temperatures of 37 °C. These proteins, together with p62^{c-myc}, appear to constitute a discrete subset of nuclear proteins. The nature of this insoluble complex is unclear. We know that it can form in the presence of chelating agents, non-ionic detergents and thiol-containing reagents, and that the components of the complex are not covalently cross-linked. We suggest that the insolubilization process involves precipitation or polymerization of a subset of nuclear proteins which exist in a specific subcompartment of the nucleus. Perhaps the ring structures we observe by immunofluorescence microscopy (Fig. 3A) are a visualization of this nuclear subcompartment, of which p62^{c-myc} is a component.

The insolubilization of nuclear proteins observed in isolated nuclei at 37 °C clearly does not occur in intact cells at this temperature, because we do not find such complexes in nuclei prepared from fresh cells cultured at 37 °C. These complexes can, however, be found in nuclei isolated from heat-shocked cells (that is, cells exposed to a temperature of 41 °C for one hour). Formation of insoluble nuclear complexes may therefore be one of the major consequences of classical heat-shock. If the proteins making up the complexes are components of DNA and RNA synthesis and processing, this may explain why there is an abrupt cessation of these functions when cells are heat-shocked.

Association of p62^{c-myc} with nuclei

Having determined that p62^{c-myc} is readily extracted from isolated nuclei by high salt buffers, providing the nuclei have not first been exposed to temperatures above 35 °C, we were interested to know precisely how the association of p62^{c-myc} with nuclei depends on salt concentration. We therefore extracted isolated nuclei in neutral buffer containing varying concentrations of NaCl. The results (Fig. 5) show that p62^{c-myc} is readily extracted from nuclei by salt concentrations as low as isotonic (140 mM).

The binding of p62^{c-myc} to cell nuclei is thus perturbable by variations in ionic strength within the physiological range. Any significance of this finding for p62^{c-myc} function *in vivo* is unclear, but two possibilities are worth considering:

(1) Binding of p62^{c-myc} to nuclei could conceivably be reversibly modulated *in vivo* by localized variations in ionic strength that are within the physiological range.

(2) At ionic strengths prevailing in the region of the nucleus in an intact cell, the binding of p62^{c-myc} to the nucleus might simply be of low affinity.

Though it is known that the gross intracellular levels of p62^{c-myc} are largely independent of the cell cycle (Hann et al 1985), the fraction of p62^{c-myc} actively associated with the nucleus may not be so invariant. If p62^{c-myc} were to act as an intracellular messenger, perhaps instructing the cell to proceed through the cell cycle, the rapid synthesis and degradation of p62^{c-myc} observed in cells expressing the c-*myc* gene might not be surprising. A low affinity or modulated interaction between p62^{c-myc} and its active site in the cell nucleus

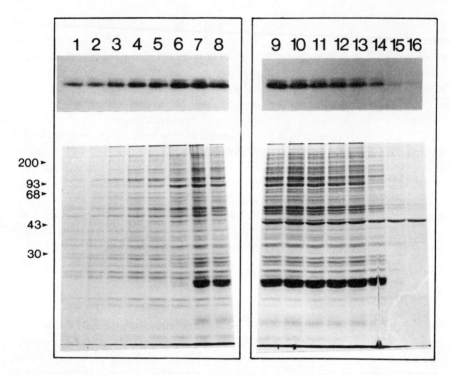

FIG. 5. Extraction of human c-*myc* protein from intact nuclei with salt. Purified Colo 320 HSR nuclei were incubated for 10 minutes at 4 °C in RSB containing varying concentrations of NaCl. The nuclei then were pelleted at $1000 \times g$ and both supernatant and pellet were fractionated on 12.5% SDS–polyacrylamide gels. Fractions were assayed for total protein by Coomassie brilliant blue staining (lower panels) and for p62^{c-myc} by immunoblotting with MAb Mycl-9E10 (upper panels). The left-hand panels show the fractions extracted from nuclei; the right-hand panel show residual nuclei. NaCl concentrations were: tracks 1 and 9, 10 mM; tracks 2 and 10, 20 mM; tracks 3 and 11, 50 mM; tracks 4 and 12, 100 mM; tracks 5 and 13, 150 mM; tracks 6 and 14, 250 mM; tracks 7 and 15, 500 mM; tracks 8 and 16, 2 M.

could be exquisitely sensitive to minor fluctuations in gross intracellular p62^{c-myc} levels—fluctuations which might be difficult to detect by standard analytical techniques. Even subtle alterations in c-*myc* expression might therefore be enough to cause the proliferative changes associated with neoplastic growth.

Acknowledgements

We would like to thank Drs J. Michael Bishop, Gary Ramsay and George Lewis for help in isolating the monoclonal antibodies described in this paper. We are also grateful to Drs Hugh Pelham, Bob Jack, Randy Schatzman and Rob White for constructive criticism and advice.

REFERENCES

Adams JM, Gerondakis S, Webb E, Corcoran LM, Cory S 1983 Cellular *myc* oncogene is altered by chromosomal translocation to an immunoglobin locus in mouse plasmacytomas and is rearranged similarly in human Burkitt lymphomas. Proc Natl Acad Sci USA 80:1982-1986

Alitalo K 1985 Amplification of cellular oncogenes in cancer cells. Trends Biochem Sci 10:194-197

Alitalo K, Ramsay G, Bishop JM, Ohlsson Pfeifer S, Colby WW, Levinson AD 1983 Identification of nuclear proteins encoded by viral and cellular *myc* oncogenes. Nature (Lond) 306:274-277

Bishop JM 1983 Cellular oncogenes. Annu Rev Biochem 52:301-354

Colby WW, Chen E, Smith D, Levinson AD 1983 Identification and nucleotide sequence of a human locus homologous to the v-*myc* oncogene of avian myelocytomatosis virus. Nature (Lond) 301:722-725

Eisenman RN, Tachibana CY, Abrams HD, Hann SR 1985 v-*myc* and c-*myc* encoded proteins are associated with the nuclear matrix. Mol Cell Biol 4:114-126

Evan GI, Hancock DC 1985 Studies on the interaction of the human c-*myc* protein with cell nuclei: p62$^{c\text{-}myc}$ as a member of a discrete subset of nuclear proteins. Cell, in press

Evan GI, Lewis GK, Ramsay G, Bishop JM 1985 Isolation of monoclonal antibodies specific for the human c-*myc* protein. Mol Cell Biol, in press

Filmus J, Buick RN 1985 Relationship of c-*myc* expression to differentiation and proliferation of HL-60 cells. Cancer Res 45:822-825

Hann SR, Thompson CB, Eisenman RN 1985 c-*myc* oncogene protein synthesis is independent of the cell cycle in human and avian cells. Nature (Lond) 314:366-369

Hayward WS, Neel BG, Astrin SM 1981 Activation of cellular *onc* gene by promoter insertion of ALV-induced lymphoid leukosis. Nature (Lond) 290:475-480

Kelly K, Cochran B, Stiles C, Leder P 1983 Cell-specific regulation of the c-*myc* gene by lymphocyte mitogens and platelet-derived growth factor. Cell 35:603-610

Lewis CD, Lebrowski JS, Daly AK, Laemmli UK 1984 Interphase nuclear matrix and metaphase scaffolding structures. In: Higher order structure in the nucleus. J Cell Sci Suppl 1:103-122

Müller R, Verma IM 1984 Expression of cellular oncogenes. Curr Top Microbiol Immunol 112:73-115

Payne GS, Bishop JM, Varmus HE 1982 Multiple arrangements of viral DNA and an activated host oncogene in bursal lymphomas. Nature (Lond) 295:209-214

Persson H, Leder P 1984 Nuclear localization and DNA binding properties of a protein expressed by human c-*myc* oncogene. Science (Wash DC) 225:718-720

Ramsay G, Evan GI, Bishop JM 1984 The protein encoded by the human proto-oncogene c-*myc*. Proc Natl Acad Sci USA 81:7742-7746

Schwab M, Alitalo K, Klempnauer KH, Varmus HE, Bishop JM 1983 Amplified DNA with limited homology to *myc* cellular oncogene is shared by human neuroblastoma cell lines and a neuroblastoma tumour. Nature (Lond) 305:245-248

Stark GR, Wahl GM 1984 Gene amplification. Annu Rev Biochem 53:447-491

Winqvist R, Saksela K, Alitalo K 1984 The *myc* proteins are not associated with chromatin in mitotic cells. EMBO (Eur Mol Biol Organ) J 3:2947-2950

DISCUSSION

Crumpton: You saw more than one band on many of your Western blots. Is this an expression of different phosphorylation states of the c-*myc* protein?

Evan: On SDS-polyacrylamide gels, the $p62^{c-myc}$ appears to be a doublet. The two components vary in their relative amounts. They are both phosphorylated and they have the same isoelectric point. Having heard the earlier discussions here, I think we ought never to have tried to make antibodies against it, because it contains many proline residues, and many people think this protein has a very defined structure. It may therefore be that the protein has perhaps two preferred conformations in an SDS gel. There is no apparent product–precursor relationship between the two components of the doublet. We can't exclude that they are covalently modified variants of one gene product.

Crumpton: There is no evidence, then, that in the cell this protein varies in the extent of its phosphorylation. So this wouldn't help to explain the change in its association with the cell nucleus?

Evan: I think that is a possibility. Many nuclear oncoproteins, however, have a half-life in cells of the order of 20 minutes, so pulse-chase labelling experiments occupy a significant proportion of the half-life, and it is difficult to show either a product–precursor relationship or the presence of subpopulations of the protein in the cell, by this sort of technique. But neither of these possibilities can be discounted. I would like to think that the protein does its job by shuttling in and out of an active site in the nucleus.

Lerner: One trick with site-specific antibodies is to synthesize the peptide with a phosphate group on it. You can raise antibodies that see the phosphorylated state of the protein. This is particularly useful in the oncogene field, where it might be interesting to make an antibody specific to the phosphorylated state of the oncoprotein.

Gupta: My question relates to your studies with the HL60 tumour cell line, where you showed that after differentiation induced by dimethyl sulphoxide, the amount of c-*myc* protein decreased. Can you differentiate the HL60 cells by using a monoclonal antibody, or $F(ab)_2$ or Fab fragments, generated against c-*myc* protein?

Evan: Probably not, because the *myc* protein in intact living cells is in the nucleus. If we were looking for a therapeutic use for these sorts of antibodies, we would not, with hindsight, have chosen a nuclear oncoprotein like *myc*. But we were interested in *myc* because it was a nuclear protein. The majority of oncoproteins are intracellular rather than expressed on the cell surface, so monoclonals specific for them are unlikely to be the basis of an immunotherapeutic strategy.

Gupta: You have been able to localize tumour cells in certain model systems, using monoclonal antibodies against c-*myc* protein, which suggests that this protein is also present on the cell membrane.

Evan: That was in a living tumour where there is a significant amount of necrosis and cell death. We are probably seeing the bits and pieces!

Lennox: Those of us who are interested in using monoclonal antibodies for the imaging and treatment of tumours will take note of this work, to see whether the *myc* protein can be used for these purposes, even though it is an intracellular protein. I wonder whether one can use intracellular proteins for imaging in general? One wonders whether your results have to do with special solubility properties of the *myc* protein and its binding to nuclear matrix material.

Ada: Could you do autoradiography on electron microscope sections to see where the binding was and what you are picking up?

Evan: We are planning to do this, but we don't know where the iodinated anti-*myc* monoclonal antibodies are binding, at present.

Corradin: Have you used fluorescence-activated cell sorting (FACS) to resolve this? There you pick up only living cells.

Evan: No. However, when we incubated, as a control, antibodies with intact Colo 320 HSR cells that express high levels of c-*myc*, they acted as a very good negative control for other antibodies that recognize surface components; so our anti-*myc* antibodies don't see anything on intact cells.

Lerner: The antibody may in fact be seeing living cells, because the *myc* protein may simply stick to cells. So perhaps the tumour cells are dying, as you say, but the *myc* protein is actually adsorbed on the surface of living cells. Thus you may well be imaging the living tumour mass as a consequence of *myc* release from the dying tumour cells.

Crumpton: Another example of this phenomenon is the presence of actin on the surface of B lymphoblastoid cells growing in culture (Owen et al 1978). The presence of actin probably reflects the affinity that Ig has for actin. An interesting question is the origin of this cell-surface actin. There is a lot of actin inside cells (about 10% of the cellular protein of lymphoblastoid cells is actin); perhaps it is released during cell division into the culture supernatant and then binds back to the B cell surface as a result of its affinity for Ig. The association of intracellular protein(s) with the surface of cells may not be uncommon.

Lachmann: Alarcon-Segovia et al (1978) studied the entry into cells of antibodies to ribonucleoprotein. Whereas these antibodies clearly could not get into most cells, they were able to enter Fc receptor-positive cells (macrophages) as immune complexes, and then react with the nucleus of the cell.

Crumpton: Dr Evan, what was the total number of hybridomas that gave your six monoclonal anti-peptide antibodies?

Evan: Roughly, out of 1000 positive-growing wells in each of the two fusions, we found these six positive anti-peptide antibodies. All the rest of the hybridoma culture supernatants that we could measure were against the carrier (KLH).

Ada: Did you compare the ability of the peptide to stick to a cell extract?

Evan: No. We just wanted a quick assay, at this stage.

Alkan: Since interferons inhibit the expression of the *myc* gene, I would like to suggest an experiment, or perhaps a collaboration. If you couple interferon to antibodies which recognize surface antigens, and then target the interferon to the cell surface, that interferon might stop the growth of cells more efficiently than interferon alone. We have demonstrated recently that this is feasible (Alkan et al 1984). Despite the doubts about the cell-surface expression of the *myc* protein, this could be tried.

Anders: Is there general agreement that immunizing with fusion proteins produced in recombinant DNA host–vector systems is not very useful for producing monoclonals? The malaria antigens containing repeats are perhaps a special case, but we have obtained excellent polyclonal antibodies by immunizing with β-galactosidase fusion proteins (Coppel et al 1983, 1984). Recently, we have produced monoclonals by immunizing with one of these fusion proteins. Most of the monoclonals produced were to the malaria antigen rather than β-galactosidase. Have you taken care to solubilize your fusion proteins or attempted to fragment them in any way?

Evan: We and others who have used this strategy agree that the problem is that one never reads about the failures in the published literature. Therefore one is forced to talk about personal experiences. There are problems associated with using bacterial antigens. There are technical problems of getting the heterologous protein expressed at high enough levels. Also, we found several extremely immunogenic components that tend to co-purify with the bacterially expressed proteins. When mice, rabbits or rats get a whiff of one of these components, they don't bother to make antibodies against the protein of interest.

When I was in Dr J. Michael Bishop's laboratory, we dealt with five or six fusion proteins against various oncoprotein sequences. These were fusion proteins with parts of human growth hormone, or with β-galactosidase. In many cases they were fused at the 3′ end of the gene, with random sequences; in one case, in the *erb*-B system, with an out-of-phase tetracycline-resistant gene sequence which terminated at a random nonsense codon. We succeeded in making monoclonal antibodies against the intact protein in only two out of about eight attempts with different bacterial proteins. In four of those cases we raised polyclonal antibodies that recognized the native protein, but in at least two of those—the two cases where we didn't obtain monoclonals—the polyclonal antibody was extremely weak in titre and not useful, apart from initial identification of the protein.

Anders: There are good examples of β-galactosidase fusion proteins being useful immunogens, apart from in malaria. For example, Beachy et al (1985) have produced antisera to *Drosophila melanogaster* bithorax complex proteins in this way.

REFERENCES

Alarcon-Segovia D, Ruiz Arguelles A, Fishbein E 1978 Antibody to nuclear ribonucleoprotein penetrates live mononuclear cells through Fc receptors. Nature (Lond) 271:67-69

Alkan SS, Miescher-Granger S, Braun DG, Hochkeppel HK 1984 Antiviral and antiproliferative effects of interferons delivered via monoclonal antibodies. J Interferon Res 4:355-363

Beachy PA, Helfand SL, Hogness DS 1985 Segmental distribution of bithorax complex proteins during *Drosophila* development. Nature (Lond) 313:545-551

Coppel RL, Cowman AF, Lingelbach KR, Brown GV, Saint RB, Kemp DJ, Anders RF 1983 An isolate-specific S antigen of *Plasmodium falciparum* contains an exactly repeated sequence of 11 amino acids. Nature (Lond) 306:751-756

Coppel RL, Cowman AF, Anders RF, Bianco AE, Saint RB, Lingelbach KR, Kemp DJ, Brown GV 1984 Immune sera recognize on erythrocytes a *Plasmodium falciparum* antigen composed of repeated amino acid sequences. Nature (Lond) 310:789-791

Owen MJ, Auger J, Barber BH, Edwards AJ, Walsh FS, Crumpton MJ 1978 Actin may be present on the lymphocyte surface. Proc Natl Acad Sci USA 75:4484-4488

Epitope mapping of human recombinant interferon alpha molecules by monoclonal antibodies

S. S. ALKAN and D. G. BRAUN

CIBA-GEIGY Limited, Pharmaceuticals Research Department, CH-4002, Basel, Switzerland

Abstract. The epitopes of six recombinant human interferon alpha (IFNα) subtypes have been analysed using 22 monoclonal antibodies (MAbs) obtained from different sources. The IFNα subtype specificity of each MAb was determined by a combined immunoprecipitation–bioassay. Eight different epitopes were identified; the number of epitopes on a given IFNα subtype varied between four and eight. Each subtype possessed a unique combination of epitopes. Using the best pair of monoclonal antibodies, predicted from epitope mapping studies, subtype-specific two-site (tandem) assays were developed. It was observed that some non-cross-reactive MAbs influenced each other's binding, indicating the flexible nature of IFN molecules. Competitive radioimmunoassay and the combined immunoprecipitation–bioassay were used to identify a common epitope, present on IFNα-A, B, C, F and J but not on IFNα-D. In neutralization studies, all MAbs that identified this common epitope inhibited the antiviral activity of all IFNα molecules tested. It was concluded that the epitope is located within the receptor-binding region of IFN molecules and is important for biological activity. A tentative localization of the common epitope and the other identified epitopes is proposed.

1986 Synthetic peptides as antigens. Wiley, Chichester (Ciba Foundation Symposium 119) p 264-278

Human interferon alpha (HuIFNα) molecules are ideal tools for investigating antigenicity and the structure–function relationships of molecules. This is because they consist of a family of 15 or more closely related, but non-identical, proteins of 166 amino acids sharing at least 77% homology. In addition, they are good immunogens in mice and several monoclonal antibodies (MAbs) are available (Alkan et al 1983, Berg 1984, Eshar et al 1983, Lydon et al 1985, Secher & Burke 1980, Staehelin et al 1981). Recently, the reactivity of selected MAbs with a few HuIFNα subtypes has been tested (Alkan et al 1985, Lydon et al 1985, Trown et al 1985). However, localization of the active site of the interferon molecule was found to be difficult. In the present study we took advantage of having a large panel of MAbs to map the epitopes of six recombinant HuIFNα subtypes, namely α-A, B, C, D, F and J. Using a liquid-phase assay, the combined immunoprecipitation–bioassay, and competitive radioimmunoassays (RIA) we identified at least eight different epitopes. The number of epitopes present on a given subtype varied between four (α-B) and eight (α-A). Each IFNα subtype expressed a unique epitope combination which helped us to develop subtype-specific and sensitive tandem assays. Using competitive RIA and the combined immunoprecipitation–bioassay we identified a public epitope which was present on all IFNαs tested with the exception of the α-D subtype. Six out of the 22 MAbs recognized this epitope. Four of these MAbs neutralized the antiviral activity of IFNα-A, B, C, F and J but not α-D. Amino acid sequence information, MAb neutralization data and the reactivity profiles of MAbs with recombinant hybrid IFNαs all indicated that this common epitope resides around position 10. We here propose that this region is the active site for some IFNα molecules.

Materials and methods

Six recombinant HuIFNα subtypes were kindly provided by the donors listed in Table 1. The production and characterization of CIBA-GEIGY (CG) MAbs have been described previously (Alkan et al 1983, 1985). The remaining MAbs were from sources listed in Table 1. Some characteristics of these MAbs have been reported previously (Berg 1984, Eshar et al 1983, Lydon et al 1985, Secher & Burke 1980, Staehelin et al 1981). The details of the combined immunoprecipitation–bioassay (Ci-Ba) were described elsewhere (Alkan et al 1983). The principle of Ci-Ba is illustrated in Fig. 1. Briefly, 10^4 units/ml

TABLE 1 List of interferon alpha subtypes and monoclonal antibodies

rIFNαs	Provided by	From
B, D, F	M. Grütter	CIBA-GEIGY
A, J	J. Davies/C. Weissmann	Biogen
C	D. Novick	Inter Yeda
Monoclonal antibodies		
CG-(1–3)	S. Alkan	CIBA-GEIGY
CT (1–2)	P. Mattock	Celltech
S (1–4)	C. Favre	Schering
IY (1–4)	D. Novick	Inter Yeda
UZ (1)	M. Aguet	Univ. Zürich
R (1–3)	T. Staehelin	Roche
KT (1–4)	W. Berthold	K. Thomae
UA (1)	K. Berg	Univ. Aarhus

Six rIFNα subtypes and 22 monoclonal antibodies are listed and their sources given. The MAbs CG, UA, S, IY, CT and R were reported earlier by Alkan et al (1983), Berg (1984), Eshar et al (1983), Lydon et al (1985), Secher & Burke (1980) and Staehelin et al (1981), respectively.

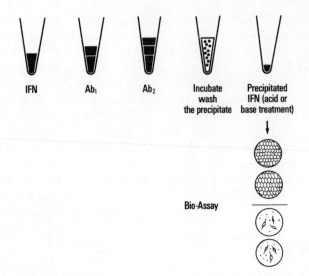

FIG. 1. The principle of the combined immunoprecipitation–bioassay (Ci-Ba) is shown schematically. Ab_1 was anti-IFN Ab; Ab_2 was pre-titrated rabbit anti-mouse Ig. For the bioassay, Hep2 cells and Mengo virus were used.

of a given IFN subtype was precipitated with a MAb and rabbit anti-mouse Ig. After washing of the precipitate, the antiviral activity of immunoprecipitated, dissolved IFN was measured in a standard IFN bioassay, as described earlier (Alkan et al 1984, Armstrong 1971). The tandem RIA and antibody neutralization assays were performed as described elsewhere (Alkan et al 1985). Immunodot assay was according to Towbin et al (1979).

Results

Reactivity profiles of monoclonal antibodies

Six rIFN subtypes, rIFNα-A, B, C, D, F and J, were tested with 22 MAbs by Ci-Ba. The results summarized in Table 2 showed that each MAb appeared to be unique in its fine specificity. However, some of the monoclonals showed very similar or identical patterns of reactivity, indicating that they recognized similar antigenic determinants or identical epitopes. When MAbs with similar reactivity profiles were put together, eight different groups were obtained. Using competitive RIA we demonstrated that extensive cross-reactions exist between the MAbs within the same group (data not shown). Reactivity patterns of some MAbs were also analysed by immunodot assay (Fig. 2). This assay yielded identical results to Ci-Ba.

TABLE 2 Antiviral activity of human rIFNα subtypes A–J immunoprecipitated with 22 monoclonal antibodies

MAbs		A(2)	B(8)	C()	D(1)	F()	J(7)	Original abbreviation
CG-1	○	+++	−	+++	+++	−	+++	1K2
-2	○	+++	−	++	++++	++	+++	2K2
-3	◑	+	++++	+++	++++	++	−	144 BS
CT-1	●	+++	++++	+++	−	+++	++++	NK2
-2	▲	+	−	++	+++	−	+++	YOK
S-1	□	+++	+	ND	++++	−	+	6N5-2
-2	◨	+++	−	ND	−	−	+	7N2-4
-3	●	+++	++++	ND	−	++	++++	7N4-1
-4	■	++++	−	+++	−	+	++++	7N4-6
IY-1	●	++	+++	ND	−	ND	++	74
-2	■	++++	−	ND	−	+	+++	23.4
-3	◨	++	−	−	−	−	++++	7.6
-4	◨	++++	−	−	+	−	++	9.3
UZ-1	●	+++	++++	++	−	+	+++	1/24
R-1	●	+++	++++	+++	−	−	ND	LI-1
-2	●	++++	++	+++	−	−	ND	-8
-3	○	++++	+	++	+++	−	ND	-9
KT-1	○	++++	−	++++	+++	−	ND	EBI-1
-2	○	++++	−	++++	++++	−	ND	-3
-3	▲	−	−	++++	++	++	ND	-4
-4	⊗	+++	++++	+++	++	+++	ND	L3B7
UA-1	⊗	++++	+++	+++	+++	+++	ND	LO.22

The original abbreviation for each MAb is given at the right-hand side. For simplicity, each MAb has been named by its producer (i.e. CIBA-GEIGY as CG) and numbered. Each symbol represents a unique MAb reactivity pattern (see also Fig. 3 below). ++++, 100%; +++, 75%; ++, 50%; +, 25%; −, 0% precipitation of IFN using Ci-Ba. ND, not determined. Normal mouse serum as negative and polyclonal mouse anti-IFN antibody as positive controls were always included in Ci-Ba.

Epitope content of IFNαs

To simplify the experimental data obtained by Ci-Ba (presented in Table 2) we designated each serologically defined epitope by a different symbol. The results are presented schematically in Fig. 3. Epitopes were assigned according to distinct MAb reactivity and placed arbitrarily in a linear order for every IFN tested. The following features emerged from this alignment. (a) IFNα-A and α-J possess the highest epitope number (eight). Although not every epitope was expressed equally on the two IFNαs, they appear to be serologically very similar. (b) IFNα-B expressed the least number of epitopes (four). However, one epitope present on α-B was also present on all

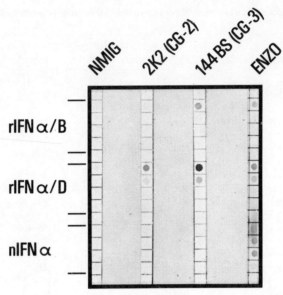

FIG. 2. Interferons were dotted on nitrocellulose paper at varying concentrations, reacted with MAb and revealed with rabbit anti-mouse Ig coupled with peroxidase. A polyclonal antibody from Enzo and normal mouse immunoglobulin (NMIG) were used as positive and negative controls respectively.

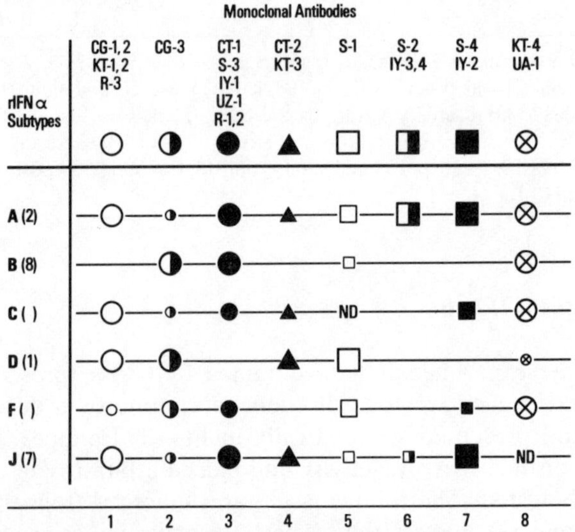

FIG. 3. Epitope distribution of IFNαs. Data were obtained from Table 2. Symbols for epitopes and abbreviations for MAbs are as in Table 2. Epitopes are ordered arbitrarily, and numbered from 1 to 8. The size of each symbol is directly proportional to the amount of IFNα immunoprecipitated by the MAb in Ci-Ba. ND, not determined.

the other IFNαs except α-D. (c) This epitope (number 3 in Fig. 3) was recognized by six MAbs obtained from five different sources (R-1, 2, CT-1, S-3, IY-1 and UZ-1). The fact that each laboratory used a different preparation of IFNα, and yet came up with MAbs of indistinguishable specificity, demonstrates the predominant nature of this epitope. (d) Despite the similarity of α-A/α-J and α-C/α-F, every tested IFN subtype was unique in its epitope content. (e) Three epitopes (numbers 2, 5 and 8) are shared by all six subtypes. However, the possibility of cross-reactions between epitopes 2 (CG-3) and 8 (UA-1) has not been tested. (f) The CG-3 MAb (epitope 2) was of particular interest, not only because of its public nature but also for its one-way cross-reactivity with CG-1,2 which was present on all subtypes except α-B. Further analysis showed that the CG-3 MAb recognized a large antigenic determinant which only partially overlapped with the CG-1,2 epitope (data not shown).

Testing the predictions

Tandem immunoassays are not only highly sensitive but are also the most specific assays, because they are based on the recognition of two different epitopes present simultaneously on a given molecule. Knowing the epitope content of a given IFNα subtype, one could predict suitable and unsuitable pairs of epitopes (MAbs pairs) for subtype-specific tandem assays. To test this prediction—and also for practical purposes—we examined several combinations of MAbs. The results of eight such experiments are presented in Table 3. As expected, the MAb CG-3/CT-1 (144BS/NK2) combination could be

TABLE 3 Selection of suitable monoclonal antibodies for tandem interferon radioimmunoassays

Solid-phase first MAbs	Iodinated second MAbs	C.p.m. obtained with 10^3 units of interferon	
		IFNα-B	IFNα-D
CG-3	CG-2	100	113
CG-3	CG-3	60	100
CG-3 (144BS)	CT-2 (YOK)	313	16 790
CG-3 (144BS)	CT-1 (NK2)	3733	80
CG-2	CG-2	52	0
CG-2	CG-3	2	50
CG-2 (2K2)	CT-2 (YOK)	0	21 680
CG-2	CT-1	0	0

The first MAb was absorbed onto macro-beads and the second MAb was labelled with [125]I. The RIA was performed stepwise and 1000 international units (IU) of interferon were used for all combinations. A Celltech kit was included as control and gave similar results. The original abbreviations of the MAbs are given in parenthesis.

used to detect the α-B but not the α-D subtype. Similarly, the CG-3/CT-2 (144BS/YOK) pair was suitable for detecting both α-B and α-D. On the other hand, the CG-2/CT-2 (2K2/YOK) combination could detect α-D but not α-B interferon, which lacks both of the epitopes (numbers 1 and 4). Detailed results of such specific and sensitive (2 pg/ml IFN) tandem RIAs are reported elsewhere (Alkan et al 1985).

Inhibition of IFN activity by monoclonal antibodies

MAbs recognizing an epitope located within the active site of any IFN molecule should interfere with receptor binding and thereby inhibit the biological activity of IFNs. When we tested 10 MAbs for their neutralization of the antiviral activities of six IFNαs, we found that not every MAb that recognized an IFN subtype could inhibit its activity (Table 4). For instance, MAb CG-2

TABLE 4 Inhibition of interferon activity by monoclonal antibodies

MAb	Neutralization of 10^3 units of rIFNαs					
	A(2)	B(8)	C()	D(1)	F()	J(7)
CG-2	−	−		+++		−
CG-3	−	++		++	+	−
CT-1	++++	+++		+	+	+
S-1				−		−
S-3	++++	++++		−		−
UZ-1	++++	++++	+++	−	++	++
R-1	++++	+++	+++	+	−	−
-2	++++	+++	+++	++	−	+
-3	++++	−	−	+++	−	−
UA-1	−	−	−	−	−	−

Neutralization of antiviral activity of six IFNαs with ten MAbs was determined using Mengo virus and Hep2 cells. ++++, full neutralization of IFN (10^3 units/ml). −, no effect. (Numbers in parentheses indicate an alternative nomenclature.)

recognized α-A, C, D and J subtypes but inhibited only α-D. Similar results with other MAbs suggested that most of the inhibition resulted probably from either steric hindrance or MAb-induced conformational changes. In fact, using CG-2, -3, CT-1 and other MAbs in tandem RIAs, we noticed that when a certain MAb was bound to IFN first, it could influence (decrease or increase) the binding of the second MAb which did not cross-react with the first MAb. These results indicate that IFNs are flexible molecules. On the other hand, a group of six MAbs (CT-1, S-3, IY-1, UZ-1, R-1,2) which recognized epitope number 3 were all found to be neutralizing antibodies, as reported by us and others (this study, Alkan et al 1985, Whitall et al 1984). We interpret these results to indicate that this common epitope is important for the biological activity of all the IFNαs tested except for α-D.

Epitope localization

In an attempt to localize some of the eight defined epitopes present on α-B, α-D and α-F IFNs we have compared the amino acid sequence of these sub-types (Fig. 4). It is clear that α-D IFN is a very different molecule from

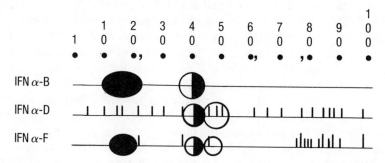

FIG. 4. Comparison of amino acid sequences of IFNα-B, D and F. Substitutions in comparison to the leader sequence of α-B were marked by vertical bars. Locations of epitope number 3 (●), number 2 (◑) and number 1 (○) are shown. Symbols for these epitopes are as in Fig. 3.

α-B, showing many substitutions scattered throughout the molecule. From the analysis of hybrid IFNs and their reactivity with neutralizing antibodies (CT-1, UZ-1, etc.) we conclude that the active site for α-B resides in the region of residues 1–23 (unpublished observations). In this region of the N-terminus, α-D IFN has five amino acid substitutions (residue positions 5, 10, 14, 16 and 22), and therefore cannot interact with any of the six MAbs which recognize α-B (see Fig. 3). IFNα-F contains only one amino acid substitution at position 22 and can bind (although sometimes weakly) to those MAbs. The first four N-terminal amino acids of these three IFNαs are identical. Together, all these results indicate that the active site of α-B (and perhaps α-F too) is situated between residues 5 and 23. Also, using the hybrid IFNs and cross-reactivity patterns of CG-1, -2 and -3, we tentatively localize epitopes 1 and 2 between residue positions 40 and 52. It is very possible that MAbs CG-1 and -2 are directed against some of the four amino acid substitutions of α-D at positions 45, 46, 50 and 52. In fact, IFNα-B, which lacks these substitutions, is the only IFN that does not bind to CG-1 and -2 MAbs.

Discussion

Until the IFNα receptors have been isolated, MAbs are probably the best
tools for elucidating the structure–function relationships of the IFNs. Our
results obtained with Ci-Ba, competitive and tandem RIAs, and neutralization
studies with a large panel of MAbs indicate that among eight identified epitopes only one appears to be of functional importance. This epitope (number
3 in Fig. 3) is present on IFNαs A, B, C, F and J but not on α-D. All MAbs
that recognize epitope 3 inhibit the antiviral activity of all the IFNαs tested.
This finding agrees with results obtained by others demonstrating the inhibition
of IFNα-A activity by MAbs (M. Aguet, personal communication 1985, Lydon
et al 1985, Trown et al 1985, Whitall et al 1984). It was further demonstrated
that MAb UZ-1 inhibits the binding of radiolabelled IFNα-A to its receptor
and that that MAb does not bind to receptor-bound IFNα-A (Aguet et al
1984 and personal communication 1985). The same group, using α-A/α-D
hybrid IFNs, demonstrated that the active site of α-A is located between
residues 1 and 63. Our finding that the active site of the IFNα-B molecule
lies between residues 5 and 23 is completely in agreement with another study
(Lydon et al 1985). This group, using CNBr-derived peptide fragments of
IFNα-A and MAbs, independently showed that the active site is located
between positions 5 and 15. However, our results do not fully agree with
those of Trown et al (1985), who concluded that the active site of IFNα-A
must be located at the C-terminal region, between residues 92 and 166. The
reasons for the discrepancy with our results are not entirely clear to us.
Although our Ci-Ba results with their MAb R-1 (LI-1) agree with theirs,
it is their data with the MAb R-2 (LI-8), that we cannot reproduce, that
may explain their proposed location of the IFNα-A active site.

From the amino acid sequence homology and MAb reactivity profiles with
authentic as well as hybrid IFNαs we have tentatively located epitopes 1 and
2 between residues 40 and 52. The positions of these two epitopes and of
epitope 3, which is located within the active site of IFNαs, are shown in
Fig. 5, superimposed on the model of Sternberg & Cohen (1982). It is interesting to note that all these MAbs (CG-1-3 and a group of six MAbs) recognize
epitopes located at or near the β-turns of IFN molecules. Since β-turns are
on the surface of molecules, they are expected to be immunogenic (Dembinski
et al 1985). Also, MAbs recognizing β-turns should be cross-reactive, as predicted by Sulkowski independently (E. Sulkowski, personal communication
1985). Having been encouraged by these results, we think that a complete
mapping of the surface topography of IFN molecules and the definitive localization of the active site(s) of the different subtypes is possible. For this, the
analysis by MAbs of hybrid IFNs and IFNs with point mutations is likely
to be of great value. This work is now in progress.

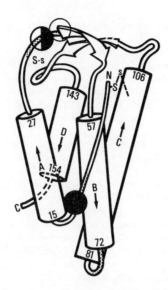

FIG. 5. Suggested locations for epitopes (1, 2 and 3 of Fig. 3) are shown using the predicted tertiary structure of the IFN molecule (adapted from Sternberg & Cohen 1982). The β-turns are marked as stippled areas. The proposed active site of IFN is between residues 5 and 23, as indicated by (●).

Acknowledgements

We are grateful to the donors listed in Table 1 for kindly providing us with their MAbs or IFNs. We thank Miss L. Küttel for her excellent technical assistance and Mrs D. Möschli for her excellent secretarial help.

REFERENCES

Aguet M, Gröbke M, Dreiding P 1984 Various human interferon alpha subclasses crossreact with common receptors; their binding affinities correlate with their specific biological activities. Virology 132:211-216

Alkan SS, Weideli HJ, Schürch AR 1983 Monoclonal antibodies against human leucocyte interferons for the definition of subclasses and their affinity chromatography. Protides Biol Fluids Proc Colloq 30:495-498

Alkan SS, Miescher-Granger S, Braun DG, Hochkeppel HK 1984 Antiviral and antiproliferative effects of interferons delivered via monoclonal antibodies. J Interferon Res 4:355-363

Alkan SS, Hochkeppel HK, Kuettel L 1985 Epitope analysis by monoclonal antibodies of five human recombinant interferon α subtypes. In: Kirchner H, Schellekens H (eds) The biology of the interferon system 1984. Elsevier, Amsterdam, p 91-98

Armstrong JA 1971 Semi micro, dye-binding assay for rabbit interferon. Appl. Microbiol 21:723-725

Berg K 1984 Identification, production, and characterization of murine antibody (LO-22) recognizing 12 native species of human alpha interferon. J Interferon Res 4:481-491

Dembinski WE, Chadha KC, Sulkowski E 1985 Purification of interferons: an ongoing endeavor. In: Dianzani MU, Rossi (eds) The interferon system (Ares Serono Symposia), in press

Eshar Z, Novick D, Gigi O, Marks Z, Friedlanter Y, Revel M, Rubinstein M 1983 Monoclonal antibodies to human leukocyte and fibroblast interferons. Protides Fluids Proc Colloq 30:491-494

Lydon NB et al 1985 Mapping of functionally important domains of alpha-2 interferon with monoclonal antibodies. In: Kirchner H, Schellekens H (eds) The biology of the interferon system 1984. Elsevier, Amsterdam, p 83-90

Secher DS, Burke DC 1980 A monoclonal antibody for large-scale purification of human leukocyte interferon. Nature (Lond) 285:446-448

Staehelin T, Durrer B, Schmidt J et al 1981 Production of hybridomas secreting monoclonal antibodies to the leukocyte interferons. Proc Natl Acad Sci USA 78:1848-1852

Sternberg MJE, Cohen FE 1982 Prediction of the secondary and tertiary structure of interferon from four homologous amino acid sequences. Int J Biol Macromol 4:137-144

Towbin H, Staehelin T, Gordon J 1979 A procedure for the electrophoretic transfer of proteins from polyacrylamide gels to nitrocellulose sheets and some applications. Proc Natl Acad Sci USA 76:4350-4354

Trown PW, Heimer EP, Felix AM, Bohoslawec O 1985 Localization of the epitopes for binding of the monoclonal antibodies LI-1 and LI-8 to leukocyte interferons. In: Kirchner H, Schellekens H (eds) The biology of the interferon system 1984. Elsevier, Amsterdam, p 69-76

Whitall TTD, King RM, Burke DC 1984 The reaction of the anti-interferon-α monoclonal antibody, NK2, with different interferons. J Gen Virol 65:629-633

DISCUSSION

Lerner: What does the Schering group find in relation to the location of the active site?

Alkan: They made CNBr fragments from IFNα-A and did inhibition and neutralization studies with the fragments. Their peptide 1–15 inhibits the binding of one of the monoclonal antibodies, which I refer to as S-3 (see Table 2, p 267). This antibody links their work with ours. However, another group have a totally different answer; they think the active site is close to residue position 90.

Lerner: One is not talking about the active site as such here, but about binding that may perturb the active site, perhaps in the way that Dr Crumpton and Dr Sela say that proteins are distorted by antibody binding. If there is a cascade or domino effect, it may be some distance from the active site.

Alkan: I agree with you, and I have no evidence against that view. But we have other antibodies which disturb IFN binding and also disturb IFN activity partially; but I think their recognition sites are not close to the active site. I think one can discriminate these two types of antibodies, in the following way. You can label interferon and do a receptor-binding study, and show that when you mix radiolabelled IFN with antibody first, it inhibits binding of IFN to the receptor. If you bind labelled interferon to the receptor first, the neutralizing antibody does not bind to that interferon any more, but the other antibodies, which are directed against other sites, will bind to the IFN which is sitting on the receptor.

Lerner: If you have a region of a protein that binds to the receptor, that is a fairly generous use of the term 'active site'.

Alkan: I agree that it is difficult to define the active site, but ours is only a suggestion.

Geysen: If you have two antibody-binding sites on a protein, and binding at one site interferes with the binding of antibody at the other, this may indicate either a steric constraint to binding both antibodies, or the transmission of an unfavourable conformational change which precludes binding of the second antibody. The same argument applies when the two sites consist of an antibody-binding site and a receptor-binding site. Therefore your results don't distinguish the relationship which applies here.

Alkan: I am not saying that we have definitely found the location of the active site of IFN.

Corradin: You say that the antibody binds to peptide 1–15, but in fact you are only saying that most binding is located in that particular segment; you cannot exclude that it is binding the C-terminal, without knowing the X-ray structure. The fact that when you remove the 1–15 fragment you lose activity doesn't exclude that it is also binding to another site on the molecule.

Alkan: I agree; in fact, we have preliminary data indicating that the interferon molecule might have more than one binding site.

Corradin: I mean that the antibody could see the N-terminal as well as the C-terminal.

Alkan: That is not so. There are truncated IFNs where I presume the last 10 residues are missing and a given neutralizing antibody still binds and neutralizes IFN activity. However, there are antibodies that do bind to the C-terminal region, and such an antibody still binds to IFN when it is sitting on the receptor.

Corradin: This doesn't exclude that once you have cleaved the first 15 amino acids, you lose only half of the binding site or more. Then, you could have some binding to another part of the protein which is dependent on the first 15 amino acids.

Alkan: Actually, there are antibodies which bind IFN and, I believe, change the shape of the molecule, because they affect the binding of a second antibody. We observed such a phenomenon during the development of tandem assays. Sometimes the binding of the second antibody is enhanced by the first antibody but sometimes it is inhibited partially. I think that interferons are flexible molecules.

McConnell: On this question of perturbing the shape of the molecule without necessarily interfering with the active site, do combinations of non-neutralizing monoclonals now neutralize?

Alkan: No. I haven't exhausted all the possible combinations, but three that I tried did not inhibit the activity of IFN.

McConnell: Were those three antibodies directed against different antigenic sites?

Alkan: Yes; two were cross-reactive and the other one was not.

Sela: Have you used Fab fragments as well as intact antibodies?

Alkan: We always used intact antibodies.

Lachmann: I gather that your antibodies don't react with mouse IFNα. What is the difference between the mouse and human molecule in the region where you believe the active site to be?

Alkan: I haven't compared mouse and human IFNαs but I have compared one human IFNα which acts on mouse cells as well as human and bovine cells. This interferon, termed IFNα-D, when compared to other human IFNα subtypes has a large number of substitutions in the region where I think the active site is.

Liu: Why don't you confirm the location of the antigenic sites with a synthetic peptide?

Alkan: People have tried to synthesize IFN fragments. None of the synthetic peptides or CNBr fragments were biologically active, so I feel that this approach to the localization of the active site of IFN is a difficult one.

Liu: Perhaps one should just make a very short peptide corresponding to the implicated regions to see if it inhibits binding between IFN and the monoclonal antibodies and to see if it will combine with the monoclonal antibodies itself.

Williams: What is the sequence of the antigenic stretch of IFNα?

Alkan: The sequence starting from residue 10 is Gly-Ser-Arg-Arg-Thr-Leu-Met-Leu-Leu-Ala-Gln. The region falls between residue positions 10 and 20. The strongest evidence for this argument comes from the following observations. IFN subtype α-D, although it is a human IFN, acts on mouse cells as well. It is like an ancestral gene product, I think. Its affinity to the human IFN receptor is much lower than that of any other human IFN subtype. By contrast, HuIFNα-B binds and acts on human cells just like IFNα-A. When hybrid molecules between D and B are made, the hybrid interferons behave like a normal human IFN (i.e. like α-B). We also know that the N-terminal region of α-D is very different from α-B. Our very recent experiments show that the activity of such hybrid IFNs can be blocked by a neutralizing antibody. On the other hand, there are antibodies which one knows recognize the C-terminal region of the IFN molecule and do not inhibit IFN's biological activity, nor its binding to the receptor, I believe (Arnheiter et al 1981).

Williams: I don't believe that the sequence between amino acid numbers 10 and 20 is a natural sequence which would give a high probability of a β-turn; that usually requires Asn, Pro, or Gly. The sequence has Gly only at position 10. The turn in the Sternberg structure may look like a β-turn, but the only reason it is shown there as a turn is that there is a strong probability for an α-helix on one side, and then he had to get round a corner. I would not assume that because this apparent requirement for a β-turn has come up before, there is a strong possibility that such a turn is strongly antigenic.

Alkan: I am suggesting that the active site may be located near a β-turn but not exactly at the β-turn.

Lerner: A nice way to select a peptide for making anti-peptide antibodies is to first treat a protein with a proteolytic enzyme such as trypsin. If trypsin cleaves at a site, there is a high probability that an antibody would reach the site as well. If I wanted to make anti-peptide antibodies to a protein, I might first look for all the basic residues where trypsin is able to cleave. Those cleavable sites are usually good candidates for choosing synthetic immunogens. In foot-and-mouth disease virus, for instance, there is a single cleavage point, and that is the target site. In certain strains of poliovirus there is a tryptic site and antibody binds very well there.

Alkan: My thinking is that to define the active site of the IFN molecule the best way is not to make peptides, mainly because IFN is a very flexible molecule, but to make hybrid molecules which are biologically active. Another approach would be to make point mutations which destroy binding to the IFN receptor.

Ada: The best way, finally, is to make the peptide.

V. Nussenzweig: Interferons are very species-specific. Is this related to the active site, or to some other area of the molecule? How is the species-specificity explained in terms of structure?

Alkan: I think both are possible—differences in the active site and differences in other sites affecting the stabilization of IFN on the receptor. Perhaps there are differences in receptor structures as well. As I said, IFNα-D doesn't bind the human receptor as well as other subtypes but binds to the mouse receptor and in fact to bovine cells very well. I haven't compared the amino acid sequences of all the other interferons, but I think that certain subtypes of human IFN (such as subtypes A,B, etc.) may have similar binding sites and similar sequences in their active sites. One exception I know is α-D. I still think that mouse IFNα will have a different sequence. But we should not exclude the role of other regions of the IFN molecule in the induction of a full antiviral or antiproliferative effect. Multiple-point binding is a possibility. We know that interferons have to sit on the receptor for hours to induce an antiviral effect.

REFERENCE

Arnheiter H, Thomas RM, Leist T, Fountoulakis M, Gutte B 1981 Physicochemical and antigenic
    properties of synthetic fragments of human leukocyte interferon. Nature (Lond) 294:278-280

Final general discussion

Reactivity of anti-peptide antibodies with the parent proteins

Ada: A number of topics remain for further general discussion. They include the proportion of monoclonal antibodies which react to the different types of epitopes in a polymeric protein, ranging from linear determinants to quaternary structures; the roles of high versus low affinity antibodies; and antigen presentation with T-dependent and T-independent antigens. But first we should discuss the question of antibodies to linear peptides reacting with the native proteins. This is a crucial aspect if peptides are to be used as the basis of future vaccines. Members of the group may be prepared to quote from their own experience, as I have the feeling that there is considerable variation in the literature.

Geysen: In our approach, we first show that a particular epitope was recognized by analysing the anti-protein response; the corresponding peptide is then synthesized, and the subsequent anti-peptide response has in all cases reacted with the original protein. That this is so is not surprising, as there was no prediction involved in the choice of which peptide to use. More importantly, we also determine the specificity of the antibodies induced by either antigen— protein or peptide. This looks past the superficial aspect of whether the anti-peptide response recognizes the protein; that is, whether each antigen induces antibodies interacting with the same contact residues.

Skehel: In the influenza system a remarkable feature of antibodies against peptides equivalent to regions of the haemagglutinin is that although all the antibodies appear to react with the peptide used to induce them, none seems to neutralize virus infectivity, and although they interact with haemagglutinin in procedures such as immunoblotting they don't immunoprecipitate native haemagglutinin. I wonder how common that is. One would imagine from such results that attempts to use peptides as vaccines against influenza would be a waste of time.

Crumpton: Let me underline this important point by referring to some results of work carried out in Mike Waterfield's laboratory of ICRF in collaboration with José Schlessinger at the Weizmann Institute, and Axel Ullrich at Genentech (Gullick et al 1985). Fifteen peptides of EGF receptor were synthesized, coupled to KLH and used to immunize rabbits; six peptides were located in the receiver's extracellular domain. All antisera contained high titres of antibodies against the homologous peptide, but only five peptides gave antisera which reacted with the native receptor, as judged by immunoprecipitation. All of the latter five peptides were located in the receptor's cytoplasmic domain. So there was a contrast between the responses induced by peptides from the extracellular and cytoplasmic domains, as judged by the reactivity of the antisera with the native receptor. The reason for this is not known. The most striking feature was the relatively small number (33%) of anti-peptide sera which reacted with the native EGF receptor.

Stevens: I think you are talking about peptides sequences where a structure has to be recognized in order for elicited antibodies to react with the receptor. That may be quite different from when an epitope consists of linear sequences in a soluble protein.

Our experience with making antibodies to peptides for reacting to an intact protein suggests that an antibody made to a peptide *per se* will not necessarily be of high reactivity, but if you can locate a peptide region that is on the surface of the parent protein molecule, there is a good probability of getting cross-reactivity. I don't think you necessarily have to look for the immunodominant site of the native protein to use for immunization. As Dr Sela's laboratory has shown, you can select a region that is not immunogenic in the native molecule and prepare a peptide to that region, so long as it is on the surface; after immunization with the peptide, you can obtain a high degree of recognition of the whole protein.

Geysen: It depends how you choose the peptide. If you just look at the sequence of the protein, choose a stretch which has, say, four arginines next to two glycines, and decide to make a peptide corresponding to that, the chances of the anti-peptide response reacting with the native antigen are almost zero. It comes down to how you select the peptide, which determines the frequency of finding that the anti-peptide response reacts with the protein.

Crumpton: One of the common rules that many people use for selection of such peptides is hydrophilicity.

Lerner: Many experiments have been published in which people have made anti-peptide antibodies that see proteins. There are also some which don't work. But anti-peptide antibodies are a site-directed technology with none of the circularity usually inherent in immunological procedures. There, one says: 'Let's screen for an antibody which neutralizes'. You let the selective system churn for you, until you get such an antibody. No surprise! In contrast, in the anti-peptide approach, we say: 'if I make an antibody to a certain shape at a certain point, I think it will do something'. In the absence of knowledge of the three-dimensional structure we must to some extent depend on guesswork.

Skehel: From these many peptides that work and the many that don't work, you would hope by now to have some clue about what makes them work.

Lerner: Why? Do you have a clue about how proteins fold, with only 20 amino acids?

Skehel: So the answer is that it is still a hit-and-miss process.

Geysen: It's more like marksmanship. If you are a good marksman you hit the target 99 times out of 100. If you are a very poor marksman, you never hit the target.

V. Nussenzweig: What are the rules of marksmanship, though?

Geysen: Just that some are better than others!

Sela: I would like to come back to what Richard Lerner called a paradox. What exactly are we talking about here? Some of the sequences in a protein are in a form in which they are very rigid and the related free peptides have a completely different conformation from the sequence within the native protein. The chance that such a peptide will transconform into the shape within the native protein is small. There are other regions in that protein which are more flexible and the chance that a peptide related to such a region may transconform into a shape similar to that present in the native protein is much better. I would like to stress, too, that the question is *not* whether there are cross-reacting antibodies. One should distinguish between 'reaction' and 'useful reaction', because a weak cross-reaction is not interesting for practical purposes, such as vaccination.

When you look at the proteins, my view is that those proteins that need disulphide bridges for their three-dimensional structure use them as crutches, otherwise their structure collapses readily. On the other hand, the coat proteins of viruses, for example, most of the time lack disulphide bridges, and segments of the complete protein are probably already in a shape much more similar to that in the intact molecule.

Corradin: My experience of making anti-peptide antibodies that cross-react with their native proteins is restricted to cytochrome *c*. I have made either polyclonal or monoclonal antibodies against both the C-terminus and the N-terminus, which contain many lysine residues and are flexible by definition. On ELISA, the antibodies cross-react well with native cytochrome *c*. The antibodies cross-react also with other peptides on ELISA. If we determine whether cross-reactivity is present in solution, they don't cross-react at all. So the method of determining cross-reactivity is important. Again, I have two cross-reacting peptides which give the same binding constant on a plastic plate, and in solution one is 10^5 or 10^6 less strong. On that criterion, there is no cross-reactivity. If we put that same low cross-reacting peptide on a macrophage, the monoclonal antibody binds to it as well as to the peptide with a high binding constant. So the notion of cross-reactivity depends on the assay used.

Rothbard: In comparing the ability of anti-peptide with anti-protein antibodies to bind the protein we should consider the thermodynamics of the process. I believe the limitations of the anti-peptide antibodies are due to the lack of a single, well-defined conformation in the peptides used as immunogens. Peptides lacking a defined conformation are capable of stimulating a large number of B cell clones, only a small fraction of which recognize the peptide in the conformation it adopts in the intact protein. How effective the peptide will be in eliciting a cross-reactive response will depend on the likelihood that either the peptide adopts the 'native' conformation, or the particular section of the protein has as much conformational freedom as the peptide. Consistent with this is the evidence that regions of high flexibility, for example the N- and C-termini of proteins, will obviously cross-react better than regions of rigid structure. The likelihood of the adoption of a particular conformation will be related to the energy requirements for adopting the structure.

There have been several reports of antibodies inducing conformational change (summarized in Habeeb 1977 and Celada 1983). Such induction of conformation is not without consequence. Thermodynamic arguments dictate that the energy necessary to induce a peptide to adopt a particular conformation will directly result in a lower affinity constant. If the energy requirements for induction are too severe, the B cell will not be stimulated to differentiate and the population of antibodies recognizing that particular conformation will not be present in the humoral response against the peptide.

One system for which I have data is a disulphide loop in pilin isolated from *Moraxella bovis*. The experiment I did is very similar to what Dr Sela and Dr Arnon did previously on lysozyme (Arnon et al 1971). I examined the ability of an antibody raised against the intact protein to recognize the amino acids composing the loop, depending on whether the cysteines were oxidized or reduced and alkylated. This experiment was possible because the loop is naturally highly immunogenic. As can be seen from Table 1, the antisera bound the oxidized loop twice as well as the reduced and alkylated material in a solid-phase binding assay.

Having shown that there are nearly identical amounts of peptide on the solid phase, I conclude that the differential binding is due to their different con-

TABLE 1 (Rothbard) Ability of antibodies elicited by intact Moraxella bovis pili to cross-react with peptides corresponding to the disulphide loop of pilin

Dilution of sera	Bovine serum albumin (BSA) (c.p.m.)	$\overset{\frown}{S\text{-}\text{-}S}$ -- BSA (c.p.m.)	RS—SR -- BSA (c.p.m.)
1 : 50	785[a]	13 904	7373
1 : 100	527	9529	2661
1 : 500	431	2611	956
1 : 1000	155	1386	506

[a] ^{125}I protein A bound to immunoglobulins in solid-phase binding assay

formations. I can relate this difference to free energy by using the differential binding as an equilibrium constant, k_{eq}, and using the following equation:

$$\Delta G = -RT \ln k_{eq}$$

$$k_{eq} = \frac{\text{counts bound to oxidized material}}{\text{counts bound to reduced and alkylated material}}$$

$$k_{eq} = 2$$

$$\Delta G = -0.4 \text{ kcal/mol}$$

As can be seen, a relatively small difference in free energy will result in a large difference in cross-reaction. An analysis of this logarithmic relationship between free energy and binding constants shows that when the differential binding equals ten, $\Delta G = -1.2$ kcal/mol and when $k_{eq} = 100$, the free energy difference is only -2.4 kcal/mol.

Therefore, if a peptide requires 2.5 kcal/mol to adopt the conformation that it has when part of the intact protein, then (i) when it is used as an antigen, antibodies against the protein directed at this sequence will bind the peptide with a binding constant two orders lower in affinity than the corresponding region of the protein, and (ii) when it is used as an immunogen, the anti-peptide antibodies will bind the intact protein with two logs lower affinity than they do the peptide. I believe that in order to elicit antibodies against relatively rigid regions of proteins, peptides must be designed to more closely resemble the intact proteins.

Williams: How many flexible pieces are there in these molecules?

Rothbard: The loop is quite big, 20 amino acids.

Williams: In that case, the difference in the weighted probability between the disulphide-bridged and the open-chain peptides due to conformational restriction should have been many thousand. The fact that you obtained only a difference of two suggests that the open form, through its lack of restriction, can match the receptor better than the closed form. The reason for this is relatively simple. The peptide loop in the closed form has a problem in presenting itself to the antibody in some conformations. The selection between open and closed forms then need not be an entropic problem, but is a ΔH problem. The free energy of binding equation has two terms, one to do with the binding energies and the other with entropies. The overall problem is that the closed loop had to get into some state which was energetically difficult for it, to make it sufficiently antigenic, but it was restricted in stereochemical terms. This disadvantage is partially offset by the gain of binding strength due to entropic restriction. The restrictions on the open form are in the opposite order.

Evan: On one occasion at least, we have isolated a monoclonal antibody that recognizes an intermediate state of naturation. This antibody recognized the c-*myc* protein only when it was on the Western immunoblotted nitrocellulose filter. It did not recognize native material or totally denatured material. There may be something of interest which people should consider there.

The second point is that on several occasions now, polyclonal antisera, raised against a given synthetic peptide, have not been shown to have good cross-reacting activity against the intact protein. Yet on many of these occasions, a high proportion of the monoclonal antibodies against that peptide did cross-react. Perhaps we should be aware that in a solution of a monoclonal antibody the concentration of the binding site is enormously higher than the concentration of individual binding sites in any polyclonal serum, even one raised against a small synthetic peptide.

Sela: This is not of great help for making a synthetic vaccine, because you cannot induce people to make monoclonal antibodies as a result of immunization with vaccines.

Evan: That is right. The question is: how many different antibody combining sites are there in a polyclonal serum against a given synthetic peptide? If there are 1000, the concentration of the antibody combining site is a thousandth of the concentration of total antibody. Moreover, if each of those combining sites recognizes, or prefers, a specific sort of conformation of that flexing sequence in the intact protein, then the concentration of the antigen is a great deal lower as well. Has anyone asked what happens if we leave a polyclonal anti-peptide antibody for a long time with the intact protein containing the peptide antigen sequence? Will it bind then? Without this kind of information, it is difficult to compare monoclonal with polyclonal antibodies.

Rothbard: We have done that in solid-phase binding assays. Many anti-peptide antibodies which have high titres for the homologous peptide fail to cross-react with the corresponding protein on solid-phase assays when they are incubated together for only an hour. However, if the serum is allowed to incubate for long periods (24 hours) a strong signal is apparent when the plate is washed and subsequently incubated with either a second antibody or Protein A. The easiest explanation is that the protein on the plate is in equilibrium between a fully folded state and a series of partially unfolded states. The anti-peptide serum has a high concentration of high affinity antibodies that recognize the particular region in 'non-native' conformations. As the protein 'breathes', the antibodies can bind and subsequently prevent that region from refolding. Over a period of time the antibody–protein complex increases in concentration, resulting in a large signal after long incubation times. We know that this is not the result of non-specific binding because the signal specifically appears in the well containing the corresponding protein and not with alternative proteins.

Evan: This observation could explain, on its own, why there is greater success with monoclonal than polyclonal antibodies when one tries to produce anti-peptide antibodies which recognize intact proteins.

Klug: We have to distinguish the different purposes to which anti-peptide antibodies are put. Dr Evan is talking about *recognizing* a protein and it doesn't matter what state of folding it is in. Other people are concerned with making an effective neutralizing vaccine. The work on c-*myc* illustrates a case of simple recognition, which is what most cell biologists want. They are not concerned with success in vaccination. Each approach has its purpose, and I would like to hear from those making anti-peptide antibodies just what fraction of their antibodies are neutralizing. Of course, it may be too early to ask this. And what really is a neutralizing antibody?

Ada: That is precisely the point. It depends on the number of sites on the protein which are important for neutralization. That is, the number of sites which bind antibody and infection by the virus is prevented.

Lerner: Perhaps we are trying to describe a diversity system of the order of 10^{11}, one member at a time! Perhaps all we can say is that there are many possibilities.

Ada: If we are going to use peptides as the basis of a vaccine against, say, a virus, what is the frequency and efficiency with which antibodies to the peptides will react with the original protein or the virus, so that infection by the virus is prevented?

Sela: The numbers available are much too small, and the diversity of the system much too big, for a statistical analysis. In the case of one viral coat protein, we prepared two peptides of 20 amino acids each. There was no reason why one should be efficient in provoking neutralizing antibodies, and the other one not at all. In the case of the cholera toxin B subunit, out of six peptides, only two peptides led to the production of antibodies that neutralize the toxin.

Ada: Perhaps because in many cases we don't know the regions of the proteins that are important for neutralization, we should try to concentrate on the question of how efficiently antibodies to peptides will bind to the parent protein.

Stanworth: In our experience, if we put ε-chain peptides on KLH as carrier using glutaraldehyde, we can produce good anti-peptide antibodies which react with parent rat IgE. If we put the same peptides onto BSA using the same method, we still get good anti-peptide antibodies but they do not react with the parent Ig. You can't evoke here some stronger antigenicity of KLH than of BSA, because we are producing antibody responses to the peptide in both cases. So is there some difference in presentation, in terms of the relationship of the peptide to the carrier? Are we referring here to different carriers? Others have also had this problem, for instance in using BSA as a carrier, in relation to other carriers.

Ada: So there are other factors, apart from the peptide itself, that have an important role in determining the specificity of the anti-peptide response.

Lennox: If it is all so obvious, as Richard Lerner implies, what advice does he give John Skehel about how to go about using peptides to make neutralizing antibodies? I think it is premature; you don't know what to tell him to do next.

Lerner: Yes. As Aaron Klug once said to me in discussing the anti-peptide antibody results: 'It is amazing that the dog speaks at all—we shouldn't expect an opera yet'.

Lachmann: In comparing antibodies for their degrees of cross-reactivity, one needs to know their affinity for various ligands in real units. This needs proper quantitative assays, rather than the excessive reliance on ELISA tests which give only arbitrarily quantitative data.

The proportion of monoclonal antibodies reactive to conformational or other linear sequences

Ada: May we now consider the question of the proportion of monoclonal antibodies that react to the various types of epitopes in polymeric proteins?

Williams: When we come to think about the different modes of antigenicity of a protein surface, we must distinguish the differences between the sequence and the conformational structure. The sequence gives you a linear pattern (A,B,C,D etc.). That is one possible source of antigenicity (type 1) that may be a recognition point for an antibody. Another (type 2) is a β-strand or helix, which is related to the sequence but the exposed surface may reveal amino acid A, then miss two or three (B,C), then reveal D or G on the surface. (I presume that some of the amino acids have to be on the surface to be recognized by the antibody at all.) Both of these recognitions depend on the sequence. When you are thinking of designing peptides, just from knowledge of the DNA, you have virtually no choice except to design from the linear sequence, but you can still design in these two ways. Once there is a three-dimensional structure, you have another possibility, to design antigenic peptides by deliberately looking at adjacent amino acids in space, not in sequence. This approach (type 3) is much more difficult to use, since it gives too many possibilities. People have suggested that perhaps the strongest antigenicity will arise from adjacent strands in space, one part of the antigenic site coming from one helix, and the other from a nearby strand, or helix.

What I find difficult is this. Running through all the discussions has been the motif of flexibility. If we think about flexibility in terms of these three possibilities for antigenicity, we see that they are very different. In the first type (sequence A,B,C,D is antigenic), flexibility would mean that groups A,B,C and D must all be revealed. Presumably, every now and again all four must appear together on the outside of the protein. This would need flexibility of the protein, because in protein structures it is not usual for all the side-chains in a sequence of about five amino acids to appear on the surface in what we could call the most stable, or ground-state, protein structure.

Similarly, if the helix is to be antigenic (A,D,G is antigenic; type 2), flexibility is helpful. It is better if the protein can breath a bit, because then the surface of the helix is more revealed, without undoing the helix. The antigenicity remains in the secondary structure. However, tertiary structure is required by the third (type 3) kind of antigenicity, but tertiary structure is removed by flexibility. Flexibility opposes tertiary structure, because groups not in sequences move away from one another, so they lose close contact. Thus it would be hard to understand type 3 antigenicity in terms of flexibility. The more flexibility you have in the fold, the less the definition of such a site; whereas the flexibility in type 2 antigenic regions will reveal the site.

I believe that some exposure must be necessary for antigen–antibody binding to be obtained, but it may start by weak binding, when, in general, the first two types are more likely to be the ways for the antibody to search. In this case, too, it is right to start from the sequence and not to wait for the structure in order to probe antigenicity. It is also correct to look for hydrophilic sequences—that is, sequences on the surface. If type 3 antigenicity is common, so many possibilities come up, not connected to the flexibility argument in the same way, that it is difficult to see how to proceed.

Sela: Perhaps for the sake of symmetry you should add quaternary structure; in multi-subunit proteins where each subunit is completely native, even without any allosteric change you will often have some antibodies that are not adsorbed by the native subunit, and react only with the intact multi-subunit protein.

Williams: I accept that. I want also to point out that it is possible to create an antibody to almost anything if you let the antibody be weak enough, so I am not talking about very poor antibodies. It is pointless to say that everything is antigenic; the question is whether there are some sequences that are more antigenic than others.

Sela: The cross-reaction between a polymer of Pro-Gly-Pro and collagen is a typical example where it is not the detail of the sequence, but the helical shape, which controls the cross-reaction.

Ada: Mario Geysen perhaps has an instance of the third mode of antigenicity.

Geysen: I can at least say that our epitope (the foot-and-mouth disease virus mimotope) is not an example of type 1 or 2, because our defining monoclonal antibody was tested against all peptides, from six to 10 residues long. So we can exclude modes 1 and 2. However, I think that types 1 and 2 are the same, and types 3 and 4 are also the same. Perhaps the symmetry would be improved by removing the second mode, because a sequential determinant in fact includes spacer and contact residues; therefore to synthesize an example of the second mode you still need to include spacers, which makes it indistinguishable from mode 1.

Sela: I would define an epitope as the juxtaposition of atoms in space, which in one case (sequential determinant) are contiguous within the sequence, whereas in the other cases the juxtaposition of the same number of atoms may come from amino acid residues which are quite far removed from each other in the primary sequence (conformational determinant).

Williams: I don't think the foot-and-mouth disease virus mimotope is a clean example of a non-contiguous antigenic site because of the way you searched in order to find a successful antigenic site. The question arises as to what your sequence is antigenic against, on the original protein; we do not know that.

Geysen: Then how do we interpret the absence of reaction of the monoclonal antibody with all the linear peptides based on the sequence of the viral proteins?

Anders: Would you classify any monoclonal that failed to react with an antigen when it was Western-blotted but reacted with the native protein in the same way?

Geysen: No! A Western-blotted antigen may fail to react with a monoclonal (intrinsically against a continuous epitope) by virtue of the protein being either in the wrong conformation, or absorbed on the cellulose nitrate support in an orientation which sterically precludes the interaction.

Klug: The fact is that there are many more examples of type 3 than of the others. If you look at an arbitrary patch in the surface of a protein, the chances of finding residues that are far apart in the sequence coming together is greater than residues contiguous in the sequence. Thus, on the whole, the monoclonals that are raised do *not* react with continuous peptides. *A priori*, you would expect type 3 recognition to be the most important case, but it is not reproducible with continuous peptides.

Crumpton: My experience with monoclonal antibodies against class I and class II histocompatibility antigens may be relevant here. Antibodies were selected on the basis that they react with the antigen as expressed on the cell surface. These monoclonal antibodies generally do not react by Western blotting against the reduced, SDS-treated antigen, although they immunoprecipitate very well the homologous antigen. Interestingly, some antibodies reacted by Western blotting with the SDS-treated antigen, provided it was not reduced, which argues for some retention of shape. Most other people's experience is the same. In other words, in this system monoclonal antibodies are rarely selected which recognize sequential determinants.

Sela: We ask all the time whether synthesized peptides react with antibodies to native proteins, but we haven't mentioned the in-between situation. If we take, for example, native ribonuclease or lysozyme, and see the extent to which antibodies prepared against the native protein react with the complete sequence of the same protein after denaturation, there will be essentially no cross-reaction; so why worry whether a peptide cross-reacts? The very fact that when a native protein is injected, the totality of the antibodies against it are not able to react with the open chain, when the disulphide bridges have been opened, means that all the antibodies are against a conformation.

Williams: This proves only that shape is required for antigenicity.

Altschuh: Again, it is a question of the relative affinity of the antibody for the peptide compared to the protein. The fact that a large molar excess of peptide over protein is needed in inhibition experiments means that anti-protein antibodies which have a reasonable affinity for the native protein have a low affinity for peptides. The serum may also contains a fraction of antibodies against the denatured antigen which bind well to peptides. If they bind weakly to the native protein, they will not be scored in competition experiments, but can be detected by direct binding assays with peptides. These antibodies are probably not significant in virus neutralization.

Lerner: With any method, what is the damnation of that method to one individual is its elegance to another. To me, the elegance of the anti-peptide technology is that it is site-specific. To those who want to neutralize all viruses, that is the damnation of the method. But unless you have a *general* site-specific technology, you probably won't have a lot of success in getting antibodies that neutralize viruses, because the sites that you need to hit on the surfaces of viruses to neutralize them are limited in number.

The site-specific nature of these antibodies is their essence. They may be used for perturbing protein structure, for localizing the products of genes, for carrying out structure–function studies, for domain mapping, for determining reading frames; and so on. The method is not however appropriate for generating broadly reactive sera.

Ada: There is increasing evidence that many antibodies are formed which recognize tertiary structures. If this is a general finding, what are the implications for antigen presentation and processing? Would such structures be seen only by B cells?

Lachmann: B cells see antigen in entirely native form so, whatever one's model for antigen processing, it cannot require that B cells look at processed antigen. It is known that there are hidden determinants inside IgG and C3 molecules to which antibodies are not made unless the native molecules are proteolysed before injection. These native proteins must therefore be seen by the B cell very much as they are.

Sela: When you inject the native protein, you can discover antibodies to proteolytic fragments, because of proteolysis by the body.

Lachmann: For plasma proteins like IgG and complement components (particularly C3), the immune response seems to look at the protein in the form in which it is given.

Humphrey: It is clear that B cells recognize the native configuration. Whether they can elicit T cell help by presenting that configuration is another matter, as we discussed earlier. From the repertoire of shapes of the Ig receptors on B cells can be selected some which bind to proteins in their native tertiary or even quaternary configuration (when a complex of two proteins is involved). What keeps the B cell clone going is another question.

Anders: Once again, it depends how you look. We initially detected expression of malaria antigens in *E. coli* by probing Western blots with antisera raised against β-galactosidase. We found that early bleeds gave clean Western blots, but antisera obtained after multiple boosts reacted with many fragments of β-galactosidase.

Ada: The message, though, seems to be that the immune system can cope with all these possibilities.

High and low affinity antibodies and their roles

Lerner: Dr Bill Jencks would say that the work of the cell is done by low affinity reactions!

Rothbard: As Dr Sela has stated, we must specify what our particular needs are. I have been attempting to raise antibodies with defined specificity with sufficiently high affinity for the intact protein to allow me to assign functional roles to particular structural domains. However, from our work with the gonococcus I am well aware that relatively low affinity antibodies can be useful in biological assays. I am also very interested in how peptides interact with T cells in biological protection.

Lachmann: It is the product of the concentration and the affinity of antibody which gives an effective signal. For a monoclonal antibody, at its very high concentration, a low affinity can be effective in giving a signal, whereas polyclonal antibody of the same affinity would be quite inactive. There is good evidence that animals that make large amounts of low affinity antibodies to certain viruses (e.g. lymphocytic choriomeningitis virus) *in vivo* are prone to develop immune complex disease (Soothill & Steward 1971). So, while all the cell's work may be done by low affinity antibodies, some of this work one doesn't wish to encounter in immunized animals or humans.

Williams: There is one big distinction between high and low affinity systems. A high affinity system is a better recognition system, but it doesn't come apart easily. So if there is a second stage in the biochemistry which depends on the system coming apart rapidly, tight binding in the first stage could be detrimental. If the antigen has to enter the B cell and some part of it has to be separated off, a low affinity system may be better because this process will be quicker. The system might get stuck if it were a high affinity reaction. This is a well-known distinction between a kinetic and a thermodynamic equilibrium pathway. Bill Jencks is for this reason interested in low affinity biology. However, not all biological effects should be of low affinity or readily reversible. Some systems, like the blocking of proteases by trypsin inhibitors, must have binding constants as high as 10^{10} and the inhibitors are nearly perfect matches for the protease surfaces. High affinity stops systems, very often; low affinity in early steps allows a system to go in subsequent stages rapidly.

Anders: Would we accept that there may be circumstances, for example the malaria merozoite or sporozoite surface, where on-rates, and therefore affinity, could be critical in determining whether the antibody is effective?

Williams: Yes; the ratio of on-rate to off-rate is critical.

Lerner: Ordinarily we are talking about antibodies, which are replicating proteins, as it were, because there is a system to replicate them; whereas the antigen in a test tube (BSA, say) is a non-replicating protein. In a virus infection, though, you have a replicating antigen up against a replicating protein. A feature of a low affinity system is that you may use your antibodies over and over again.

Lachmann: The effector actions of the antibody will also be important here. Whether it is IgM or IgG and whether it fixes complement may be even more important than its affinity. The monoclonal antibody CAM-PATH-1, which kills T cells and prevents graft-versus-host disease (Waldmann et al 1984), is of low affinity (apparent affinity, $4-7 \times 10^7$ M^{-1}; G. Hale, personal communication), but because it is IgM and an excellent complement fixer, it is highly effective biologically.

Evan: It is also worth mentioning that with monoclonal antibodies in particular, the assay used to screen for positive antibodies has affinity parameters that one never bothers to think about, let alone define; yet these parameters may well limit the type of antibodies eventually selected.

Rothbard: Again, with vaccination, the concentration of antibodies in a particular site may be more critical than affinity. In mucosal immunity the problem is how do we particularly stimulate IgA. This is still poorly understood.

Lerner: That is a problem for any antigen, synthetic peptide or otherwise.

T-dependent and T-independent antigen presentation

Humphrey: There are certain instances where you can attach epitopes to a carrier, inject the conjugate in small amounts into human beings, and get a prolonged antibody response against the epitope. As I said, there are linear or non-linear polysaccharides which, if you put enough epitopes on, stimulate thymus-independent antibody responses. At least in mice, rats and man, the antibodies appear to be made by a subset of B cells which is relatively sessile and resides in the marginal zone of the white pulp of the spleen. The evidence for this is that if you take the spleen out, the response is greatly diminished, and cannot be restored simply by supplying large numbers of spleen cells as a cell suspension (Amlot et al 1985). So the architecture of the spleen as well as the subset of B cells, and probably also the marginal zone macrophages as antigen-presenting cells, are all needed.

Polysaccharides such as Ficoll, hydroxyethyl starch or linear dextran with attached rhodamine, fluorescein or dinitrobenzyl groups and injected into mice or rats elicit antibody within one or two days. The response is maximal at five days but declines very slowly and persists for many weeks. The antibody is exclusively against the attached epitope. Perhaps, if peptides were attached to such carriers, or better still to lipopolysaccharide, you would get a prolonged antibody response. This would be worth testing, because one of the problems is how to keep the immunogen around. However, you get no detectable B memory cells by this method. We should remember the importance of the carrier, in respect of the kind of response we want to get. Victor Nussenzweig, for instance, wants to immunize with the circumsporozoite peptide on a carrier, and wants to be sure that if the mosquito injects sporozoites later on, the sporozoite antigen will stimulate the appropriate memory cells. I think that he should avoid using a carrier, if he can, or rather make the antigen become its own carrier by—perhaps—extending the peptide and polymerizing it.

Lachmann: Do you get any antibody other than IgM by this method?

Humphrey: Yes. In humans you also get IgG and IgA. In a rat it would be IgG2c mainly, and in the mouse IgG3. These classses of Ig are expressed on a sizeable proportion of the sessile population of spleen marginal zone B cells.

Ada: If you use a polymerized small epitope where you have essentially a similar repeating pattern, would you risk finding a significant proportion of an outbred human population who might respond poorly?

Humphrey: I suppose that one might. I think it would be wise to extend the peptides by using adjacent amino acid sequences, and perhaps to introduce some block to rapid degradation by peptidases—for example, a short polyproline sequence.

Sela: N.A. Mitchison showed that some (T,G)-A–L was compartmentalized, not in the lysosomal pockets in which it would be readily digested, but in another compartment in which it was preserved intact for many months.

Lerner: There is a problem with polymers. One tends to think that if one takes a seven-amino acid peptide and polymerizes it, this is the same as an equal number of multimers of the free peptide; but it isn't. Except for the two ends, each block of seven has the wrong neighbours, even though they are 'self' neighbours, and you greatly change what is going to happen. So, what experiment would you like us to try?

Humphrey: A simple experiment is to attach a peptide to a carrier such as Ficoll. I have tried this with luteinizing hormone-releasing hormone (LHRH), but I obtained only a small antibody response in mice. I perhaps did not attach enough epitopes, because I have since found that the antibody response is better when the epitope density is greater (unpublished); and I shall try again. It would probably be sensible to use a carrier such as lipopolysaccharide which can activate macrophages as well. Liposomes and micelles have already been mentioned (in my Introduction) as vehicles which increase antibody responses, and they are largely targeted towards macrophages. The thing to do is to try out different approaches, since we still do not really know what to do for the best!

Lachmann: Liposomes sound a very good idea. However, the extreme immunodeficiency in the acquired immunodeficiency syndrome (AIDS), which is believed to be due exclusively to failure of the T-helper system, suggests that without T cell help, a response adequate to provide immunity may be impossible. AIDS patients do not become hypogammaglobulinaemic and they do make antibodies, presumably largely by this T-independent system. But these antibodies fail to prevent all the AIDS-related infections.

REFERENCES

Amlot PL, Grennan D, Humphrey JH 1985 Splenic dependence of the antibody response to thymus-independent (T1-2) antigens. Eur J Immunol 15:508-512

Arnon R, Maron E, Sela M, Anfinsen CB 1971 Antibodies reactive with native lysozyme elicited by a completely synthetic antigen. Proc Natl Acad Sci USA 68:1450-1455

Celada F, Schumaker V, Sercarz E (eds) 1983 Protein conformation as an immunological signal. Plenum Press, New York

Gullick WJ, Downward J, Parker PJ, Whittle N, Kris R, Schlessinger J, Ullrich A, Waterfield MD 1985 Proc R Soc Lond B Biol Sci, in press

Habeeb A 1977 Influence of conformation on immunological properties of proteins. In: Atassi MZ (ed) Immunochemistry of proteins. Plenum Press, New York, vol 1:163

Soothill JF, Steward MW 1971 The immunopathological significance of the heterogeneity of antibody affinity. Clin Exp Immunol 9:193-199

Waldmann H, Or R, Hale G et al 1984 Elimination of graft-versus-host disease by *in vitro* depletion of alloreactive lymphocytes using a monoclonal rat anti-human lymphocyte antibody (CAM-PATH-1). Lancet 2: 483-486

Chairman's summing-up

GORDON L. ADA

Department of Microbiology, The John Curtin School of Medical Research, Australian National University, PO Box 334, Canberra City, ACT 2601, Australia

1986 Synthetic peptides as antigens. Wiley, Chichester (Ciba Foundation Symposium 119) p 294-296

The success of meetings like this one can doubtless be judged in many ways, such as by the excellence of the presentations and the depth of the ensuing discussions. Other criteria are equally important. Have the proceedings either made us think differently, or sharpened our understanding of particular points? Can we see more clearly what further work needs to be done and what additional questions might be raised by this work? Has the meeting catalysed collaborative projects between participants? I think there is evidence of success in this meeting on all these grounds.

It has been said that the 1960s was the decade of T and B cells, and the 1970s, the decade when antigen presentation was recognized to be of prime importance. The indications are, however, that antigen presentation will remain of central importance throughout this decade. John Humphrey reported on recent findings and proposals that in addition to acknowledged mechanisms, antigen may also be presented to T cells by B cells which first concentrate and then process the antigen. The precise mechanisms involved have yet to be established. As was pointed out in the symposium, B cells presumably recognize epitopes ranging from short linear sequences to those formed by quaternary structures but, especially in the latter case, what message does the T cell receive? What are the relative contributions of 'traditional' antigen-presenting cells, such as macrophages and dendritic cells?

The nature of the carrier is extremely important and Peter Lachmann raised our hopes for a 'universal' carrier by showing that PPD in BCG-sensitized hosts provides a powerful way of inducing T cell help. It would seem to be advantageous to couple PPD to the two 'B cell' peptides which are the closest to forming the basis of future human vaccines, namely the CS epitope from the malaria parasite and the 37-amino acid C-terminus peptide from hCG.

In my introductory remarks, I expressed the hope that we might now be nearer than we were to predicting those amino acid sequences of a protein that can induce the formation of antibodies capable of binding well to the parent protein molecules. I attempted during the discussion of papers in the second section, and in the final discussion, to obtain a degree of consensus on guidelines for this purpose. But although properties such as segmental mobility, and findings with some proteins that immunodominant peptides occur at the 'corners' of the molecules, can all be regarded as 'guidelines', it now seems unlikely that a single criterion for predicting the regions of a protein which will elicit antibodies reactive with the native parent molecule will be universally applicable. In this connection, it may not be coincidence that with both the CS and the hCG peptide—the two preparations which seem likely to be developed as the basis of human vaccines—the importance of the size of the effective peptides was stressed. This may indicate a requirement for more than one sequence in the peptide to be recognized, or it may mean that peptides of these sizes more readily assume conformations which facilitate immunogenicity. Aaron Klug also pointed out that where 'long' peptides could be used to assign regions of antigenicity, additional epitopes might be found corresponding to more structural areas of the molecule, including α-helices.

Though protein chemists may have predicted this for some time, Allen Edmundson's pictures clearly showed that the binding site of the Ig light chain dimer (and presumably it will be found for Fab fragments too) is also flexible and adjusts to the surface contours of a peptide. The concept held for many years that antigen–antibody interaction was comparable to a rigid die-template binding is no longer tenable.

Traditionally, peptides corresponding to a sequence in a protein molecule have been synthesized once the sequence is known, or have been derived by cleavage of the protein; it seems, as discussed above, that we are still some way from predicting the sequences we need to make or isolate. Mario Geysen has possibly provided us with an alternative procedure. First, pick a monoclonal antibody with the desired property, such as viral neutralization. Then synthesize a priori the peptide which binds to the highest titre to that antibody. Though this paper and the ensuing discussion clearly excited most of us, two further experiments need to be done. First, if Allen Edmundson could prepare a crystalline Fab for which the eliciting epitope was known and its fit was 'mapped', it would be most interesting if Mario and his colleagues could a priori- synthesize their 'best' fit. A comparison of the 'natural' and 'engineered' epitopes could be very enlightening. Secondly, if the antibody possessed some activity such as neutralization of infectivity, would the engineered peptide, when appropriately presented, induce the same activity?

Considerable enthusiasm has been generated for the use of peptides as important biological tools and as the basis of vaccines. The formal papers and the discussions in this symposium have gone some way to support this enthusiasm. There is no doubt about the former use. In two to three years time, we may have two peptide-based vaccines ready for Phase II human trials. If by then there are several more at the stage represented now by the CS and hCG peptides, great progress will have been made.

Index of contributors

*Entries in **bold** type indicate papers; other entries refer to discussion contributions*

Ada, G. L. **1**, 21, 22, 45, 47, 48, 49, 50,
51, 52, 54, 55, 71, 72, 88, 89, 90, 91, 105,
120, 123, 124, 125, 126, 127, 128, 146,
148, 161, 176, 179, 181, 195, 196, 219,
222, 223, 224, 261, 277, 279, 285, 286,
287, 289, 290, 292, **294**
Alkan, S. S. 23, 46, 51, 52, 146, 182, 198,
261, **264**, 274, 275, 276, 277
Altschuh, D. 46, **76**, 85, 87, 89, 90, 289
Anders, R. F. 21, 41, 106, 120, 124, 125,
149, 162, 163, **164**, 175, 176, 177, 178,
179, 180, 181, 182, 262, 288, 290, 291
*Arnon, R. **184**

*Braun, D. G. **264**
Brown, F. 148, 162, 176, 197, 198, 223, 224
*Brown, G. V. **164**
*Burt, D. S. **226**

*Coppel, R. L. **164**
Corradin, G. 21, 45, 49, 51, 52, 54, 74, 88,
90, 161, 182, 198, 261, 275, 281
*Cross, K. J. **58**
Crumpton, M. J. 40, 47, 48, 50, 55, 71, 72,
86, 87, **93**, 102, 105 106, 120, 121, 122,
128, 144, 149, 161, 179, 180, 181, 240,
241, 259, 260, 261, 279, 280, 288

*Dyson, H. J. **58**

Edmundson, A. B. 86, **107**, 119, 120, 121,
122, 123, 124, 125, 126, 127, 242, 243
*Ely, K. R. **107**
Evan, G. I. 25, 47, 49, 128, **245**, 260, 261,
262, 283, 284, 291

Geysen, H. M. 43, 70, 72, 74, 87, 88, 122,
123, 127, 128, **130**, 144, 145, 146, 147,
148, 149, 180, 181, 221, 222, 241, 275,
279, 280, 281, 287, 288
Gupta, S. K. 41, 42, 161, 197, 216, 217, 221,
222, 260

*Hancock, D. C. **245**
*Hastings, G. Z. **226**
Heusser, Ch. 149, 163, 198
*Houghten, R. A. **58**

Humphrey, J. H. **6**, 19, 20, 21, 22, 23, 41,
44, 45, 50, 51, 148, 178, 180, 219, 222,
225, 242, 290, 291, 292, 293

*Jacob, C. O. **184**

*Kemp, D. J. **164**
Klug, A. 20, 42, **76**, 86, 87, 88, 89, 91, 102,
105, 123, 124, 125, 128, 178, 180, 285, 288

Lachmann, P. J. 19, 21, **25**, 40, 41, 42, 43,
44, 45, 46, 47, 51, 54, 55, 72, 90, 91, 146,
147, 175, 195, 196, 198, 220, 241, 242,
261, 276, 286, 289, 290, 291, 292, 293
*Leach, S. J. **164**
Lennox, E. S. 22, 41, 54, 261, 285
Lerner, R. A. 21, 43, 44, 47, 48, 55, **58**,
70, 71, 72, 73, 74, 87, 88, 90, 102, 105,
119, 122, 123, 124, 125, 126, 128, 145,
161, 175, 179, 181, 182, 183, 196, 197,
218, 219, 220, 221, 224, 244, 260, 261,
274, 275, 277, 280, 281, 285, 286, 289,
290, 291, 292
*Littlewood, T. **245**
Liu, Y. 20, 45, 148, 276

McConnell, I. 44, 45, 125, 145, 197, 220, 276
*Mason, T. J. **130**

Nussenzweig, R. S. **150**, 162
Nussenzweig, V. 21, 73, 87, 90, 125, 126,
150, 160, 161, 162, 163, 176, 179, 180,
182, 183, 196, 216, 277, 281

*Ostresh, J. **58**

*Pauza, C. D. **245**

*Rodda, S. J. **130**
Rothbard, J. B. 43, 73, 91, 120, 126, 145,
160, 161, 243, 281, 283, 284, 290, 291

*Scanlon, D. B. **164**
Sela, M, 20, 43, 47, 48, 49, 50, 54, 71, 73,
88, 146, 176, 178, 180, 181, **184**, 196, 197,
198, 219, 222, 224, 276, 281, 284, 285,
287, 288, 289, 292

*Non-participating co-author
Indexes compiled by John Rivers

Subject index

Date Due

JAN 18 1989			
			UML 735